# Understanding Youth Mental Health

## Causes, Interventions, and Policy Perspectives

snova
New York

# Mental Illnesses and Treatments Series

**Hoarding Disorder:**
**Insights and Implications for Health and Safety**
Paul M. Singleton (Editor)
ISBN: 979-8-89530-506-5
eBook ISBN: 979-8-89530-521-8

**A Desperate Asylum:**
**Crisis in a Canadian Psychiatric Hospital During Wartime**
Anne Marie Creamer, PhD
ISBN: 979-8-88697-696-0
eBook ISBN: 979-8-88697-863-6

**More information about this series can be found at**
https://novapublishers.com/product-category/series/mental-illnesses-and-treatments/

**Michael A. Post**
Editor

# Understanding Youth Mental Health

## Causes, Interventions, and Policy Perspectives

snova
New York

**Library of Congress Cataloging-in-Publication Data**

ISBN: 979-8-89530-700-7 (Hardcover)
ISBN: 979-8-89530-874-5 (eBook)

*Published by Nova Science Publishers, Inc. † New York*

# Contents

# Preface

Mental health is important for everyone and encompasses our emotional, psychological, and social well-being. It affects how we think, feel, and act, as well as how we cope with stress, relate to others, and make decisions. For children and youth, mental health also includes reaching developmental and emotional milestones and learning skills to cope with challenges and function well at home, school, and in their communities.

Mental health is a component of behavioral health, which includes choices or actions that affect overall well-being. Young people with mental health problems need a place to go to receive the care they really need in a supportive environment. This book reports on ways to improve access to quality mental health care for young people.

Chapter 1

# Why Are So Many American Youth in a Mental Health Crisis? Exploring Causes and Solutions*

## Committee on Health, Education, Labor, and Pensions

Thursday, June 8, 2023
U.S. Senate,
Committee on Health, Education, Labor, and Pensions,
Washington, DC.

The Committee met, pursuant to notice, at 10:01 a.m., in room 430, Dirksen Senate Office Building, Hon. Bernard Sanders, Chairman of the Committee, presiding.

Present: Senators Sanders [presiding], Casey, Baldwin, Murphy, Kaine, Hassan, Smith, Markey, Cassidy, Murkowski, Braun, Marshall, Romney, Tuberville, and Budd.

### Opening Statement of Senator Sanders

The CHAIR. The Senate Committee on Health, Education, Labor, and Pensions will come to order. And we are delighted to welcome our panelists that we are going to hear from in a few minutes.

But let me begin by telling everybody what they already know, and that is it is no great secret that in America today we have a mental health crisis, and the crisis has been exacerbated by the horrific COVID pandemic which we have experienced.

This is a crisis that has hit all of us, but I think especially the younger generation. In America today, 40 percent of parents report being either very or extremely worried that their child is struggling with anxiety or depression.

According to a recent survey by the Centers for Disease Control, nearly one out of every three teenagers in America reported that the state of their mental health was poor. Two out of

---

* This is an edited, reformatted and augmented version of Hearing of the Committee on Health, Education, Labor, and Pensions, United States Senate, One Hundred Eighteenth Congress, First Session on Examining the American Youth Mental Health Crisis, Focusing on Causes and Solutions, Publication No. S. HRG. 118–202, dated June 8, 2023.

In: Understanding Youth Mental Health
Editor: Michael A. Post
ISBN: 979-8-89530-700-7

every five teenagers felt persistently sad or hopeless, and tragically, one out of every five teenagers in our Country has seriously considered suicide.

How frightening is that? Tragically, suicide was the second leading cause of death for young people between the ages of 10 and 14, and it was the third leading cause of death among teenagers. All of us understand that the pandemic has had a huge and lasting impact on the mental health and well-being of our Country and our young people.

Let us never forget, and sometimes it is easy to forget, we remember the million people who died during the pandemic. But over 200,000 children, often children of color by the way, lost one or both of their parents to COVID.

Think about the impact that had on their lives. Further, and I think we are going to hear more about this later, our kids have become less connected humanly to each other, and this is kind of a new phenomenon.

Dr. Murthy has written about this, and I am sure will be speaking about it this morning. Instead of building trusting healthy, and strong relationships with their friends, their teachers, their mentors, an increasing number of kids are turning to their phones and social media to feel connected.

What type of impact does social media have on the mental health of our Nation's youth? That is an issue that we have got to really explore at great length as a Nation. According to a recent study, 32 percent of teen girls said that when they felt bad about their bodies, Instagram made them feel worse.

More than 40 percent of Instagram users who reported feeling unattractive said the feeling began on Instagram. About 25 percent of teenagers who reported feeling not good enough, inadequate, said it started on Instagram. But we are not here to single out Instagram alone, certainly, and I am sure that the same can be said about other social media platforms.

Let's be clear, and something I think this Committee in the months ahead will get into, we are up against some of the best minds in the world who keep coming up with new ways to get teenagers addicted, addicted to their websites in order to sell them more products and make more money, and that is what we are going to have to address.

But it is not just social media, as dangerous as that may be. Kids in Vermont, and I have been around to a lot of high schools and some community colleges in my state, but around this country as well, worry about the kind of future that awaits them.

They wonder if their political leaders in this country and around the world will address climate change, or whether the world that they and their kids will grow up in will be increasingly unhealthy and uninhabitable.

I really do wonder, walking here today through the smog and the smoke that Washington, DC. is experiencing right now, the horror in New York City, yes, it is a bad day, but you wonder what impact it has on the kids who wonder, is this the future—and what that does to them psychologically.

Yesterday on another issue, I had the occasion to meet with people who came to the Capitol who lost loved ones as a result of gun violence in schools. And I was stunned, in Vermont, where kids worry, when we were young, you went to school. It was a safe haven.

Now they really wonder that some terrible thing might happen. And when we talk about the anxieties facing young people, we can't ignore economics. Everything being equal, if we don't get our act together, the young people will have a lower standard of living than their parents.

Right now, some 60 percent of our people are struggling paycheck to paycheck. So, all I would say is the pandemic has exacerbated a bad situation. It is there. As political leaders in this country, it is our job to address it. Senator Cassidy, the mic is yours.

## Opening Statement of Senator Cassidy

Senator CASSIDY. Thank you, Mr. Chairman. Everybody here knows a fellow American struggling with mental health issues. Everybody watching knows, school closures, isolation from the COVID–19 pandemic exacerbated, almost concentrated this among those who are younger.

According to the CDC, from 2021 to 2022, the percent of teenagers feeling sad or hopeless increased from 37 percent to 42 percent. Those seriously considering suicide, seriously considered suicide, goes from 19 percent to 22. To say it is troubling is to kind of not have an adequate adjective.

This is terrible. The goal of this hearing is how do we improve access to quality mental health care for young people? Now, we must highlight that Congress has done a lot in recent years to improve mental health care and access for children and all Americans. We have walked this ground.

We need to see what our recent work has accomplished, need to measure its effectiveness, and then to figure out what gaps remain. Now, just for context, we have know this for decades, the Nation's mental health system was dysfunctional, under-resourced, not getting crucial services to Americans facing mental health issues, especially those in underserved areas. I worked in a hospital for the uninsured and the under-insured for 25 years.

I worked with this. Now, before I go on, let me give a shout out to Senator Chris Murphy. He and I in 2015 led the Mental Health Reform Act, an historic bill that overhauled our mental health system to increase access to quality mental health care for all Americans.

I remember Chris at that time saying, Bill, there are some things we agree on, a lot of them, and a few that we disagree. Let's focus on that which we agree and leave the other for another day.

By that, we did something which Lamar Alexander, then the Chair of this Committee, said he didn't think two freshmen Senators could do. There is both an insult and a praise in there.

[Laughter.]

Senator CASSIDY. But we accomplished it. And Lamar went on to say it was the most profound—the most profound reform of mental health law in the previous 30 years. He and I were both honored. Now, we teamed up again this past year to reauthorize this and to reform it to better address the needs of Americans.

We increased funding for mental health block grants to better serve children at risk for serious mental illness, expanded telemental health care, and promoted the integration of mental health providers into primary care, increased mental health workforce programs, focusing on treating children and underserved populations, and I could go on.

Now, additionally, and again I am going to give a shout out to Murphy once more, in response to the tragedy in Uvalde, Congress passed the bipartisan Safer Community Act, which invested billions of dollars so that every child and every American had access to mental health care no matter whether they are in a pediatrician's office, their school, an emergency room, or a community health center.

Chris was the lead on that, I had the privilege to work with them, but Congress passed it. The legislation invested $8.6 billion to expand certified community behavioral health clinics to all 50 states, offering 24/7 crisis intervention services, outpatient mental health, and substance abuse services, case management, increasing access to primary care for Americans, especially those who are lower income and uninsured.

It provided $2 billion for school based mental health treatment, to train school personnel to better help students through a crisis, to increase care for children suffering from trauma, to fund prevention programs, to decrease bullying and violence in schools, and much more.

Additionally, the Safer Communities Act instructing the Department of Education and the Department of Health and Human Services, both represented here today, to improve guidance to schools, particularly those in local—excuse me, in small or rural communities, to more easily build Medicaid for school based mental health services. And we will talk and hear more about that during the first panel.

I am proud of the work that Congress put into this legislation and signed into law, and these achievements show that there is a strong bipartisan support for addressing youth mental health issues.

But, and I say this all the time at home, these grants and programs only make a difference if state and local Government are aware of them, and apply, and show local leadership in order to participate. We need this local leadership to use these resources to make sure the assistance reaches those who need it most.

What we can't do is pretend that Congress hasn't done anything and that we must start anew. That, sweeping the debt clean, so to speak, in our minds, not acknowledging the basis upon which we build will create duplicate, inefficient programs, wasting dollars and wasting effort.

By the way, the Chair, just echoing the Chair, made the point, and I agree wholeheartedly, as you might guess, that the resources Congress appropriates should not be wasted. Now, Congress can't solve this on its own. Throwing money at an issue without accountability is not the solution.

There has to be complete buy in from the executive, from states, local Government, tribal leaders, and community organizations, among others, to make sure these programs work as Congress intended. There is, however, existing legislation up for reauthorization that requires attention.

As I mentioned in last week's hearing, the Committee has nine health care reauthorizations are waiting for programs that expire in September. One of these is the Support Act which helps individuals dealing with substance abuse disorder and increases support services for children suffering from trauma.

There are more than 50 individual provisions in the Support Act that fall in this Committee's jurisdiction. The fact that the Committee has 2 months left to reauthorize the programs and we have not formally considered bipartisan text, let alone marked them up, is concerning. I reiterate that reauthorizing the Support Act and these eight other health related bills on time, bipartisan must be the Committee's top priority.

As Ranking Member of the Committee, improving our Federal programs so they are more effective and having greater reach is crucial. So let me finish by saying I look forward to hearing from our witnesses as to how we can better address the mental health crisis to make sure that more young people have access to quality mental health and that the resources already allocated are used effectively.

Thank you, I yield.

The CHAIR. Thank you, Senator Cassidy. Now we are going to hear from our witnesses. And our first witness will be Vice-Admiral Vivek Murthy, who is the Surgeon General of the United States of America.

In my view, Dr. Vivek has done an extraordinary job in talking about the mental health crisis and the crisis of loneliness and many, many other issues. Dr. Vivek, thanks very much for being with us.

## Statement of Vice Admiral Vivek H. Murthy, U.S. Surgeon General, U.S. Department of Health and Human Services, Washington, DC

Admiral MURTHY. Thank you so much, Chairman Sanders. And thank you so much, Ranking Member Cassidy, for your leadership as well on issues related to mental health. To all the Members of the Committee who are here today, I am Dr. Vivek Murthy.

I have the privilege of serving as Surgeon General and as Vice Admiral of the U.S. Public Health Service Commission Corps, but I am most importantly here, as a father of two young children who is concerned about their future and the future of kids across America.

I am here to speak about what I believe is the defining public health issue of our time, and that is a youth mental health crisis. It now threatens the foundation for health and well-being for millions of our children.

In 2021, more than two in five high school students, including almost 60 percent of girls and 70 percent of LGBTQ youth, reported feeling persistently sad or hopeless. Nearly one in five high school students reported making a suicide plan, and this followed a 57 percent increase in the suicide rate among young people in the decade prior to the pandemic.

In response to this crisis, in December 2021, I issued a Surgeon General's advisory on protecting youth mental health, and I did this to call our Nation's attention to this urgent issue and to the need to act.

Over the last 2 years, I am grateful that Congress, on a bipartisan basis, and the Biden administration have made unprecedented investments to strengthen the mental health care system and to connect more youth to care.

These investments have already started to help children and families. But as all of you know, we have much more to do. Last month, my office released two new Surgeon General's advisories, and one on our epidemic of loneliness and isolation, and the other on social media and youth mental health.

Together, they explore two important drivers of the youth mental health crisis. Regarding loneliness and isolation, we now understand that social disconnection is both exceedingly common and profoundly consequential.

About one in two adults are reporting measurable levels of loneliness, and social disconnection is associated with an increased risk of not only depression, anxiety, and suicide, but also heart disease, dementia, stroke, and premature death.

The loneliness epidemic has hit young people particularly hard, and they have the highest rates of loneliness across age groups. The time young people, ages 15 through 24, spend in-person with friends declined by more than 50 percent from 2003 to 2019.

Furthermore, there has been a decline in participation over the last half century in community organizations that have traditionally brought us together, including faith organizations and recreational leagues.

Second though, I am increasingly concerned about the harmful impact that social media is having on youth mental health. Despite near universal users' inadequate evidence to conclude that social media is sufficiently safe for our kids, and while social media may provide some benefits for some children, there is a growing body of research associating social media use with potential harms.

This is especially concerning during adolescence, which is a highly sensitive period of brain development for kids and when they are particularly susceptible to peer comparison. The data show that youth who spend more than 3 hours a day on social media face double the risk of experiencing symptoms of depression and anxiety.

This is deeply worrisome because on average, teenagers are spending 3.5 hours a day on social media. And excessive social media use can also disrupt activities that are essential for healthy development, like physical activity, sleep, and in-person interactions. For example, a third of adolescents are telling us that they stay up until midnight or later on weeknights in front of their screens, and much of that is, in fact, social media use.

In addition, too often kids on social media are exposed to extreme, inappropriate, and harmful content. Indeed, nearly half of adolescents are saying that social media now makes them feel worse about their bodies. Now, two other drivers of youth mental health crisis that I just want to note briefly.

One is trauma, which has become all too common in young people's lives, particularly from violence and abuse, and the loss of loved ones to incarceration, addiction, and death. When young people go through such adverse childhood experiences, we know it has a negative impact on their mental and physical health.

Additionally, for many young people, their confidence in the future has been undermined by the serious challenges they are set to inherit, from economic inequality, and climate change, to racism, and gun violence.

This is what they say to me time and time again when I meet with young people around the country. The bottom line is our kids can't afford to wait longer for us to address the youth mental health crisis.

We have to expand our efforts to ensure every child has access to high quality, affordable, culturally competent mental health care. But we also must tackle the root causes by addressing the potential harms of social media through age appropriate health and safety standards and data transparency requirements, by investing in school based programs that equip children with the tools to manage their emotions, adversity, and their mental health, by addressing trauma, particularly violence, and by embarking on a generational effort to rebuild social connection and community in America.

Finally, we can all play a role in addressing the ongoing shame and stigma that still surround mental health and prevent young people for asking from help. Now, our obligation, finally to act is not just medical, it is moral.

It is about fulfilling our most sacred responsibility to care for our children and to secure a better future for them. I thank you for giving this critical issue the attention and the action it deserves, and I look forward to your questions.

[The prepared statement of Mr. Murthy follows:]

## Prepared Statement of Vivek H. Murthy

Chairman Sanders, Ranking Member Cassidy, Members of the Committee. I'm Dr. Vivek Murthy, and I have the privilege of serving as Surgeon General of the United States; as Vice Admiral in the United States Public Health Service Commissioned Corps; and, most importantly, as the father of two young children, a 5-year-old girl and a 6-year-old boy. They are the primary reason I am grateful for this opportunity to speak with you today.

Over the next few years, both of my children will enter an important stage of their education and development, where they'll learn how to build friendships, deal with adversity, and develop the values that will guide them throughout their lives. They and millions of their peers will start down the path to adulthood. Each path will be different. All will be filled with challenges along the way.

It's these challenges that I want to talk about today. I'm deeply concerned, as a parent and as a doctor, that many of the obstacles that this generation of young people face are unprecedented and uniquely hard to navigate. The resulting impact on the mental health of millions of our children has been devastating.

In 2021, more than 2 in 5 high school students reported feeling persistently sad or hopeless almost every day for at least 2 weeks in a row—so much so that they stopped their regular activities.[1] This is an increase of 14 percent from 2019 and 50 percent from the previous decade. We also know that, in 2021, nearly 1 in 5 high school students reported making a suicide plan, a 13 percent increase from 2019.[2] And, within these numbers, we know that disparities exist. For example, nearly 60 percent of high school girls reported persistent feelings of sadness or hopelessness—a figure that was double the share of boys and the highest in a decade.[3] Students who identified as lesbian, gay, bisexual, questioning, or another non-heterosexual identity were approximately two times more likely than their heterosexual peers to experience persistent feelings of sadness or hopelessness too (69 percent vs 35 percent).[4] And also, in 2021, 3.7 percent of youth ages 12–17 had both a Major Depressive Episode (MDE) and a substance use disorder (SUD).[5]

The pandemic exacerbated this problem, but these challenges started well before the pandemic began and have many other contributing factors. From 2011 to 2015, youth psychiatric visits to emergency departments for depression, anxiety, and behavioral challenges

---

[1] Centers for Disease Control and Prevention. (2023). Youth Risk Behavior Surveillance Data Summary and Trends Report: 2011–2021. Retrieved from *https://www.cdc.gov/healthyyouth/data/yrbs/pdf/YRBS-Data-Summary-Trends-Report2023-508.pdf.*

[2] *Id.*

[3] *Id.* at 1.

[4] *Id.* at 1.

[5] Substance Abuse and Mental Health Services Administration. (2022). Key substance use and mental health indicators in the United States: Results from the 2021 National Survey on Drug Use and Health (HHS Publication No. PEP22–07–01–005, NSDUH Series H–57). Center for Behavioral Health Statistics and Quality, Substance Abuse and Mental Health Services Administration. *https://www.samhsa.gov/data/report/2021-nsduh-annual-national-report.*

increased by 28 percent.[6] And between 2007 and 2018, suicide rates among youth ages 10–24 increased by 57%—a total of 65,026 young people lost.[7]

Many mental health challenges first emerge early in life—half of all lifetime mental health issues begin by age 14, and 75 percent begin by age 24.[8] We need to do more to give young people and their families the tools to prevent and treat these mental health challenges. The average delay between the onset of mental health symptoms and treatment is 11 years—11 long, isolating, confusing, and painful years.[9]

We have the opportunity, the responsibility, and—as evidenced through my travels across the country and my conversations with many of you—the desire to address the youth mental health crisis in America. In 2021, I released The Surgeon General's Advisory on Protecting Youth Mental Health, which outlines the policy, institutional, and individual changes it will take to treat and prevent mental health challenges. Just last month, my office released two new advisories. First on Our Epidemic of Loneliness and Isolation: The U.S. Surgeon General's Advisory on the Healing Effects of Social Connection and Community. And second, The U.S. Surgeon General's Advisory on Social Media and Youth Mental Health. Together, these Advisories explore what's contributing to the mental health crisis among youth and how to address it.

One of the key barriers to addressing mental health is the stubborn and pervasive stigmatization of mental health that tells people they should be ashamed if they are struggling with depression, anxiety, stress, or loneliness. It's isolating and further separates people experiencing mental health challenges from their loved ones and from sources of support. This stigmatization prevents kids from seeking help and receiving the long-term recovery supports they need.

I felt that stigma myself, growing up in Miami as a child who didn't look the same as the other kids, and who too-often was bullied and called racial slurs by classmates who told me I didn't belong. Not surprisingly, that left me feeling lonely and anxious about going to school—and I felt a deep sense of shame as well. Like it was somehow entirely my fault that I was hurting. Even though I knew my family loved me unconditionally, the embarrassment I felt prevented me from asking them for help.

Even when children are able to summon the courage to ask for help, we do not always have sufficient resources to meet their needs. I am grateful that, in recent years, Congress and the Biden administration have made unprecedented investments in expanding access to mental health care and treatment for kids. In 2022, President Biden announced his Unity Agenda for the Nation—calling on us all to work together to tackle the mental health crisis, particularly for our youth. He released a comprehensive strategy to transform how we understand, treat and integrate mental health in America. And, already several actions have been taken to strengthen

---

[6] Kalb, L. G., Stapp, E. K., Ballard, E. D., Holingue, C., Keefer, A., & Riley, A. (2019). Trends in Psychiatric Emergency Department Visits Among Youth and Young Adults in the US. Pediatrics, 143(4), e20182192. *https://doi.org/10.1542/peds.2018-2192.*

[7] Curtin, S. C. (2020). State suicide rates among adolescents and young adults aged 10–24: United States, 2000–2018. National Vital Statistics Reports; 69:11. Hyattsville, MD: National Center for Health Statistics.

[8] Kessler, R. C., Berglund, P., Demler, O., Jin, R., Merikangas, K. R., & Walters, E. E. (2005). Lifetime prevalence and age-of-onset distributions of DSM-IV disorders in the National Comorbidity Survey Replication. Archives of general psychiatry, 62(6), 593–602. *https://doi.org/ 10.1001/archpsyc.62.6.593.*

[9] Wang, P. S., Berglund, P. A., Olfson, M., & Kessler, R. C. (2004). Delays in initial treatment contact after first onset of a mental disorder. Health services research, 39(2), 393–415. *https:// doi.org/10.1111/j.1475-6773.2004.00234.x.*

system capacity and connect more youth to care, including unprecedented investments to increase access to school-based mental health services with a focus on high-need school districts; to harness technology to bring virtual mental health services to where young people are; and to increase the number of peer support workers across the country. And historic investments have been made to enhance crisis response through the 988 Suicide and Crisis Lifeline to ensure that anyone experiencing a mental health crisis receives faster access to mental health services and trained mental health professionals. Significant investments have also been made to expand proven models of care like Certified Community Behavioral Health Centers (CCBHC) to provide comprehensive behavioral health care—including crisis care—to the most vulnerable Americans regardless of their ability to pay.

These are tremendous steps and many children now have access to care that they didn't previously have. However, more action is needed to help the millions who still lack adequate access. This means training providers, expanding peer support programs, enabling widespread use of technology to provide remote care, integrating behavioral health care with primary care and other settings, and strengthening and enforcing health insurance parity laws to ensure that insurers do their part to provide fair, equitable access to mental health services.

In addition to investment in treatment, it's crucial we do more to address the root causes of the youth mental health crisis. Today, I'd like to highlight three drivers that impact the mental health of today's kids and that I am particularly concerned about: loneliness, the impact of social media, and profound concerns about the state of the world.

First, increasing rates of loneliness. Across many measures, Americans appear to be becoming less socially connected over time. This is a problem that preceded the COVID–19 pandemic, though it certainly worsened for many people over the last 3 years. Social networks have been getting smaller, and levels of social participation have been declining. For example, objective measures of social exposure obtained from 2003–2020 find that social isolation, measured by the average time spent alone, increased from 2003 (285-minutes/day, 142.5-hours/month) to 2019 (309-minutes/day, 154.5-hours/month) and continued to increase in 2020 (333-minutes/day, 166.5-hours/month).[10] This represents an increase of 24 hours per month spent alone. At the same time, social participation across several types of relationships has steadily declined. For instance, the amount of time respondents engaged with friends socially in—person decreased from 2003 (60-minutes/day, 30-hours/month) to 2020 (20-minutes/day, 10-hours/month).[11] This represents a decrease of 20 hours per month spent engaging with friends. This decline in total time spent in-person with friends was starkest for young people ages 15 to 24. For this age group, time spent in-person with friends has declined by nearly 50% over the last two decades, from roughly 150 minutes per day in 2003 to less than 70 minutes per day in 2019.[12] This is concerning because, for children and adolescents, loneliness and social isolation in childhood increases the risk of depression and anxiety both in the short-term and well into the future (up to 9 years later).[13]

---

[10] Kannan, V. D., & Veazie, P. J. (2022). US trends in social isolation, social engagement, and companionship—nationally and by age, sex, race/ethnicity, family income, and work hours, 2003–2020. SSM—population health, 21, 101331. *https://doi.org/10.1016/j.ssmph.2022.101331*.

[11] *Id.*

[12] *Id.* at 9.

[13] Loades, M. E., Chatburn, E., Higson-Sweeney, N., Reynolds, S., Shafran, R., Brigden, A., Linney, C., McManus, M. N., Borwick, C., & Crawley, E. (2020). Rapid Systematic Review: The Impact of Social Isolation and Loneliness on the Mental Health of Children and Adolescents in the Context of COVID–19. Journal of the

Second, as discussed in the recent U.S. Surgeon General's Advisory on Social Media and Youth Mental Health, we have reason to be concerned about the impact of social media[14] use on youth mental health. Social media use by youth is nearly universal. Up to 95 percent of youth ages 13–17 report using a social media platform, with more than a third saying they use social media "almost constantly."[15] Although age 13 is commonly the required minimum age used by social media platforms in the U.S., nearly 40 percent of children ages 8–12 use social media.[16] Despite this widespread use among children and adolescents, there is insufficient evidence to conclude that social media is sufficiently safe for kids. Instead, there is a growing body of data associating social media use with potential harms to kids. There are also widespread concerns among parents and caregivers, young people, health care experts, and others about the impact of social media on youth mental health.

While social media may have benefits for some children and adolescents, such as serving as a source of connection, information, and support, especially for youth who are often marginalized, we must acknowledge and better understand the growing body of research about potential harms associated with social media use and urgently take action to create safe and healthy digital environments—ones that minimize harm and safeguard children's and adolescents' mental health and well-being while also maximizing the potential benefits of social media on health and well-being.

We are especially concerned about social media use among children because adolescence represents a highly sensitive period of brain development that can make young people more vulnerable to harms from social media. During this period, we know that young people are more prone to engage in risk-taking behaviors, their overall well-being (in terms of mood, physical health, etc.) fluctuates the most, and mental health challenges begin to emerge. We also know that, in early adolescence, when identities and sense of self-worth are forming, brain development is especially susceptible to social pressures, peer opinions, and peer comparison. As such, adolescents may experience heightened emotional sensitivity to the communicative and interactive nature of social media.

Social media platforms may contribute to youth mental health concerns in a number of ways. Excessive social media use can disrupt activities that are essential for healthy youth

---

American Academy of Child and Adolescent Psychiatry, 59(11), 1218–1239.e3. *https://doi.org/10.1016/j.jaac.2020.05.009*.

[14] The definition of social media has been highly debated over the past few decades. As a result, there isn't a single, widely accepted scholarly definition of social media. (Aichner et al., 2021) The definition may vary from the cited research in this document based on the methods used in each study. In making conclusions and recommendations, this document regards social media as "internet-based channels that allow users to opportunistically interact and selectively self-present, either in real-time or asynchronously, with both broad and narrow audiences who derive value from user-generated content and the perception of interaction with others." (Carr & Hayes, 2015). For the purposes of this product, we did not include studies specific to online gaming or e-sports. Aichner, T., Grunfelder, M., Maurer, O., & Jegeni, D. (2021). Twenty-Five Years of Social Media: A Review of Social Media Applications and Definitions from 1994 to 2019. Cyberpsychology, Behavior And Social Networking, 24(4), 215–222. *https://doi.org/10.1089/ cyber.2020.0134*; Carr, C. T., & Hayes, R. A. (2015). Social Media: Defining, Developing, and Divining. Atlantic Journal of Communication, 23:1, 46–65. *https://doi.org/10.1080/15456870.2015.972282*.

[15] Vogels, E., Gelles-Watnick, R. & Massarat, N. (2022). Teens, Social Media and Technology 2022. Pew Research Center: Internet, Science & Tech. United States of America. Retrieved from *https://www.pewresearch.org/internet/2022/08/10/teens-social-media-and-technology2022/*.

[16] Rideout, V., Peebles, A., Mann, S., & Robb, M. B. (2022). Common Sense Census: Media use by tweens and teens, 2021. San Francisco, CA: Common Sense. Retrieved from *https://www.commonsensemedia.org/sites/default/files/research/report/8-18-census-integrated-report-final-web-0.pdf*.

development like physical activity and sleep and reduce time for positive in-person activities. The content on social media platforms can reinforce negative behaviors like online harassment, abuse, exploitation, and exclusion, perpetuate body dissatisfaction and social comparison, and undermine the safe and supportive environments kids need to thrive. Research suggests that social media use can be excessive and problematic for some kids; that children and adolescents on social media are commonly exposed to extreme, inappropriate, and harmful content. The research also shows that those who spend more than 3 hours a day on social media face double the risk of experiencing poor mental health outcomes, such as symptoms of depression and anxiety.[17] This is deeply concerning as a survey of teenagers showed that, on average, they spend 3.5 hours a day on social media, with one in four spending 5 or more hours per day and one in seven spending 7 or more hours per day on social media.[18] Over half of teenagers report that it would be hard to give up social media, and on a typical weekday, nearly one in three adolescents report using screens (most commonly social media) until midnight or later.[19,20]

When asked about the impact of social media on their body image, nearly half (46 percent) of adolescents ages 13–17 said social media makes them feel worse, 40 percent said it makes them feel neither better nor worse, and 14 percent said it makes them feel better.[21]

This increase in social media use may also contribute to the bombardment of messages that undermine this generation's sense of self-worth—messages that tell our kids with greater frequency and volume than ever before that they're not good-looking enough, not popular enough, not smart enough, not rich enough.

Third, many young people are grappling with challenges that impact their present-day experience and the world they'll inherit, including economic inequality, climate change, racial injustice, discrimination against individuals who identify as LGBTQI+, the opioid epidemic, and gun violence. And they feel progress is too slow. The COVID–19 pandemic further exacerbated the stresses young people already faced. As of December 2022, more than 275,000 children lost a primary or secondary caregiver due to COVID–19 and many more worried about losing loved ones who fell sick.[22] With the support of Congress, the Administration has taken actions to support this population of youth who have been affected by COVID–19 and other disasters, such as the Children and Youth Resilience Prize Challenge which will fund innovative community-led solutions to promote resilience in children and adolescents. Millions of children experienced increased food insecurity, instability, and economic stress at home, and were isolated from friends and family during an extraordinarily stressful period. The collective

---

[17] Riehm, K. E., Feder, K. A., Tormohlen, K. N., Crum, R. M., Young, A. S., Green, K. M., Pacek, L. R., La Flair, L. N., & Mojtabai, R. (2019). Associations Between Time Spent Using Social Media and Internalizing and Externalizing Problems Among US Youth. JAMA psychiatry, 76(12), 1266–1273. *https://doi.org/10.1001/jamapsychiatry.2019.2325.*

[18] Miech, R. A., Johnston, L. D., Bachman, J. G., O'Malley, P. M., Schulenberg, J. E., and Patrick, M. E. (2022). Monitoring the Future: A Continuing Study of American Youth (8th-and 10th-Grade Surveys), 2021. Inter-university Consortium for Political and Social Research [distributor]. *https://doi.org/10.3886/ICPSR38502.v1*

[19] *Id.* at 14.

[20] Bickham, D.S., Hunt, E., Bediou, B., & Rich, M. (2022). Adolescent Media Use: Attitudes, Effects, and Online Experiences. Boston, MA: Boston Children's Hospital Digital Wellness Lab. Retrieved from *https://digitalwellnesslab.org/wp-content/uploads/Pulse-Survey-Adolescent-Attitudes-Effects-and-Experiences.pdf.*

[21] *Id.*

[22] Imperial College London. (14 February, 2022). Global Orphanhood estimates real time calculator. Imperial College London. Retrieved from *https://imperialcollegelondon.github.io/orphanhood-calculator/#/country/United%20States%20of%20America.*

impact of these challenges and the absence of a clear, unified path to progress has undermined young people's confidence in the future that awaits them.

It is imperative that we act now. Our children do not have the luxury of time— their childhoods and developments are happening now.

Out of the many recommendations in the recent Surgeon General's Advisories, I'd like to highlight four overarching recommendations today:

First, ensuring that every child has access to high-quality, affordable, and culturally competent mental health care. To do this, we must make sure that children are enrolled in health coverage—far too many children in our Country are eligible for coverage under Medicaid and the Children's Health Insurance Program, but aren't enrolled. We need to do better here, especially as pandemic-era provisions to support coverage have come to an end, which could leave gaps in coverage for countless families and children.[23] We also need to expand our mental health workforce, from clinical psychologists, school counselors, and psychiatrists, to recovery coaches and peer specialists—and that includes making sure these professionals can serve in, and provide services at, schools. We have too few providers to meet the growing demand. And we need to make sure that care is delivered at the right place and time, whether that's in health care settings like primary care practices, or community-based settings like schools, and whether it's in person or through telehealth. The Departments of Education and Health and Human Services are collaborating to help make it easier for schools to file Medicaid claims for crucial mental and physical school-based health services, with potential to unlock additional supports for millions more students nation-wide. This is on top of the from the American Rescue Plan Elementary and Secondary School Emergency Relief Fund and the Bipartisan Safer Communities Act that we know states and schools districts are already using to provide more counselors, other mental health providers, and nurses in schools. More than 14,000 new mental health professionals—including school psychologists, counselors, and social workers—are projected to be placed in U.S. schools.[24] Those funds, coupled with Medicaid funding, are available now to help meet our young peoples' critical mental health needs.

Second, focusing on prevention, by investing in school-and community-based prevention, promotion, and early intervention programs that have been shown to improve the mental health and emotional well-being of children at low cost and high benefit. Every dollar we spend on prevention represents multiple dollars we won't have to spend on treatment—in fact, one study estimated that investment in early prevention offered a fourfold return down the line.[25] We've seen the extraordinary potential of certain strategies and programs—Project AWARE and What Works in Schools, for example, which help communities develop a sustainable infrastructure for school-based mental health programs and services. The recent Surgeon General's Advisory on Our Epidemic of Loneliness and Isolation lays out a set of recommendations for schools,

---

[23] Centers for Medicare & Medicaid Services. (n.d.). Unwinding and Returning to Regular Operations after COVID–19. Retrieved from *https://www.Medicaid.gov/resources-for-states/ coronavirus-disease-2019-covid-19/unwinding-and-returning-regular-operations-after-covid-19/ index.html*.

[24] U.S. Department of Education. (15, May 2023). Press Release: Biden-Harris Administration Announces Nearly $100 Million in Continued Support for Mental Health and Student Wellness Through Bipartisan Safer Communities Act. Retrieved from *https://www.ed.gov/news/press-releases/today-biden-harris-administration-announcing-more-95-million-awards-across-35-states-increase-access-school-based-mental-health-services-and-strengthen-pipeline-mental-health-professionals-high-needs-school-districts-t*.

[25] Karoly, L.A., Greenwood, P.W., Everingham, S.S., Houb, J.S., Kilburn, M.R., Rydell, C.P., Sanders, M.R., & Chiesa, J. (1998). Investing in Our Children: What We Know and Don't Know About the Costs and Benefits of Early Childhood Interventions.

including developing a strategic plan for school connectedness, building social connection into health curricula, implementing socially based educational techniques such as cooperative learning projects, and creating supportive school environments that foster belonging.

These programs support families, teaching parents how to recognize challenges as they emerge, find available resources, and offer support and care. They also give kids tools to manage their emotions in healthy ways, build supportive relationships, and get help when they need it. We need to invest in scaling these programs, and programs like them, across the country. And that must go hand-in-hand with continuing to advance comprehensive public health approaches such as preventing adverse childhood experiences, promoting positive childhood experiences, and addressing the systemic economic and social barriers, like safety, housing, food, and economic insecurity, that contribute to and create the conditions for poor mental health for young people, families, and caregivers.[26]

Third, we need to take action now to protect children against the potential harms of social media. The recent Surgeon General's Advisory on Social Media and Youth Mental Health describes the current evidence on the impacts of social media on the mental health of children and adolescents. It details how there are critical gaps to understanding the full extent of mental health risks posed by social media—including a lack of evidence that social media is sufficiently safe for children and adolescents. There are critical steps policymakers can take to address the complex issues related to social media use and protect youth from the risk of harm, including by strengthening safety protections, developing age-appropriate health and safety standards, limiting access in ways that make social media safer for children of all ages, requiring platforms to better protect children's privacy, supporting digital and media literacy curricula within schools and in academic standards, and supporting research on both the benefits and harms of social media use. The Administration has taken actions to help us fill critical knowledge gaps such as the establishment of the National Center of Excellence on Social Media and Mental Wellness, which will develop and disseminate information, guidance, and training on the impact— including risks and benefits—of social media use on children and young people and examine clinical and social interventions that can be used to prevent and mitigate the risks. It's crucial that these platforms are designed to maximize the benefits and minimize the harms to the mental health of our youth and with the health and well-being of all users, especially children, in mind.

The final recommendation I will highlight today concerns individual and community engagement to cultivate a culture of connection—a culture in which we prioritize cultivating healthy relationships with family, friends, neighbors, coworkers, and community members. A strong culture of connection shapes not only our individual experience but also how we design our school and work environments and the investments we make in community organizations that bring us together. Such a culture rests on core values of kindness, respect, service, and commitment to one another. As leaders, parents, friends, and fellow Americans, it is up to us to build this culture by reflecting these core values through our actions, our words, and our example. We can do it by investing in local-level programs, policies, and physical elements of a community that facilitate bringing people together, by reaching out to people in our lives who are having a hard time to offer our support, by choosing to understand someone's intention and

---

[26] Centers for Disease Control and Prevention. (22 September, 2022). Preventing Adverse Childhood Experiences: Data to Action (PACE:D2A). Retrieved from *https://www.cdc.gov/violenceprevention/aces/preventingace-datatoaction.html*.

choosing not to demonize them because of our differences, and by sharing our own stories and struggles with mental health, recognizing that there is great power in our authenticity and vulnerability.

A nation with a strong culture of connection is one where people feel a sense of community and belonging, where people recognize that we are defined not by our differences and disagreements but by the hopes we share for our kids, our community, and our Country.

I look forward to discussing these recommendations and possibilities with you today. Mitigating this crisis is urgent, but it will take a bipartisan, all-of-society coalition of governments, community organizations, employers, technology and social companies, schools and health care systems, and young people and their families alike. I thank you for recognizing this, and for your shared commitment to action.

Our obligation to act is not just medical—it's moral. It's not only about saving lives. It's about fulfilling our sacred obligation—to care for our children and secure a better future for them. Throughout our history, progress has been born in the wake of tragedy. I'm eager to partner with you to make it happen again.

Thank you for having me, and for giving this critical issue the attention it needs and deserves.

* * *

The CHAIR. Let me turn to Senator Cassidy, who will introduce our next witness.

Senator CASSIDY. It is an honor to introduce Mrs. Katherine Neas, Deputy Assistant Secretary of the Office of Special Education and Rehabilitative Services at the U.S. Department of Education.

In her role, Mrs. Neas works to improve the educational and employment outcomes for students with disabilities. Today, she will discuss the Department's broader work to support the mental well-being of all students. Mrs. Neas.

## Statement of Katherine Neas, Deputy Assistant Secretary, Office of Special Education and Rehabilitative Services, U.S. Department of Education, Washington, DC

Ms. NEAS. Chairman Sanders, Ranking Member Cassidy, and distinguished Members of the Committee, thank you for the opportunity to share the Department of Education's work on youth mental health and promising interventions.

The Youth Risks Behavioral Survey, released this past February by the Centers for Disease Control and Prevention, conveyed alarming findings of the prevalence of mental health or substance use disorder among our Nation's youth.

The report advances the critical need for schools to expand school based services and to connect youth and families to community based sources of care. Simply put, schools are a gateway to needed services that otherwise might be inaccessible to many young people. The report also emphasizes the responsibility of schools to ensure that all learning occurs in a safe and supportive environment.

The Department's work is focused on three top priorities, increasing the skill and knowledge of existing school personnel to support the mental health needs of students, increasing the supply of mental health professionals who can work with students, and increasing funding through the Medicaid program to support school health services, including mental health services.

One year ago, Congress provided new funding under the bipartisan Safer Communities Act that significantly bolstered Federal, state, and local efforts to address student mental health needs. I am pleased to provide you with an update of our work to implement this law.

Last September, the Department awarded $1 billion to state educational agencies to competitively award sub-grants to high needs school districts for activities to support safe and healthy students. This Stronger Connections Grant Program will support school districts to develop, implement, and evaluate comprehensive programs and activities that foster safe, healthy, supportive, and drug free environments that support student academic achievement.

The bipartisan Safer Communities Act also provided $1 billion over 5 years to be equally divided across two programs to increase the supply of school based mental health service providers. The response to these two grants has been enthusiastic. Under the school based mental health services grant, 12 states and the District of Columbia and 229 school districts across 41 states submitted applications.

The Department was able to fund nine states, the District of Columbia, and 94 school districts across 31 states. Under the Mental Health Services Professional Demonstration Grant Program, 266 school districts applied, and the Department was able to find 160 grants.

To support this $280 million of Federal support across 264 grantees that will train 14,000, sorry, school based mental health professionals, the Department will fund a mental Health Personnel Technical Assistance Center later this year.

This past January, the Department awarded $86 million in grants to local communities through the Promise Neighborhood and the Full Service Community Schools Program. The bipartisan Safer Communities Act also directed the Departments of Health and Human Services in collaboration with the Department of Education to issue guidance to increase access to school based health services to children enrolled in Medicaid and the Children's Health Insurance Program.

This guidance was released on May 18th of this year. Medicaid and CHIP provide health coverage to more than half of America's children, roughly 41 million children. These programs are administered by state according to Federal requirements.

Children are eligible based on family income or unique health care needs, such as having a disability or a serious mental illness, or if they are in foster care. Under Medicaid's Early Periodic Screening Diagnostics and Treatment Program, eligible children can receive comprehensive primary health, mental health, and behavioral health services.

Medicaid enrolled children who need services in school can fall into two categories, eligible children who need general health care services and students with disabilities who receive services under the Individuals with Disabilities Education Act.

In 2021, schools receive nearly $6 billion in total payments for school based health care to Medicaid students. Schools also received about $14 billion in Federal IDEA funding. In 2014, the Centers for Medicare and Medicaid Services issued a letter to state Medicaid directors clarifying reimbursable services in a school based setting.

The CMS letter explained that schools can seek payment for all Medicare covered services provided to all students enrolled in Medicaid, not just for students with disabilities. As of May

2023, 21 states have used this policy to expand their school based Medicaid programs. Most states use these funds to hire and sustain essential personnel who can deliver or facilitate the delivery of health and mental health services.

As you can see, the Department is actively engaging in efforts to address the mental health crisis facing our Nation's youth. We are committed to ensuring that students' needs are met, that they are ready to learn, and that they have the full access to learning opportunities. Thank you for the opportunity to be here, and I look forward to answer your questions.

[The prepared statement of Ms. Neas follows:]

## Prepared Statement of Katherine Neas

Chairman Sanders, Ranking Member Cassidy, and distinguished Members of the Committee, thank you for the opportunity to share the Department of Education's (Department's) work to meet the needs of the 49.5 million students enrolled in public schools across the country and the 25.3 million students enrolled in colleges and universities.

While I serve as the Department's Deputy Assistant Secretary for the Office of Special Education and Rehabilitative Services, mental health is a deep personal and professional area of interest to me, and a priority issue across the Department. Mental health affects the well-being of every student, educator, school, and community in America; and the Department is committed to creating the conditions for all students to thrive academically and personally.

The *National Survey on Drug Use and Health* released in January by the Substance Abuse and Mental Health Services Administration and the *Youth Risk Behavioral Survey* released this past February by the Centers for Disease Control and Prevention (CDC) conveyed alarming findings of the prevalence of mental health or substance use disorders, or co-occurrence of both among our Nation's youth.[27] The *Youth Risk Behavioral Survey* also included recommendations on how schools can be part of the solution. The report advances the critical need for schools to expand school-based services and to connect youth and families to community-based sources of care. Simply put, schools are a gateway to needed services for many young people. As trusted community partners, schools can provide critical behavioral and mental health services directly or establish referral systems to connect those in need to community sources of care that might otherwise be inaccessible. The report also emphasized the responsibility of schools to ensure that all learning occurs in a safe and supportive environment.

The Kaiser Family Foundation highlights several factors that limit schools' current ability to effectively provide mental health services to students.[28] These factors include insufficient mental health professional staff coverage; inadequate access to licensed mental health professionals; inadequate funding; concerns about reactions from parents; requirements that schools pay for the services, and a lack of community support for providing services.

We know the COVID–19 pandemic exacerbated certain pre-existing challenges to student wellness and academic success, and the ongoing impacts of the pandemic continue to hinder

---

[27] Centers for Disease Control and Prevention, *Youth Risk Behavior Survey: Data Summary and Trends Report 2011–2021*, *https://www.cdc.gov/healthyyouth/data/yrbs/yrbs-data-summary-and-trends.htm*.

[28] Nirmita Panchal, Cynthia Cox, Robin Rudowitz, "The Landscape of School-Based Mental Health Services," Kaiser family Foundation, September 6, 2022, *https://www.kff.org/other/issue-brief/the-landscape-of-school-based-mental-health-services/*.

some state and local recovery efforts.[29] Moreover, suicide was the second leading cause of death among people age 20–34.[30] Additionally, college students who experience basic needs insecurity experience significantly higher rates of depression, anxiety, and suicidal ideation, planning, or attempt.[31] The Department embraces the opportunity to reflect on what we have learned and move forward with a renewed energy to support the field in accelerating learning and supporting the mental health of preschool to postsecondary students and school personnel.

The Department is actively engaged in efforts to accelerate recovery. These efforts have been supported by historic investments that continue to raise the bar so students can recover academically and access critical supports for their mental health and well-being. Raising the bar means recognizing that our Nation already has what it takes to continue leading the world—if we deliver a comprehensive, rigorous education for every student; boldly improve conditions for learning; and ensure every student has a pathway to multilingualism and to college and careers. When the bar is raised in education, all our Nation's students will build the skills to succeed inside and outside of school. Our students will reach new heights in the classroom, in their careers, and in their enriched lives and communities, making a positive difference in the world, for generations to come.

While the work is far from over, I am pleased to share what is underway.

## Department of Education Priorities

The Department's work aligns with the President's Unity Agenda, the CDC and the Kaiser Family Foundation findings and is focused on three top priorities: (1) increasing the skills and knowledge of existing school personnel to support the mental health needs of students; (2) increasing the supply of mental health professionals who can work with students; and (3) increasing funding through the Medicaid program to support school health services, including mental health services.

One year ago, Congress provided new funding under the Bipartisan Safer Communities Act (BSCA) that significantly bolstered Federal, state, and local efforts to address student mental health needs. I am pleased to provide you with an update on our work to implement this legislation.

## Funding of School Based Mental Health Services

Through BSCA, the Department received four categories of funding, reflecting a comprehensive approach to supporting States, Local Educational Agencies (LEAs), and schools in creating safe and healthy learning environments.

This includes:

---

[29] U.S. Department of Education. "Education in a Pandemic: Disparate Impacts of COVID–19 on America's Students." Retrieved from: *https://www..ed.gov/about/offices/list/ocr/docs/20210608-impacts-of-covid19.pdf.*

[30] Centers for Disease Control and Prevention. Facts About Suicide. *https://www.cdc.gov/suicide/facts/index.html.*

[31] Katharine M. Broton, Milad Mohebali, Mitchell D. Lingo. *Basic Needs Insecurity and Mental Health: Community College Students' Dual Challenges and Use of Social Support*. 2022. *https://journals.sagepub.com/doi/abs/10.1177/00915521221111460.*

- $1 billion through Title IV, Part A of the Elementary and Secondary Education Act of 1965 (ESEA) to enable State Educational Agencies (SEAs) to competitively award subgrants to high-need LEAs for activities to support safe and healthy students under ESEA section 4108. The Department has designated this component of BSCA the *Stronger Connections Grant Program*. States are in the process of running Stronger Connections grant competitions. ESEA section 4108 allows funds to be used to "develop, implement, and evaluate comprehensive programs and activities" that foster safe, healthy, supportive, and drug-free environments that support student academic achievement. Therefore, Stronger Connections funds may be used to hire professionals who are necessary to implementing such programs.
- An additional $50 million in formula funding for the 21st Century Community Learning Centers, which provides academic enrichment opportunities to students during non-school hours.
- $500 million for competitively awarded School-Based Mental Health (SBMH) Services Grants designed to increase the number of credentialed school-based mental health services providers delivering school-based mental health services to students.
- $500 million for competitively awarded Mental Health Services Professionals (MHSP) Demonstration Grants to support innovative partnerships involving states, school districts, and institutions of higher education (IHEs) to train and increase the number and diversity of high-quality school-based mental health services providers available to address shortages of such providers in schools within high-need districts. Nearly half of the new MHSP awardees included a partnership with a Minority Serving Institution, Historically Black Colleges or Universities or Tribal Colleges.
- $280 million across 264 projects projected to train approximately 14,000 school-based mental health professionals.
- $86 million in grants to local communities awarded in December 2022. Under the Promise Neighborhood Grants, six communities received $23 million to provide coordinated support services and programs to students from low-income backgrounds at every stage of their education from early childhood through their careers. These grants will also focus on preventing and reducing community violence that too often impacts low-income communities. Under the Full-Service Community Schools program,
- $63 million in new awards went to 42 LEAs, non-profits, and IHEs across 18 states, the District of Columbia, and Puerto Rico.

To support grantees funded under the SBMH and MHSP grant programs, later this year, the Department will fund a first of its kind school-based mental health professional development technical assistance center. This center will provide support and resources to grantees, help ensure accurate data-collection and reporting to gauge progress, and disseminate best practices in credentialing, recruiting, training and developing, and retaining school-based mental health services providers. This will include best practices for establishing and sustaining partnerships with IHEs to create and provide innovative high-quality training and credentialing options and maintain a robust pipeline of school-based mental health services providers.

IHEs have also worked creatively on the ground to utilize funding from the Higher Education Emergency Relief Fund to address mental health at colleges and universities around the country.[32]

Some examples include:

- North Carolina Central University created a suicide prevention coordinating committee. The committee has worked to develop on-campus resources and a suicide response plan.
- The University System of Georgia created a system-wide task force to develop a comprehensive plan for long-term solutions to address mental health challenges and provide mental health services at their institutions.
- The University of Alabama provided centers for students from underserved or marginalized groups and communities, open for all students, including a Safe Zone for LGBTQ+ students, a Collegiate Recovery and Intervention Services Center for students with substance use disorders, and a Women and Gender Resource Center for students who are survivors of violence.
- Lac Courte Oreilles Ojibwe College in Wisconsin partnered with a mental health platform to allow all students and faculty on-demand, 24/7 access to counselors.

## Interagency Collaboration and Capacity Expansion through Medicaid

BSCA also directed the Department of Health and Human Services, in collaboration with the Department of Education to issue guidance to state Medicaid agencies, LEAs, and school-based entities to support the delivery of medical assistance to Medicaid and the Children's Health Insurance Program (CHIP) beneficiaries in school-based settings. This guidance, *Delivering Services in School-Based Settings: A Comprehensive Guide to Medicaid Services and Administrative Claiming* was released on May 18, 2023.[33]

Medicaid and CHIP provide health coverage to millions of people living with disabilities and low-income families, children, pregnant individuals, adults, and seniors, including over half of American children (57 percent = 41.9 million children enrolled in Medicaid and CHIP / 73.1 million children in the U.S.).[34] These programs are administered by states, according to Federal requirements. Children are eligible based on their family income or unique health care needs (such as a disability or serious mental illness), or if they are in foster care. Under Medicaid's Early Periodic Screening, Diagnostic and Treatment (EPSDT) benefit, eligible

---

[32] U.S. Department of Education. *Using Higher Education Emergency Relief Fund (HEERF) Institutional. Portion Grant Funds to Meet the Mental Health and Substance Use Disorder Needs of Students*. May 19, 2022. *https://www..ed.gov/about/offices/list/ope/ heerfmentalhealthfaqs.pdf.*

[33] The Centers for Medicare and Medicaid Services, *Delivering Services in School-Based* Settings, 2023, *https://www.Medicaid.gov/Medicaid/financial-management/downloads/sbs-guide-Medicaid-services-administrative-claiming.pdf.*

[34] The Centers for Medicare and Medicaid Services, *Delivering Services in School-Based Settings*, 2023, *https://www.Medicaid.gov/Medicaid/financial-management/downloads/sbs-guide-Medicaid-services-administrative-claiming.pdf.*

children under age 21 should receive comprehensive physical health, mental health and behavioral health services.[35]

Medicaid-enrolled children who need services in school can fall into two categories: eligible students who need general health care services and students with disabilities who receive special education services under the Individuals with Disabilities Education Act (IDEA). School-based services delivered to children with disabilities are at no cost to their families. The Medicaid Budget and Expenditure System (MBES) expenditures reports for 2021 show more than $5.98 billion in total computable payments for school-based health care services to Medicaid students. Schools also received $14.1 billion in Federal IDEA funding in 2023.[36]

Medicaid can support schools to sustain essential services for eligible students.[37] In 2014, the Centers for Medicare & Medicaid Services (CMS) issued a letter to State Medicaid Directors clarifying reimbursable services in a school-based setting. The CMS letter explained that schools can seek payment for all Medicaid-covered services provided to all students enrolled in Medicaid.[38] As of May 2023, 214 states have used this policy to expand their school-based Medicaid programs. Most states use these funds to hire and sustain essential personnel who can delivery or facilitate the delivery of health and mental health services. The actual amount of additional Medicaid funding varies across school districts based on a wide variety of factors, including: (1) the number of students who are eligible for Medicaid in a district; (2) the unique needs of each child with a disability; and (3) State Medicaid payment rates;

Here are a few examples of how states have leveraged this opportunity to date to leverage Medicaid payments to hire key staff to provide essential health and mental health services to youth:

- Louisiana was the first state to expand its program, focusing solely on school nursing services. The State's financial analysis showed a 35 percent increase in Federal revenue. The program was such a success that the State did a second school Medicaid expansion to include all eligible providers and services.[39]
- Colorado ran a pilot project to better understand the financial impact of expanding its program. The state began by examining the impact of adding additional Medicaid eligible providers and, with the inclusion of additional school behavioral providers, estimated an increase of around $8 million, Michigan expanded its program to allow claiming for all Medicaid-enrolled students and added a number of additional providers, including masters-level school psychologists and behavioral health analysts.

---

35 The Centers for Medicare & Medicaid Services, *CMCS Informational Bulletin: Information on School-Based Services in Medicaid: Funding, Documentation and Expanding Services*, August 18, 2022, *https://www.Medicaid.gov/Federal-policy-guidance/downloads/sbscib081820222.pdf.*

36 The Centers for Medicare and Medicaid Services, *Delivering Services in School-Based Settings*, 2023, *https://www.Medicaid.gov/Medicaid/financial-management/downloads/sbs-guide-Medicaid-services-administrative-claiming.pdf.*

37 Healthy Schools Campaign, "State Data on Medicaid-Eligible School Health Services and Providers," *https://healthystudentspromisingfutures.org/map-school-Medicaid-programs/.*

38 Centers for Medicare & Medicaid Services, *SMD# 14–006 Medicaid Payment for Services Provided without Charge (Free Care) https://www.Medicaid.gov/Federal-policy-guidance/downloads/smd-Medicaid-payment-for-services-provided-without-charge-free-care.pdf.*

39 *https://healthystudentspromisingfutures.org/state-successes/examples/.*

Billing for masters-level school psychologists alone is projected to lead to an increase of $14 million to the school system.

- Voices for Georgia's Children estimates that Georgia's pending expansion to allow claiming and payment for school nurses would bring in an additional $48.6 million in Federal revenue to the school-based Medicaid program.

## Conclusion

The Department's mission is "to promote student achievement and preparation for global competitiveness by fostering educational excellence and ensuring equal access." This mission is urgent now more than ever as members of the educational community work together to address the learning gaps and increased mental health needs, fueled by the pandemic, that affected all students, particularly students from historically underserved groups.

As described above, we are actively engaging in efforts to accelerate recovery. We note throughout this testimony how the Department prioritizes work to address the mental health crisis facing our Nation's youth. We are committed to ensuring that students' needs are met, that they are ready to learn, and that they have full access to learning opportunities.

Thank you. I look forward to answering your questions.

## [Summary Statement of Katherine Neas]

Mental health affects the well-being of every student, educator, school, and community in America; and the Department is committed to creating the conditions for all students to thrive academically and personally. The Department's work is focused on three top priorities: (1) increasing the skills and knowledge of existing school personnel to support the mental health needs of students; (2) increasing the supply of mental health professionals who can work with students; and (3) increasing funding through the Medicaid program to support school health services, including mental health services. The Department also is engaged in robust delivery of technical assistance through funded technical assistance centers.

One year ago, Congress provided new funding under the Bipartisan Safer Communities Act (BSCA) that significantly bolstered Federal, state, and local efforts to address student mental health needs. Here is an update on our work to implement this legislation.

$1 billion through Title IV, Part A of the Elementary and Secondary Education Act of 1965 (ESEA) to enable State Educational Agencies (SEAs) to competitively award subgrants to high-need LEAs for activities to support safe and healthy students under ESEA section 4108. The Department has designated this component of BSCA the *Stronger Connections Grant Program*. States are in the process of running Stronger Connections grant competitions. ESEA section 4108 allows funds to be used to "develop, implement, and evaluate comprehensive programs and activities" that foster safe, healthy, supportive, and drug-free environments that support student academic achievement.

$280 million across 264 projects projected to train approximately 13,500 school-based mental health professionals and hire approximately 14,000 more under the School-Based Mental Health Services Grant and the Mental Health Services Professionals Grants.

$86 million in grants to local communities under the Promise Neighborhood Grants and the Full-Service Community Schools program.

A new competition for a mental health professional development technical assistance center is underway. services providers.

BSCA also directed the Department of Health and Human Services, in collaboration with the Department of Education to issue guidance to State Medicaid agencies, LEAs, and school-based entities to support the delivery of medical assistance to Medicaid and the Children's Health Insurance Program beneficiaries in school-based settings. This guidance, *Delivering Services in School-Based Settings: A Comprehensive Guide to Medicaid Services and Administrative Claiming* was released on May 18, 2023.[40]

**Additional Resources from the US Department of Education**

Bipartisan Safer Communities Act—Office of Elementary and Secondary Education

Safe and Supportive Schools—Office of Elementary and Secondary Education Center to Improve Social and Emotional Learning and School Safety—Office of Elementary and Secondary Education

Supporting Child and Student Social Emotional Behavioral and Mental Health Medicaid School Based Services information

www.ed.gov/raisethebar

The CHAIR. Mrs. Neas, thank you very much. Let me start off with Dr. Murthy. Senator Cassidy mentioned what is true, that the Congress has taken some action. But I will tell you, as I go around Vermont and talk to teachers and principals, they tell me they need more help.

In your judgment, do we have at this moment the kind of mental health infrastructure, from psychiatrists, the social workers, the counselors that this country needs?

Admiral MURTHY. Well, thank you, Senator. And I do appreciate the significant historic investments that have been made over the last few years. I think they have helped, but we do need more to help build the infrastructure.

When we think about care, for example, mental health care, there are several pieces of the infrastructure that still need to be expanded. No. 1 is the mental health workforce itself.

I am talking here not only about psychologists and psychiatrists and others in the traditional mental health delivery model, but I am also thinking about peer support models and others, which we know can help kids, and we need to think more broadly about that workforce.

The CHAIR. Let me ask you this, we have talked a lot about the problems. Talk about some of the solutions. Are there communities or schools in America that are doing something that is effective in addressing the crisis we are talking about?

Admiral MURTHY. The good news is that there are successful models around the country. Many of them do not know about each other and hence are not learning from each other, and we have to invest in studying and scaling them.

But a few that I will mention. One is the Becoming a Man Program, which has been a very powerful program, started in Chicago and now spread to some other cities, which has worked

[40] Medicaid, *Medicaid and School Based Services: Overview of Medicaid and School-Based Services*, May 18, 2023, *https://www.Medicaid.gov/resources-for-states/Medicaid-state-technical-assistance/Medicaid-and-school-based-services/index.html*.

in high schools with helping young people, essentially be sources of support to one another, and it has been able to demonstrate actual benefits in trials that were run by the University of Chicago.

We also know the Afterschool Matters Program has been another one, which has brought community organizations together to be with kids and provide the mentorship, support, and safe spaces to play and learn after school. And that has also demonstrated positive benefits.

The CHAIR. Let me ask you this, because you have written about this. What is—you write about loneliness, and yet people spend half their lives on these things. What is the difference, in your judgment, between human interactivity and activity on social media, and how does that impact the well-being of Americans?

Admiral MURTHY. Well, Senator, this has been an important point of concern for me. There is no substitute for in-person interaction. As human beings, we evolved over thousands of years to perceive not just the content of what someone says, but also interpret their body language, to sense nonverbal cues.

We take all of that in, and that contributes to a rich human interaction. When you strip a lot of that away, you lose richness, you lose quality of connection. That is not to say there is never a place for texting or for online connection.

But what I worry about is that the balance has shifted dramatically toward online connection and away from in-person connection, particularly for our kids. But the other concern, Senator, is not only what kids are missing out on as a result of social media, but what they are being exposed to on social media.

We—I talk to parents all over the country who—and to kids as well, who say that they are exposed to content that is violent and sexual in nature, that they are often bullied and harassed online. Six out of ten adolescent girls are telling us that they have been approached by strangers on social media in ways that have made them feel uncomfortable.

These are—I am concerned both about what is not happening as a result of social media in our kids' lives, but also about some of the toxic effects of what they are being exposed to.

The CHAIR. Mrs. Neas, you spoke about the impact that Medicaid is having on providing services to kids who desperately need it. We are now, as a result of the end of the pandemic and the cessation of the funding,—the many billions of dollars we put into funds and increasing Medicaid,—what impact will hundreds of thousands of millions of people losing their Medicaid have on mental health in this country?

Ms. NEAS. Senator, thank you for that question. The work that we have done with the Department of Health and Human Services to make it easier for schools to access the Medicaid program for school based services is one that we are very proud of because we think it is going to make it easier for schools to hire and sustain necessary people.

At the same time, we have been working hand in glove with the Department to get word out to our school leaders about this time of re-enrollment and hoping that those children who have to re-enroll in Medicaid are found eligible.

That those that are found not eligible can be directed to another source of insurance. But it is something that I think the Administration is very concerned about and wanting to do everything we can to make sure that children who are eligible can stay on the program.

The CHAIR. But is it a concern that if hundreds of thousands of millions of families lose their Medicaid, it is going to make it harder for people to get the mental health services they need?

Ms. NEAS. Without question, sir.

The CHAIR. Senator Cassidy.

Senator CASSIDY. Although I am tempted not to because my fellow Southerner did not wear a seersucker today, I am going to defer to Senator Tuberville.

[Laughter.]

Senator TUBERVILLE. I have got two suits, I just forgot.

[Laughter.]

Senator TUBERVILLE. Thank you, Mr. Chairman, for having this hearing. I spent 35 years with the youth of this country as a coach, educator, and this is not just a crisis that we have, mental health, it is an emergency. We got huge problems. This is probably the biggest problem we have in this country. It is getting worse every day.

I saw it change in just a short period of time. The No. 1 commodity that we have in this country is not gold and silver, it is our young people, and we are destroying them, and we are sitting back and watching it happen. I have seen prescription drugs take over our youth, especially a lot of kids that I work with.

We have ruined the nuclear family, and that is where a lot of this has got to come from. I counted up yesterday 32 mental health programs that we have in this country—32. We spend tens of billions of dollars. We are not making any progress. We are going the opposite way. We have all kinds of addiction.

I talked to a sheriff last week in Montgomery, Alabama, and he said, coach, I had never heard the word fentanyl till 2 years ago. Now, that is 95 percent of the drugs that we have in our schools and on the streets. The biggest drug we got is this right here. We all got it. There is not a person in here that doesn't have one of these.

I am guilty like everybody else, and I stay on it. I think everything on it is true, but it is not. But our young kids think that it is. That is the problem, and we have got to get control of that. And a lot of it, that is what we are talking about here today, is loneliness. And we can agree on some of that.

We have a program in Alabama that is called Harsha that our state mental health Department is running through our children's hospital. It works to connect interested primary providers with mental health specialists across the state and operates a sort of a command center at the hospital in Birmingham. Kids experiencing these—all the issues that they have, they are connected with providers that are close to them, whether it is rural or inner city.

Money for this particular program has tripled in the last year in the bipartisan Safer Communities Act. Now, I will tell you this. We can afford a lot of things around here, but we cannot not afford to fund mental health.

We can't. We have to be able to afford it and through situations like this. So, Dr. Murphy, are we tracking the successes and failures of the rest of the billions of dollars that we spend, or we track?

Are we tracking that, where it is working? Have you got people that are doing that in your line of work, that is helping us track the money going in? Is that money helping to the degree where we can see success?

Admiral MURTHY. Well, thanks, Senator, and I wish I could circle, underscore, star so much of what you just said, because you are right on and you are right that the most important task that we have is our kids, and we have got to do more to protect them.

I also agree with you that when we do put funds toward a cause, it is important to know, is it actually working? Is it delivering the benefit? And, while our office, the Surgeon General does not conduct evaluation trials, that is not what we are a resourced to do, we do have colleagues across the Department of Health and Human Services, at NIH and at SAMHSA, who do conduct evaluations of programs so that we understand what is working, who it is working for, and what more—what is missing.

But I think, Senator, to pick up on something else you said here as well. I think—and I like the program you mentioned in Alabama in terms of the concept of building a network and an infrastructure so that primary care doctors in particular and others aren't trying to manage all this on their own.

Programs like the Pediatric Mental Health Access Program, for example, have been very helpful in making sure that those primary care doctors can get expertise, mental health expertise, into the clinic when a patient is there, and we do need more programs like that.

But I don't think that we will be able to keep up with the sheer disturbing trends that we are seeing in terms of increased mental health concerns unless we simultaneously attack some of these root causes.

You mentioned our devices, and particular for young people, social media has become, I worry for too many of them, a contributor, an important contributor to their mental health strains. I also spent a lot of time with student athletes when I travel around the country, do roundtables specifically with student athletes.

Many of them tell me that not only are they having a hard time sometimes getting help, some of them have incredibly supportive coaches and administrations. Others do not. I had one football player who told me that after having serious thoughts of taking his own life, he approached his coach and said—and it took a lot of courage for him when he admitted to his coach what was going on and asked for help.

But as a response from the coach as well if that is how you are feeling, maybe this program is not for you. You should consider going to another university. And he was heartbroken. Now, thankfully, that is not the response that most kids get, but we still have more to do in terms of making sure kids get the help they need.

But if we can focus on making social media safer for our kids, if we can focus on rebuilding the social connection and community that our kids need, families are a key part of that, faith institutions are a key part of that, other community organizations like YMCA, boys and girls clubs, these are all play vital roles in helping connect kids to each other, families to each other, but participation in them, Senator, has been declining for a half a century, and it is leaving people lonely, isolated, and in greater risk for mental illness.

Senator TUBERVILLE. Thank you. And one thing I would like to say, I know we are over a little bit here, Mr. Chairman, but we have, unfortunately, people in this country that are born with a mental health problem, and we are trying to treat them with a lot of prescription drugs. And I think that is fine to a certain degree.

Sometimes we are overprescribing. But the problem is we are creating more mental health problems now than we are having young people born with mental health problems. And I think we all have to understand that. If we will start understanding that I think we can understand the problems that we have to overcome.

Because if we don't do this now, we are going to lose the country that we all grew up in, because mental health is the No. 1 problem in this country, the No. 1 problem, and we have to—because it leads to everything else. Leads to so many things in this country that are negative. So, thank you. Thank you for your answer. Thank you. Mr. Chairman.

The CHAIR. Senator Casey.

Senator CASEY. Mr. Chairman, thanks for having this hearing. I want to thank you and the Ranking Member for convening us. And I want to thank both of our witnesses for their testimony and their public service.

I wanted to start with Deputy Assistant Secretary Neas to talk about bullying and harassment, one aspect of this larger challenge. I think we can all agree that children deserve to go to school without any fear or intimidation.

But as we know, far too often bullying and harassment affects so many children and can have very serious consequences for the mental health that stay with them for the rest of their lives, and it undermines their ability to achieve academically.

We know that these issues are especially prevalent among students with disabilities, LGBTQ+ students, students of color, and students who are either in high school or elementary school, girls and young women.

To support the well-being of all students, I have introduced multiple times now the Safe Schools Improvement Act, which would require school districts to adopt codes of conduct that explicitly and transparently prohibit bullying and harassment based upon race, color, national origin, sex, disability, sexual orientation, gender identity, and religion, very much consistent with our civil rights statutes.

The bill would ensure that school districts take proactive action to support the safety and inclusion of all children. And Deputy Assistant Secretary, what is the value of universal prevention strategies such as legislation like I just outlined, in supporting mental health and academic achievement of every student?

[Technical problems.]

Ms. NEAS. Is that better? Here we go, sorry. Thank you for that question. The Department has partnered with the Department of Health and Human Services on a website called *stopbullying.gov*, which includes resources for schools to do exactly what you are saying.

I think one of the reasons we are so proud of the bipartisan Safer Communities Act and the work we are doing to increase the supply of mental health professionals who are in school is to make those things real. It is important to have the culture of a school be conducive to learning and safe for everyone.

We want to have those resources in schools and available to schools so that they can actually act on it. So, I couldn't agree with you more. The need for us to address the bullying, particularly of vulnerable kids, kids with disabilities, kids who may have uncertainty at home. We want school to be that safe place where they always know that there is somebody there who has their back.

Senator CASEY. Thank you. I wanted to move to a question for Dr. Murthy. One of the many pieces of data that you cite in your testimony—and I am looking at page one of your written testimony, it just kind of leaps off the page, and I am just reading a pertinent part here, "in 2021, nearly one in five high school students reported making a suicide plan."

Hard to comprehend those numbers, one in five high school students. And I wanted to not just focus on those high school years, but what happens afterwards as well. And because if that is the circumstance in high school, we can only imagine what that means down the road.

This challenge that we are all talking about here today predated obviously the pandemic but was made much worse by it. I am citing here the Kaiser Family Foundation, showing that half of young adults, ages 18 to 24, reported anxiety and depression symptoms this year, 2023—half of young adults.

Despite these rising needs, many institutions of higher education are poorly equipped to handle the mental health needs of students. I have introduced the Higher Education Mental Health Act, along with Senator Kaine.

The legislation promotes collaboration among educators, students, parents, advocates, and communities to study the mental health concerns facing college students. How can institutions of higher education better support students who are struggling with mental health today?

Admiral MURTHY. Well, thank you, Senator. And I appreciate your leadership on this issue, and with your proposed legislation. I think higher—institutions of higher learning have a huge role to play.

First of all, they are aware a lot of young people are, and we better bring the care to where people are. They can help to change culture by starting conversation addressing stigma. They can increase access to mental health services on campus and through telehealth to make it easy for kids to get care. But they can also invest in building the kind of connection and community that we know is vital to the mental health of children.

It doesn't just happen by throwing kids in a room and saying, hey, mingle and build connection. It turns out a little bit of structure, along with a little bit of time, can help kids actually build the relationships that they want. And finally, let's just keep in mind, many kids don't have what we might assume are just basic tools for managing emotions, building strong, healthy relationships.

Many of them may not have gotten that. And so, we have got to recognize that. And it is why I think programs that focus on building social skills and an emotional development so kids can manage their emotions and understand the emotions of others are really vital. That is a life skill. That, to me, is just as important as learning how to read or write.

Senator CASEY. Thanks very much.

The CHAIR. Senator Cassidy.

Senator CASSIDY. I defer to Senator Budd.

Senator BUDD. Thank you, Senator. And thank you, Chair. And thank you both for being here today. So, I sent a letter to NIH back on May 9th asking why taxpayer dollars were spent on a study entitled, Psychological Functioning in Transgender Youth After Two Years on Hormones, in which two participants tragically committed suicide. So, I am still waiting for a response from NIH on that letter, and I, Chairman, I ask for unanimous consent that I can submit my letter for the record.

The CHAIR. Without objection——

[The following information can be found on page 90 in Additional Material:]

Senator BUDD. Thank you. Now, the researchers, they concluded that the study was a success, but they admitted also that they couldn't show that cross-sex hormones improved the psychosocial functioning for minors. So clearly, it looks like this was a real waste of taxpayer dollars.

Even worse than that, it led or contributed to the suicide of two youth. So, Dr. Murthy, considering what I understand is your past support for providing cross-sex hormones to children, can you explain whether you think spending more taxpayer dollars on research into transgender procedures on minors will actually help children with the mental issues that we are discussing today?

Admiral MURTHY. Well, thanks, Senator Budd, for that question. While I was not directly involved in this study, and I am not familiar with it——

Senator BUDD. I understand——

Admiral MURTHY [continuing]. What I will say is that it is important for us to study what measures may help improve the mental health and well-being of transgender youth, because what we see clearly in the data is that as disturbing as these rates of anxiety, depression, and suicide are, they are actually disproportionately higher among LGBTQ youth, particularly transgender youth.

Studies that look to understand what interventions that work to address those psychosocial concerns I do think are important because this is a community that is struggling.

Senator BUDD. Thank you. A follow-up to that. Are you concerned about causing sterility and infertility in children who receive these cross-sex hormones, and about the negative long term impacts of these medical interventions on their mental health?

Admiral MURTHY. Well, Senator, I think whenever you have a medical intervention, it is vital to study both the short and long term impacts on physical and mental health. And I think that is where an investment of resources is needed.

Senator BUDD. Just to clarify, you said you would be concerned about the long term and short term impacts of these medical interventions on their health, their mental health?

Admiral MURTHY. Well, I think it is important for us to understand what those are through research, sir. So that is what I am saying. And I think that this is a space where, this is obviously a very complex area, and what we need to do here is what we do in other areas of medicine, which is to look to experts who have expertise in this area to put together the kind of guidelines that clinicians can then look at, and then make the best decision for patients based on that, or individual circumstance, just like we do in other areas of medicine.

Senator BUDD. Thank you. And I would just hope that the medical community and their research would be very cautious here. I mean, we have seen an NIH study which contributed to the suicide of two individuals, so please be careful, is the message. I want to shift gears just a little bit back to social media.

We know that children are being bombarded every day by unhealthy information on social media. Millions of children are suffering, as we have talked about, from anxiety and depression, and loneliness, because of the addictive content on social media.

There is an advisory, I think, that you issued on social media and youth mental health, and it discussed the increased use of social media by kids. So, to what extent, Dr. Murthy, do you agree that social media is damaging to the mental well-being of children? And how do you believe that we should address this?

Admiral MURTHY. Well, thanks for that, Senator. And my concern here is not just the Surgeon General, sir, it is as a doctor and as a parent. I have a five and 6 year old child—children, and my daughter is five. She is in preschool. And she came home a couple of weeks ago and asked my wife and me if she could post a picture on social media. She didn't have a social media account.

We have never talked to her about social media, yet all of her friends are talking about this. And I do believe that while there are some kids who get benefits from their use of social media in terms of opportunities to interact with others, in terms of the opportunity to find a community online, whereas they may not have one in person, I do worry that for many children the effects are in fact harmful and are contributing to the depression and the anxiety that we see among many young people, as well as issues with body image. In terms of what we can do, I think there is a lot we can do.

Ultimately, this isn't all about what Government can do. I think there is an important role, a critical role for parents here and for kids themselves. But I think what parents need is some support and help. And by establishing safety standards for social media that help protect kids from exposure to harmful content, and from harassment and bullying, and from features that seek to manipulate them into excessive use, I do think that we can help parents.

We also need, as policymakers, I think there is also a role to require data transparency here. And researchers around the country, Senator, tell me that they have had a hard time getting the data from companies to fully understand the extent of the impact of social media.

I will just say this, Senator, when our child—when our children get old enough to drive a car, or when they are small like mine were a few years ago and we needed to get a car seat for them, we don't tell parents, go inspect the tires yourself, check out the engine, make sure the frame is adequately strong, because we know that not all parents have the expertise to do this.

They rely on us establishing standards and then enforcing those with manufacturers. These are incredibly complex platforms that are rapidly evolving, fundamentally changing how our kids see themselves and interact with the world, and parents need help here to interpret and understand their safety.

Senator BUDD. Good. Thank you both.

The CHAIR. Thank you.

Senator Murphy.

Senator MURPHY. Thank you very much, Mr. Chairman. Thank you for holding this very important hearing. I am so proud of this Congress and many on this Committee for passing the bipartisan Safer Communities Act, and I am glad to get an update today on how that money is being impactful to help our kids. It is part of a trend. We are spending more money today on mental health than ever before.

We have gone from about $155 billion in 2010 to $238 billion in 2020, and it is still not enough. But I think this hearing is so important because I think we have come to the conclusion that unless you get at the root causes of unhappiness and isolation and loneliness, there is almost no amount of money that can make up for that inattention.

Dr. Murthy, I wanted to continue this conversation about social media, in part because I think it is the most immediate public policy concern that this Congress can tackle, and because I think there is easy agreement between Republicans and Democrats, but not because I think it is the whole story.

I think, frankly, we probably spend more time than we should talking about this narrow but very important problem that our kids are facing. But I think we can do something about it, so let's not lose the opportunity. I know the Administration hasn't endorsed any specific policy proposals, but just give us your take on which direction we should head.

Senator Schatz, and Cotton, and Britt, and I have a piece of legislation that says, you have got to do age verification and make sure that you can't get on before you are 13. You can't use algorithm boosting on younger kids, and parents have to have a say. Other legislation says you should have a standard that applies to social media companies so that they are only putting healthy content online. As you look at the sort of cornucopia of policy options that Congress is looking at here, what direction would you point us in to best protect our kids?

What are the tactics that the social media companies are using that are most disturbing to you? And I will just give you maybe the statistic that is most worrying to me. There is a recent study that shows within 2 minutes of establishing a TikTok account, a teenager can be fed information glorifying suicide.

Within 4 minutes of establishing a TikTok account, a teenager can be sent content celebrating eating disorders. That is how quickly really damaging, really dangerous content can get to kids who are in crisis, who are in trouble. And it just compels us, in this Congress, to do something about it. So, give us a little bit of advice.

Admiral MURTHY. Well, thanks, Senator. And I just want to also appreciate your leadership on the issue of loneliness and isolation. It has been an honor to work together with you on addressing this. And I agree with you that there are multiple drivers of the mental health crisis. Social media is one of them, and I agree it is an important one for us to address.

A few things I would say in terms of avenues of focus on, recognizing that social media has been around for almost two decades. During that time, there has been a lot of evolution in the platforms, a lot of different ways in which it is affecting our kids' lives. And so there is actually a lot to do here if we truly want to make them safe.

I think one certainly is around enforcement concerning age. Many platforms established 13 as the age at which kids can use social media. By the way, that is not based on health grounds, the age of 13.

Although many people think it is. But it—40 percent of kids 8 through 12 are on social media. So whatever rules the platforms have in place are very poorly enforced. I think the second area is we need to protect the privacy, data privacy of kids. Kids at this point do not have sufficient control over their data, neither do their parents.

This data is often used in direct ads to them, and other content is driven by the algorithms. We need to give kids and parents control over that data. The third is actually around data transparency. Companies are not fully disclosing the data they have about the health impacts of their platforms to our kids, to kids, to parents, to researchers, and to the public at large.

This is what researchers tell us all the time. And without that transparency, we don't even know the full extent of the problem and which kids are more most affected, and so it is hard to target interventions. But finally, I would say when it comes to safety standards, this is a place where I do think we can build models off of other products where we establish safety standards.

Whether it is for cars, car seats, medication, baby formula, whatever you want to consider as a parallel, but the bottom line is, we need to have standards that push companies to assure us and to be able to demonstrate through data that they are not exposing our kids to harmful content, that they are not in fact allowing kids to be bullied and harassed online, particularly by strangers, and also that they are not promoting the use of features that lead to excessive use.

We know that kids are in a vulnerable stage here of development and they are particularly susceptible to some of these features. We can't have companies taking advantage of those. So, these are some areas that I think are essential for.

I would be happy to work with you and other Members of this Committee as you develop legislation around this, because I think this can't come soon enough.

Senator MURPHY. I appreciate our partnership. I appreciate your guidance to this Committee. The only thing we cannot afford to do is to stand pat. There is a consensus here that we can find with your help. Thank you very much, Mr. Chairman.

The CHAIR. Thank you.

Senator Cassidy.

Senator CASSIDY. I defer to the sartorially splendid, Dr. Marshall.

Senator MARSHALL. Well, thank you, Senator Cassidy. And thank you, Chairman Sanders. We have to stop the hemorrhaging. We have to stop the hemorrhaging. When a patient comes to the emergency room when they are bleeding out, we don't start pumping blood into them. The first thing we have to do is stop the bleeding. Most of our solutions today seem to be pumping more blood into people.

We got to go back and start over. The greatest health care mistake the NIH and CDC ever did was locking our youth out of schools, and that has launched this mental health epidemic that we have. Irrefutable damage to our children's mental health, and I hope the CDC will own that someday.

Instead of our children talking to their friends, their colleagues, their teachers, their coaches, they talk to social media. That became their best friend. So how do we stop that hemorrhaging? I think we have to go back and think about, I look at social media today it is worse than pornography.

My young sons were exposed to pornography when they were very young because of social media, and I think the addictive pressures coming from social media today are worse than pornography. And just like we had to set parameters around pornography, we need to do the same thing with social media.

I wish we didn't have to. I think we need to start over on what the solutions are. Dr. Murthy, would you support some type of an electronic Surgeon General's warning on a statement on mental health and the impact of social media?

Admiral MURTHY. Well, thank you, Senator Marshall. And it is always good to be here with a fellow clinician as well. I know you have seen this from different angles.

I do worry about social media, as you do, and what I have tried to actually do in the advisory we just issued 2 weeks ago was to put in writing clear as day what our concerning was. Our concern was about social media, and to issue that warning to the American public.

I don't think it is the last thing, though, that we need to do. I think it is a start.

Senator MARSHALL. Much like when I was growing up, we put a Surgeon General's warning on tobacco. And it had an impact. I think, when we put a Surgeon General's warning on alcohol for pregnant women, it has an impact. Are you willing to use your bully pulpit and say, we need a Surgeon General's warning on what is the biggest threat to our youth right now when it comes to their health.

This is the No. 1 threat to our children's health right now. It is not cancer. It is not osteoporosis. It is not a whole lot of things. This is the No. 1 threat. Are you willing to use your pulpit and put your reputation on the line and say, we need a Surgeon General's warning on social media for youth?

Admiral MURTHY. Well, Senator, I do think it would be appropriate to have a warning on social media to warn parents and kids. And if Congress is willing to provide the legislative or regulatory authority to put that label on, then I would certainly be willing to partner.

Senator MARSHALL. Does it take legislation for you to put that label on? I don't know the answer to that.

Admiral MURTHY. Yes, it takes either a legislative or regulatory authority to do that.

Senator MARSHALL. Okay. Another issue I want to talk about are—is fentanyl or drug cartels, that they are selling fake Adderall. This, of course, laced with fentanyl. You are well aware of this. And they are using social media.

Of course, the top buyers are children. Senator Shaheen and I wrote legislation with leaders on the Judiciary Committee to hold social media companies accountable for illegal drug sales happening on their platforms.

Does this have the support—it does have the support of the White House and the DOJ and would love to add your continued efforts with this. Any comments on that?

Admiral MURTHY. I want to highlight the word you use, accountability, because there has been an utter lack of that when it comes to how we have been addressing the impact of social media on our kids.

What you mentioned, which is the use—the platform is being used to expose our kids to drugs and other harmful content is one example of that. So yes, I would support measures to ensure there was more accountability for the platforms.

Senator MARSHALL. Okay. The last thing we need to do is go back and study this and form committees and pray about this. We know social media is preying on our youth. We know it as surely as alcohol causes infant problems for moms as well. We know it. We don't need to study this more.

As black and white as you can make this, what would be your recommendations to stop this from happening? What—if you were—if you owned the social media company, why wouldn't you take the responsibility yourselves? Why does it take an act of Congress to do the right damn thing? What would you recommend that they do?

Admiral MURTHY. Well, do you mean this company specifically?

Senator MARSHALL. Yes.

Admiral MURTHY. Yes. So, what I laid out on the advisory is a series of checks for the tech companies specifically. One is to apply age appropriate design to their platform, so they are not exposing young kids to harmful content.

Second is to be transparent with their health impacts and the data that they are collecting that—so everybody can see how these platforms are impacting our kids' health. But the truth is, Senator, these social media platforms have been around for nearly 20 years. If we are going to just rely on them to fix this problem, I think we are waiting for something that is not going to happen.

Because while they have made some efforts to put safety measures in place, it is not nearly enough, and it is not happening nearly fast enough.

Senator MARSHALL. Greed is a horrible thing. Using greed to take advantage of our youth is a horrible thing. I just call on the social media companies to take self-accountability and to do something about this. Don't wait for Congress to do it. They know what the right thing is to do. They are taking advantage of our youth. They are poisoning our youth. They are killing our youth.

Admiral MURTHY. Senator, I would just say, when you and I have practiced medicine and we have prescribed medicines to people, to patients, we have been able to generally tell them what the evidence is if something works or doesn't work, and what the evidence is around safety.

I think it is very reasonable for us to expect a company to demonstrate similar data to us, so that parents like we can take that into account as we make decisions for our kids on when to start using social media and whether or not to even use it.

The CHAIR. Senator Kaine.

Senator KAINE. Thank you, Mr. Chair. And to our witnesses, what an important hearing. And my colleagues have asked a lot of good questions that I was thinking about asking, but I have decided I would like to just take my time to speak to any young person that is watching this hearing, here in the room, or watching it live, or maybe watching it streamed.

Young people feeling depressed about the future of the world, feeling hopeless has many causes, but to some degree you probably feel that way because you think adults have let you down, climate change, gun violence—a couple people were killed in my hometown at a high school graduation the other day.

Both my kids graduated from that building. My wife and I both spoke in that building. That is where we do all the graduations in Richmond. So, I think young people's part of this sense of hopelessness is this feeling that adults have let us down, whether it is on climate, or guns, or political polarization, or kids getting kicked around by adults for political purposes if they are marginalized.

I look in my own life, I have a Social Security card now, but I look at my own life to can I even remember what it was like to be a 5 to 18 year old? And I want to tell you, I had the same feeling when I was 5 to 18, that the adults in the world were letting us down. I came home from kindergarten in November 1963.

I saw my mother crying for the first time in front of the television because JFK had been assassinated. I picked up the newspaper in April 1968 and the news of RFK—of MLK being assassinated. And then in June of 1968, RFK being assassinated. You saw protests about the Vietnam War.

You saw protests about civil rights issues. I was 16 when our President was forced to resign because of corruption. So, my formative life from 5 to 16 was a time of chaos. War, nuclear weapons, drills in the classroom.

It was a time of chaos and there was a palpable feeling that I had, and that a lot of my friends had, that the adults in the world were letting us down. And that was a creator of confusion and anxiety and even depression.

We weren't so open about talking about mental health and mental health stresses then, but I could just remember that feeling. But what I want to say to young people watching, and Dr. Murthy, your focus on loneliness and isolation really gets at something really important, young people have the power—young people have the power to change the reality if you link arms and band together, and to reduce some of the things that might make you feel hopeless or depressed right now.

Because in all of that confusion, I saw young people a little older than me, I wasn't into it, but I saw young people protesting against the war and helping lead to its end. I saw young people in the civil rights movement helping battle to get voting rights done and civil rights laws passed.

I saw young people who are now eligible to vote at age 18, becoming deeply engaged in events that led to improvements, that led to a Congress willing to hold the President accountable for impeachable behavior, forcing his resignation.

The lesson that I learned from 5 to 16 was the adults were screwing a lot of things up, and if we waited for adults to solve those things, we would wait for a very long time. But when the young high schoolers and college kids that I was looking up to as a younger person linked arms and said, well, we are not going to just wait for adults to fix it, we are going to get engaged, when young people do that, young people change the direction of the country.

I guess what I would just like to say to any young person watching this is you might not think you have the power to change the conditions that you find depressing. I think an awful lot of young— well, I am not even on up to vote yet, or what does one vote matter the system is rigged so that we don't matter.

Our history shows the opposite. Things get worse when young people don't engage. Things get better when young people do engage. And not only do they get better in society, but the therapeutic value of linking arms with colleagues to battle for improvements in climate or reductions in gun violence, that very act of forming community among young people has a positive impact not only on society but on one's sense of well-being. You have a purpose on the table right before you.

If you look at us and you think we are not responsive to you, you can link arms and you can change the world and feel a lot better about the world that you are living in. So, with that, Mr. Chair, I yield back.

The CHAIR. Thank you, Senator Kaine.

Senator Cassidy.

Senator CASSIDY. Thank you, Mr. Chair. In Senator Sanders, opening questions of Dr. Murthy, he suggested, yes, we have done a lot, but we need to do more. But Mrs. Neas, you made it clear that we were actually on a trajectory to do more. Yes, we have put in these programs. For example, you mentioned in your testimony a school in Louisiana that has very successfully instituted a Medicaid based clinic for those with mental health.

Now there is another one opening. And presumably there will be another, and another, and another. So sometimes it is the potential of that which is being realized, which is more important to allowed to be realized, than creating a whole new program.

I say that, though, my question is, are my assumptions correct, that the programs that we put in place, for example, to help schools use Medicaid to pay for services, is that increasing in terms of its implementation, and do you suspect that it will continue to increase?

Ms. NEAS. Senator, thank you so much for that question. And we certainly hope that with this Medicaid guide and a new technical assistance center that will be announced shortly, that we are going to make it easier for more and more school districts to figure out how to access Medicaid so they can, in fact, do just the things that you are talking about. We have seen a number of great examples across the country of partnerships. We were just in Delaware——

Senator CASSIDY. Let me stop, because I understand you have got these examples, but are you getting—what I am really asking is, do you have the interest being shown to expand upon these examples to make this even more widely used?

Ms. NEAS. Absolutely.

Senator CASSIDY. The potential is being realized. And I think that is the point I want to emphasize.

Ms. NEAS. Yes, sir.

Senator CASSIDY. Now, let me speak to something which perhaps is not being realized, and maybe you can speak to it directly. But in the bipartisan Safer Communities Act passing because of Republican support, there was $1 billion for funding physical safety of schools. In one says we are trying to address the front end.

How do we keep kids from having a problem? But we are also trying to address the back end. If a kid does have a problem and comes in and tries to commit violence or someone else does. And as far as I know, the rules to tell schools districts how to implement physical hardening of their schools has only been promulgated into three different states.

Why have those rules not been promulgated? Okay, this is what is allowed to physically harden your school in case there is somebody who attempts to commit violence. Why have those not been promulgated to all 50 states?

Ms. NEAS. Senator, thank you for that question. The Stronger Connections Grant that we released the funds to states last September and states are—we are doing listening sessions with key stakeholders on what kinds of things they wanted to use those funds for.

Our guidance that was put out in November, and again revised this past March, does help schools understand what are allowable activities. What we are hearing from——

Senator CASSIDY. Let me stop you, again to being specific with my question——

Ms. NEAS. Yes, sir.

Senator CASSIDY. I was called by my state Superintendent that they were being told that they could not use the money to physically harden the school. I spoke with the Secretary, and he said he would correct that. But I am told, maybe I am wrong, that the correction that says that schools may use the money, as is Congress intended by the way——

Ms. NEAS. Correct.

Senator CASSIDY [continuing]. To physically harden was only promulgated with three states, Louisiana being one of them. Is that— am I correct in that or am I wrong?

Ms. NEAS. Senator, I am not aware of—my understanding is, from what we have heard from states, that they have used these funds for things to increase the physical security of schools.

Senator CASSIDY. Now, that is different from hardening. So, if I can ask, can you get back with me on the particulars of that most updated information?

Ms. NEAS. Yes, sir, I would be happy to do that.

Senator CASSIDY. Next. It has been suggested several times that there are things which subject children to ridicule that can otherwise make them prone to these episodes of depression, etcetera. I am very concerned about the issue of dyslexia.

I think anyone that as a child stands up that can't read in front of a class and is ridiculed because she can't read understands that pain. Now, there is a lot of money put out in these bills to help school districts do catch up learning. And I mentioned dyslexics because they are particularly vulnerable.

Here is an article, though, from The Times from 3 days ago. Schools receive billions in stimulus funds that may not be doing enough. Pandemic aid was supposed to help students recover from learning loss, but results have been mixed. And it points out that there was little guidance given to schools beyond, you shall spend 20 percent of it.

There are some schools that have put in very good programs, small, focused learning, and others that apparently have not. Any comments on that? And specifically, what can Congress—knowing the money is about to run out, but what can we do now to try and get schools to use best practices as opposed to just frittering dollars away?

Ms. NEAS. Right. Senator, one of the key elements of the Federal special education law is child find. And one of the things that states have struggled with that we are working very closely with them on to address is making sure they are identifying and serving any eligible child. And certainly, students who have dyslexia are among those kids that we want—

Senator CASSIDY. I get that but there are best practices. It does not appear as if they are universally adopted.

Ms. NEAS. That is correct, sir. We are—and we are working on specific guidance on these specific issues so that states can fully understand what their responsibilities are, so they can make, so that we can have a different situation.

Senator CASSIDY. Okay.

The CHAIR. Senator Hassan.

Senator HASSAN. Thank you very much, Mr. Chairman, Ranking Member for this hearing. Thanks to our witnesses not only for being here today, but for the work that you do. And I just want to start by following-up a little bit on what Senator Kaine was talking about.

I think we all have been hearing from constituents about concerns about mental health, in particular children's mental health. I will tell you that in the spring of 2021, when schools in New Hampshire began to reopen more fully, I went and visited in one of my local school districts with a mix of students, and teachers, and administrators. Students from first grade all the way through high school.

I was struck toward the end of the discussion when we had been talking about how kids were doing, how their families were doing, what the schedule in school felt like. Did they feel that they were keeping up with their learning?

How the year had been, when a girl who must have been about ten turned to me and said, so, Senator, what are you doing about mental health? And I had been kind of dancing around it. I am from a generation where we didn't talk about mental health in the same way we talked about so-called physical health.

Then recently, another one of my constituents, Loreley, who is 18 years old, raised awareness about mental health because she was driving with a friend 1 day and the friend had a panic attack, and Loreley didn't know what to do.

Now Loreley is working to help students get that kind of understanding for mental health first aid—what can kids do to help each other in these moments where they need to be supported and until they can get professional help.

I also want to encourage young people to know that when you speak up, your representatives hear it, and we are doing our best to listen, and we are trying to make progress. And I want to ask a couple of questions to our witnesses about some of the progress we have made.

Sometimes it doesn't seem enough, fast enough, but it is really important to understand the building blocks that maybe are in place. So let me start with a question to Dr. Murthy. I really enjoyed our discussion, doctor, in my office yesterday, and my team appreciated it very much, too.

Last year, my colleague, Senator Ernst and I, led something called the Stand Up Act, which was passed into law. And it is a law that helps ensure that schools are using suicide prevention policies that are actually evidence based. So, Dr. Murthy, why is it important for schools to adopt policies that are evidence based?

Senator Cassidy was just talking about our schools using the resources we are giving them in the right way. Why is it important that they are evidence-based, especially given the increased mental health risks that our youth face from social media?

Admiral MURTHY. Well, thank you, Senator. And Loreley's story will remain with me, and I have something I want to say about that at the end. But specifically, to your question, having evidence based practices is important because sometimes, even with the best of intentions, our programs may not have the desired effect, either in terms of the extent of impact, or in terms of who they are impacting.

They may leave certain people behind. The only way we really know that is to study them. The other piece is that sometimes when we study programs well, we realize that there may be unintended consequences of those programs. They may help in some areas and actually harm in others.

That is the whole point of studying these programs and then making sure that people know what the evidence tells us so that the program, when they do finally invest resources, time, and effort, they can do it in programs that we have greater confidence will actually help.

Senator HASSAN. Yes. Good. So let me then ask a question to you, Mrs. Neas. This is another example coming out of New Hampshire. Our University of New Hampshire and Manchester School District, which is our biggest school district in New Hampshire, they are leveraging funds from the bipartisan Safer Communities Act to train and place 80 graduate students studying social work in high school—in high needs schools—high schools, and elementary, and middle schools.

These graduate students will benefit from a yearlong internship with on the job training while public school students receive needed services. So, Mrs. Neas, in addition to this innovative example from my state, what other innovative local solutions are you seeing school districts deploy to address the school mental health personnel shortage?

Ms. NEAS. Senator, one of my favorite questions. We have seen some really innovative things across the country. We were just in a school in Delaware where the children's hospital runs a clinic that is on the campus of the school.

The majority of these children in this elementary school are homeless and live in nearby shelters. The year before the clinic was on staff, they had more than 1,000 instances of this disruptive behavior that resulted in suspensions. The first year of the center, that 1,000 number went down to 100, and now there are virtually none.

It is a great partnership. The children's hospital staffs it, does all the billing, and the school provides the physical space. What the principal said to me, I said, what keeps you up at night? And he said, learning loss. He said, we have got the support for kids and the teachers don't have to be both therapist and teacher.

Senator HASSAN. Right.

Ms. NEAS. That the staff there help teachers figure out how to get through the day to support kids so that they are emotionally Okay and learning. And I think that is one of the greatest things that we are seeing, is that partnership between educators and mental health providers on behalf of children, where children are.

Senator HASSAN. Well, thank you very much. Thank you, Mr. Chair, for your indulgence. I have some other questions, too, including the importance of providing services in summer programs and summer camps, which is something I think I will follow-up with our witnesses on.

Last, again, to the young people watching, this hearing probably wouldn't be happening if young people hadn't been speaking up, so thank you all very much for that.

The CHAIR. Senator Smith.

Senator SMITH. Thank you, Chairman Sanders and Ranking Member Cassidy. And thanks so much to both of you for being here. So, when I was in—a sophomore in college, I was really struggling.

I, thanks to my roommate who recognized some of the signals and signs of somebody who is dealing with depression, she suggested that I go to a school counselor at my university. And man, that made a huge difference.

I don't think I would have done that on my own, and I can see now that I was struggling also in high school, but having access to that care in my school setting made a huge difference because the barriers and the stigma that I would have experienced were sort of stripped away.

I share this story often, especially with young people, because I can see them kind of go, finally somebody is being real about this with me. This is one of the reasons why I have been so focused on expanding access to school based care.

Ms. Neas, I am really excited about the support that we have put behind school based services. I have heard from places in Minnesota where we are doing this, especially in places, this is something I have been working on, helping schools partner with community based organizations to get those services in schools.

It makes a huge difference. But here is the thing. In Minnesota— and Minnesotans we are go getters. All of this money. Three higher education institutions focus on training. That is fantastic. One school district has pursued this so far. So can you talk to us just a little bit about—because I have this feeling that we are sort of constantly putting grant opportunities in front of school districts.

Some of them, especially rural districts, just do not have the capacity to even know about these opportunities, let alone act on them. Could you talk a little bit about that issue, and how we are putting resources out there that is actually not that accessible to a lot of schools?

Ms. NEAS. Absolutely. And thank you very much for that question. And we hear that all the time about capacities, especially small districts not able to write for these opportunities. It is one of the many motivators to our Medicaid work.

Senator SMITH. Right.

Ms. NEAS. Where we are really trying hard to make it possible for people that are in schools to work with their Medicaid agencies so that—we know we have got lots of kids.

Half the kids in our public schools——

Senator SMITH. Right.

Ms. NEAS. Are eligible for Medicaid. If we can help schools figure out how to recoup some of those payments——

Senator SMITH. Exactly.

Ms. NEAS. They can sustain things. They don't have to write a grant.

Again, we know that with the 21 states that have access to free care rule, that they are—that is resulting in an almost $6 billion of revenue to schools for services they want to provide. And that is to me, how do—we need the more people, and the people—we need to train more people.

Senator SMITH. Yes.

Ms. NEAS. We need to train more people. And that is something that you can do with grants. But I want this to be sustainable for the long term—

Senator SMITH [continuing]. They need sustainable funding. Yes, exactly——

Ms. NEAS. For small school districts to not be left out of that. That is really what we hope TA center and the guidance and in our efforts to shine a light on this opportunity, that we can have more of that happen.

Senator SMITH. Let me just ask for clarification. How many states did you say are participating in this right now?

Ms. NEAS. 21.

Senator SMITH. 21. So only—less than half of the states are participating. And that is a decision essentially of the Governor and the legislature. So, this is another problem we have, Mr. Chairman, is that in some places there is opportunity, in some places there are not based on the calculations that state leaders have. Vice Admiral Murthy—I am used to calling you Vivek, so——

[Laughter.]

Senator SMITH. You and I have had some really terrific conversations. I am so grateful for your leadership on issues of social isolation, both for our elders, as well as for young people.

Now, I have had people say to me, Tina, like, you can't legislate away loneliness, but you have done research that really shows how we can think about this as a social determinant of people's health, and that can make a huge difference. Could you just speak briefly to that, because I think it is really important.

Admiral MURTHY. Absolutely. And I think, I agree that you can't legislate away loneliness, but I don't think that is the solution here.

Senator SMITH. Right.

Admiral MURTHY. But I think there are steps Government can take to help support community organizations, to invest in research, to understand more deeply the drivers and solutions of loneliness.

But we also need community organizations, families, individuals to recognize that this is an important priority for all of us. I worry that we have become a lonely and disconnected nation, and that has massive consequences for our mental health, for our physical health, for economic prosperity, for our ability to pull together in the face of adversity, whether that is a pandemic or another hardship.

For all of those reasons, I believe that addressing loneliness is a strategic and critical priority for our Country. It is something I think we can do, and the people who give me the most faith that we can do that are young people.

Because when I talk to them around the country, they are not waiting for others to step in, they are building programs at their schools to help connect one another. They are reaching out to support each other.

They are talking more openly about mental health and issues like loneliness than any prior generation. And I think their leadership is going to be vital in us addressing this challenge.

Senator SMITH. Thank you. Thank you so much, Mr. Chair.

The CHAIR. Thank you.

Senator Murkowski.

Senator MURKOWSKI. Thank you, Mr. Chairman. And thank you for the hearing this morning. I think it is somewhat telling that with everything that is happening this morning, there is a significant overflow room just down the hall.

I have been back and forth between a couple of different committee hearings this morning and there continues to be a line of young people, of young people trying to get into this Committee hearing. And so, I stopped and talked to them. Why are you standing in this line today? Why is it important to you?

One of the young men said, it is personally important to me. I am curious to know, as a—apparently as a young immigrant, the intersection, the services that are available for those in—from other areas. Another one indicated that she was interested in education, but she wanted to understand more how people who had adverse incidents in their lives as young kids as she had, what more support could be provided in schools? Young people are paying attention to this as an issue.

They are paying attention to what we as legislators do. And I have listened to some of my colleagues, and yes, we can't legislate loneliness going away. It is hard enough to; how do you legislate against bullying? How do we do the reach out? I appreciated your comments to Senator Tuberville when he mentioned that as a coach he interacted directly with these young people.

Your comment that you sat down at roundtables with students, particularly student athletes. What more are we doing to ask young people what the solutions are? We had a hearing in this—

in the HELP Committee last year on youth mental health. We invited an extraordinary young Alaskan by the name of Claire Rainier.

I think Claire at the time was 19. She gave testimony and presented the youth perspective and what she had done as one individual that had gone through real crisis, what she had done within her school community to engage more.

I remember Claire's story and how strong she was in sharing that with us. But what are we doing to ask the young people what we can do to help? And I will throw that out to you, Surgeon General.

Admiral MURTHY. Well, thanks so much, Senator——

Senator MURKOWSKI. I understand you are coming to Alaska soon, and I hope those conversations are going to take place.

Admiral MURTHY. I am. Thank you. Yes, I am really looking forward to it. And it is actually relevant, like when I first came to Alaska, when you and I met there in 2016, that was an opportunity.

We did a lot of roundtables, including with young people. And the goal there was to really understand how they are being impacted by substance use disorders, and more broadly by behavioral health concerns.

To involve young people, to answer your question, I think there are a few things we have to do and that we are doing more and more. No. 1 is we have got to bring young people to the table to understand and hear their concerns and go to where they are.

That is part of what my office has been doing, is having roundtables with young people in communities across the country. The second thing we have to do——

Senator MURKOWSKI. Can I just stop you there?

Admiral MURTHY. Of course.

Senator MURKOWSKI. Because it takes extraordinary strength for a young person to say, no, I am going—I want to be part of this public dialog and engagement.

The ones that are really hurting are the ones that are just struggling to get up out of bed that morning, much less go to a roundtable. How do we get them?

Admiral MURTHY. That is exactly right. And that is why what we are also doing is recognizing that it is not easy for everyone to come to those tables, to be open. It is easier often when they are doing that with folks they know with trusted institutions, trusted organizations.

We are also working with faith organizations, with universities, and others to help them pull roundtables and other such listening sessions together with young people to create opportunities for them to give input that don't necessarily involve showing up at a roundtable—that may involve more commenting on a survey or share their input anonymously.

We want to create as many channels as possible for young people to be heard on this. And then using that input, we are encouraging mayors as well as the institutions I mentioned to then formulate their plans.

My belief is that if we want to do something that is going to help young people here, we need them at the table throughout the process, before we developed a solution, as we work on execution, and when we do evaluation to understand whether it is working or not. And that is what we are encouraging localities to do, from Mayors to non-Governmental organizations like YMCAs, educational institutions, and others.

But, Senator, it is not—I will just say this, it is not easy to do this, right. It takes time, effort, and focus, and continued attention. The easiest thing is just to go into a closed room and come up with your own solutions and try to implement them, but I just don't think that is what is going to get us the best result here.

Senator MURKOWSKI. Agreed. Recognize that we just need to be doing more to be inclusive of these young people. I am going to have a question for the record for you, Mrs. Neas.

This is relating to the fact that of the bipartisan Safer Communities Act funding through the mental health services grant, professional demonstration grant programs, apparently only 17 percent of these grants were awarded to rural districts.

I am trying to understand what more we can be doing to make sure that these grant resources are going out to all areas of the country, including rural. Thank you, Mr. Chairman.

The CHAIR. Thank you very much. Senator Baldwin.

Senator BALDWIN. Thank you, Mr. Chairman. In June, we celebrate pride. It is a time for folks to gather and lift up and celebrate LGBTQ Americans, the movement for the fight for equality. And we also reflect upon the challenges.

There is an intersection of our conversation here. It has already come up a little bit that with the mental health crisis that kids are facing, from data last year, 45 percent of LGBTQ youth reported that they had considered attempting suicide—45 percent. Youth who live in communities that are not particularly accepting or families that aren't particularly accepting report higher rates of attempting suicide.

I am just going to note, and maybe we can introduce it for the record, there was an article last weekend in the New York Times about death investigations and the fact that we don't have complete—after suicides, we don't have complete information, because oftentimes they don't ask the question about sexual orientation or gender identity.

But in Utah, they are. And it was a fascinating piece that we should have as a part of the record, because that is data that we are lacking. But at the same time, we are celebrating pride month, we are witnessing in America a staggering number of pieces of legislation at the state level that are described as anti-LGBTQ bills. I—491 reported so far this year. At the state and local level, school board level, we see a lot of additional activity.

I don't have any numbers on that. I don't know who is aggregating those. But it is rampant. And I wonder, again, what the impact of that is on mental health of members of the LGBTQ community. Now, I want to get to a question.

We are talking about offering support in schools, but I want to also think of other gateways where people come in and get help. I was proud to co-sponsor the bill that brought us the 9–8–8 suicide prevention hotline, and it was made—it was—became operational last summer.

There is the ability with that technology to provide more customized service. I know the first thing people are asked, are you a veteran? And if so, you will get your mental health services, if you choose, from the VA.

But we, along with Susan Collins, we have provided funding for a pilot program in 9–8–8 for offering specialized support for people who call, text, or chat on 9–8–8 who are identifying as LGBTQ. So, how do we use we have school board—or sorry, school based mental health in some cases, but how do we use a gateway like 9–8–8 to provide better support for, in particular, our LGBTQ population?

Admiral MURTHY. Senator, first, just thank you for your leadership on 9–8–8. As it is a topic that I talk about often when I travel around the country, and I can't tell you how many faces I have seen turn from worry to look of relief when they know that there is some help actually available immediately when they or their child have a crisis. So, thank you for that. It is already making a difference.

I do want to say, specifically with LGBTQ youth, I agree with you that we need to look for more ways to ensure that they know help is available for them. I think schools are a natural place. I think 9–8–8 is a place where early on, if we can signal to young people that this is a place where you can get assistance, where people will understand your unique circumstance and your background, I do think that is essential.

I also think that, and I say this just as a doctor and as a father, I believe that every child deserves to know they matter, regardless of what their background is. The reason my parents came to America many years ago was because they wanted my sister and me to grow up in a country where we knew that just because we had a different color of our skin or our name sounded funny or a background was different, it didn't mean that we mattered any less than any other child. And that is a value we aspire to as a country.

We may not always have gotten there, but I think that is a place where we need to do more when it comes to making LGBTQ youth feel that they do matter, that they are valued. And too many of them tell me often that they don't feel that way. They often feel left out or bullied or attacked.

Finally, I would just urge leaders, whether they are elected leaders, whether they are leaders in the community, to include LGBTQ youth at the table when they are listening to what communities have to say, and to specifically reach out to them to understand their perspective and their life experience.

I have just learned as a doctor over the years who has had the privilege of sitting with patients and with very different backgrounds, and listening and learning to them, that there is nothing that replaces face to face contact with people, listening to someone's story, and it shifts how we think about issues.

I think that could not be more important now because too many of our LGBTQ youth are struggling, and you see it in the suicide rates. And to me, that is in—a five alarm fire that we are dealing with.

Senator BALDWIN. Yes. Thank you. Mr. Chairman, I have several questions for the record, since I have run out of time, but I thank our witnesses.

The CHAIR. Thank you very much, Senator Baldwin. And let me thank the panelists for what I think is an extraordinarily interesting hearing on a subject that I think everybody here recognizes is of enormous consequences to this country.

I just want to take a few seconds to make this point. I think we are all proud of the accomplishments that we have made, and we wanted to help them. But there is another reality, and I want you to tell me what I am missing here, if I am missing anything.

If 85 million Americans are uninsured or underinsured, and if we have a scarcity of mental health providers in this country, am I missing something in suggesting that for tens of millions of people—I know people call my office.

I am sure they call other offices. My husband is in desperate shape. I can't find the help. We can't afford the help. And on top of that, correct me if I am wrong, but I think it as a result of the ending of the public health emergency, some 17 million people are going to be dropped from the Medicaid rolls. Is that correct, Mrs. Neas? Is that correct?

Ms. NEAS. I am not—I know that it is a large number, sir. I am not exactly——

The CHAIR. The point is, yes, we want to take pride in what we have accomplished, but let's not kid ourselves. We have got to move dramatically if we are serious about protecting the mental health and helping people in this country. There is a lot of work that has to be done. So, with—Okay. Yes, Senator Cassidy. Well, let me just, with that—all right, give the mic to Senator Cassidy.

Senator CASSIDY. A lot of great things said today. In my closing, 30 seconds, I want to emphasize three things. Senator Kaine is speaking about how young people can be the drivers of change. Senator Murkowski is speaking about how folks are lined up and they are all young.

Looking at the audience here, you are young, and I suspect those watching on TV are young. And Dr. Murthy saying that we can't leave it up to Government, but we also have to have individual action.

I guess my appeal is all the young people who rightly have a concern about this, you are the ones who can introduce people to this hotline set up by Senator Baldwin. You are the ones that can advise, as Senator Smith was advised, to go seek help.

We can only do so much. You are going to do a heck of a lot more than we. So, I just finish by echoing wonderful comments from my colleagues.

The CHAIR. All right. To the witnesses, thank you very, very much. This is the end of our first panel. We are going to be going to our second panel in a moment. Thank you. Thank you all very much for being here, and we are going to continue this discussion on this issue of enormous concern to the American people.

I—Senator Murphy was going to introduce Charlene RussellTucker, but unfortunately, he is detained. So let me begin by introducing her. And that is, Mrs. Russell-Tucker was appointed Commissioner of the Connecticut Department of Education in 2021.

Previously, she served as Chief Operating Officer and Division Chief for the Department's Office of Student Supports and Organizational Effectiveness. Mrs. Russell-Tucker, thank so much for being with us.

## Statement of Charlene M. Russell-Tucker, Commissioner, Connecticut State Department of Education, Hartford, CT

Ms. RUSSELL-TUCKER. Thank you. Good morning, Chairman Sanders, Ranking Member Cassidy, and Members of the Senate Committee on Health, Education, Labor, and Pensions. I am Charlene Russell-Tucker, Commissioner of Education in Connecticut. I am honored to share critical information regarding the youth mental health crisis and Connecticut's response to support the needs of our students.

My big audacious goal is to ensure every Connecticut school has a coordinated and sustainable system of care to provide comprehensive behavioral and mental health support and services to all students and school staff. As Surgeon General Murthy mentioned and a survey of Connecticut high school students confirms, our students face unprecedented mental health challenges.

Too many of our students reported having felt sad or hopeless, and that their mental health was not good most or all of the time. Most concerning is that 14 percent said they had seriously considered suicide, and 6 percent actually attempted suicide. These data highlight the immense need to address student wellness and underscore the urgency for action at Federal, state, and local levels.

Effective solutions require teams of stakeholders, including policymakers, community leaders, parents and families, educators and students. I like to say, it can't be about them without them.

The Commissioners Roundtable for Family and Community Engagement and Education is a diverse constituent group of stakeholders, representing school staff, advocates, parents and guardians, community leaders, and students to advise me on policy and programmatic priorities.

Connecticut's Student Voice for Change Program allows high school students to propose projects utilizing state ESSER funds. Notably, 80 percent of student proposals focused on mental health, using their voice to advocate for mental health supports for their peers. They spoke and we are listening.

Our ESSER funded behavioral health pilot established a system of coordinated care for schools in seven districts. One pilot school district identified 250 students at risk of suicide and was able to provide critical and immediate responses. Our state's mobile crisis intervention services deliver a range of crisis response and stabilization services to youth and families.

Simply call in 2–1–1, or now 9–8–8, immediately dispatches clinicians to schools or anywhere a child is in crisis. The Surgeon General report on the epidemic of loneliness reinforces the importance of school attendance and engagement.

Our Governor's Learner Engagement and Attendance Program is a research based home visit initiative that improves attendance, feelings of belonging, and family, school relationships. Additionally, we invested $33 million in ESSER and ARP funding in a multiyear summer enrichment grant program, prioritizing communities disproportionately impacted by the pandemic.

Programs place a strong focus on peer relationships, wellness, and academic acceleration during the summer. In the first year, this program connected more than 108,000 students with enrichment opportunities. The Department invested $2.2 million in ESSER funds for innovation grants to support new partners in underserved communities in designing innovative, high quality afterschool programs to address students' academic and mental health needs.

Mental health is a bipartisan state priority, including addressing workforce shortages. Governor Lamont and our General Assembly directed $100 million for multi-agency mental health initiatives, including $28 million for mental health professionals in schools. Multi-state agencies are working together to expand the ranks of clinicians to meet increasing mental health needs.

Additionally, the school districts are leveraging over $183 million of local ESSER funds for student and staff well-being. We are committed to funding and sustaining what works. We also invested ESSER funds to establish a groundbreaking collaborative that brings together teams of university researchers to conduct rigorous evaluations of the many new programs and initiatives that are underway in our state to ensure programs and investments are achieving results.

Thank you for modeling bipartisan national discourse that will lead to enhanced access to needed services, and ultimately, improve academic access, supports, and outcomes for young people. Thank you very much. I am happy to take your questions.

[The prepared statement of Ms. Russell-Tucker follows:]

## Prepared Statement of Charlene M. Russell-Tucker

Good morning. Chair Sanders, Ranking Member Cassidy, Committee Members, thank you for having me here today.

My name is Charlene Russell-Tucker, and I am the Commissioner of Education in Connecticut. I am honored to appear before you all today to represent our great state and share critical information regarding the youth mental health crisis, its impact on learning, and the interventions, policies and initiatives Connecticut implemented before, during and after the pandemic to support the emotional, mental, physical, and behavioral health needs of our students. Many of the interventions that I am discussing today align with what I call my "Big Audacious Goal," which is to ensure every Connecticut school has a coordinated and sustainable system of care for all K–12 schools to provide comprehensive behavioral and mental health supports and services to students and staff.

As mentioned by Surgeon General Murthy earlier today, Connecticut, like the rest of the country, is experiencing an unprecedented need for mental, physical, and behavioral health supports among young adults and adolescents—likely stemming from and exacerbated by isolation and loneliness caused by the pandemic and its after-effects, as well as a lack of meaningful connection due to this isolation. Concurrently, consistent with national trends, Connecticut is experiencing a shortage of mental health professionals. Despite these challenges, Connecticut is leveraging substantial Federal and state resources to build a scalable system of supports to address our students' mental, physical, and emotional health through prevention and early intervention services, as well as just-in-time crisis support. Sound mental health is foundational to learning and ultimately all aspects of human development; therefore, we must continue to develop, evaluate, and provide resources to support these efforts.

Connecticut prioritized student mental health alongside academic recovery when investing the more than $1.7 billion that has been allocated to our state under the Elementary and Secondary Schools Emergency Relief (ESSER) Fund. On behalf of the State of Connecticut, we are very appreciative for Congress's critical support. The priorities we established for these funds at both the state and district levels included supporting learning acceleration and academic renewal, ensuring safe and healthy schools during and post pandemic, technology enhancements, and family and community engagement. We knew, however, that none of these investments would be successful if we did not first implement a system of supports for students' physical, social, emotional, and mental wellness, which is why we included this funding priority as well. Districts responded by earmarking over $183 million for supporting student and staff wellness through hiring additional staff, providing professional learning and technical assistance, and partnering with external partners for the provision of referral services, enhanced counseling, and care coordination. Additionally, this is also why the Connecticut General Assembly and Gov. Ned Lamont, in a bipartisan effort, allocated over $100 million in the 2022 legislative session to support mental health statewide, of which $28 million was earmarked for the Connecticut State Department of Education (CSDE) to create grant programs to support the hiring of school mental health professionals.

## The Connecticut Landscape

Connecticut has a beautifully diverse student body of more than half a million students. Across 205 districts, we have over 1,500 schools and more than 110,000 school staff devoted to helping our students thrive.

Looking more closely at our student population, more than half of students identify as nonwhite; 42.4 percent are eligible for free or reduced-price meals, 17.1 percent are students with disabilities, and 9.7 percent are English/multilingual learners with more than 145 spoken languages.

Results from the Connecticut School Health Survey, modeled after the Centers for Disease Control and Prevention (CDC) Youth Risk Behavior Survey, indicated that feelings of sadness and hopelessness in high school students have increased steadily over time, reaching a new high during the COVID–19 pandemic. In the 2021 survey, 35.6 percent of Connecticut high school students reported having felt sad or hopeless, 28.5 percent reported that their mental health was not good most or all the time. Most concerning in the survey results, is that 14.1 percent said they had seriously considered attempting suicide and 5.9 percent had actually attempted suicide.

The survey found that mental health issues are more common among female students, with 47.6 percent of female students reporting feelings of sadness or hopelessness compared to 24.2 percent of male students and 40.5 percent of female students saying their mental health was not good most or all of the time compared to 16.4 percent of male students. Suicidality in females was also much more pronounced, with 19.8 percent of female students verses 8.7 percent of male students seriously considering attempting suicide and 8.8 percent of female students verses 3.3 percent of male students actually attempting suicide. These data highlight the immense need to address student wellness and underscore the need for action at all levels—Federal, state, and local—to protect our students' mental health.

## Stakeholder Involvement and Collaboration

I want to lead with what makes Connecticut unique—what in Connecticut is referred to as "The Connecticut Difference." This is our longstanding focus on *bestin-class* collaboration, working together, and listening to one another, in search of common ground for the sake of our students.

With almost every policy or initiative, including supporting the mental, physical, and behavioral health needs of our students, Connecticut prioritizes engagement with our various partners and stakeholders—the Office of the Governor, the State Board of Education, state agencies, educators and administrators, families, students, advocates, policymakers, local health officials, and more—as often as possible to develop and implement our policies. Policies designed without hearing different perspectives, and without our constituents' input and feedback, are not likely to produce the intended and needed results.

We are staunchly committed to ensuring that family, student, and community voices are included in our decision-making processes. I like to say, "It can't be about them without them." We cannot actively gauge the impacts of isolation and the pandemic on our students' mental health without understanding their perspectives.

In Connecticut, we strongly affirm these voices, particularly when they indicate severe mental health concerns, suicidality, or other harmful thoughts because these challenges negatively impact students' overall well-being and, therefore, their ability to learn. We believe that part of addressing student learning and academic needs is the provision of mental and behavioral supports. A quote from yesteryear still rings true today—there is no curriculum brilliant enough to compensate for a hungry stomach or a distracted mind.

Listed below are structures that the CSDE has in place that are foundational to engaging stakeholders in driving our mental and behavioral health policies, practices, and initiatives.

### *1. Commissioner's Roundtable on Family and Community Engagement*

In 2017, recognizing the critical importance of family and community voice, I developed and implemented the Commissioner's Roundtable for Family and Community Engagement in Education, which is a diverse constituent group of education stakeholders representing school and district staff, advocacy organizations, parents and guardians, community members, and students, who advise the Commissioner of Education regarding policy and programmatic priorities. The Roundtable meets quarterly to bring authentic parent and community voice to CSDE products and initiatives; communicate state-level initiatives with families and communities; recommend effective practices to increase successful school and district engagement with families; and provide strategies to empower families in supporting their children's education. The Roundtable has informed many of our mental, physical, and behavioral health initiatives through active deliberation and discussions. This group developed the Connecticut Framework for Family and Community Engagement, which defined family engagement as "*a full, equal, and equitable partnership among families, educators, and community partners to promote children's learning and development form birth through college and career.*"

### *2. AccelerateCT Taskforce*

AccelerateCT Education Taskforce was launched to develop a statewide education recovery and acceleration framework and programming for students across the state beginning with enhanced learning and enrichment opportunities. The Taskforce is made up of over 30 members representing every aspect of education and focuses on six key areas: learning acceleration; academic renewal and student enrichment; family and community connections; social, emotional, and mental health of students and school staff; leveraging technology to accelerate student learning; building safe and healthy schools; and summer enrichment. As noted, mental health is a core component of the Taskforce's priorities, consistent with our statewide approach.

### *3. School Discipline Collaborative*

Understanding that students sometimes do not feel welcomed and valued in school and that exclusion from school impacts students' overall behavioral health and learning, I formed the Connecticut School Discipline Collaborative. The Collaborative advises the Commissioner of Education and State Board of Education on strategies for transforming school discipline to reduce the overall and disproportionate use of exclusionary discipline. Members reflect a diverse range of expertise in the fields of school administration, teaching and learning, public policy and legislation, education law, youth development and children's advocacy, family and student engagement, and community leadership.

### *4. Voice4Change Initiative*

In November 2021, the CSDE launched Voice4Change, the first statewide student participatory budgeting initiative in the country, to give students a direct say in how a portion of the $1.5 million of ESSER funding should be spent across Connecticut schools. Using the same five investment priorities set forth for districts, students crafted and voted on proposals for projects or supports they desired in their school community. More than 80 percent of winning proposals addressed the need for more supports for student social, emotional, and mental health. Students also saw what worked during the pandemic—best practices they wanted to make permanent in their school going forward like a mental health first aid team available to students, peer mediation, afterschool programming focused on stress reduction, and creative and innovative learning environments such as outdoor classrooms.

In addition to the structures described above, the CSDE works closely with our member associations in Connecticut to gain feedback from the field, drive policy development and implementation, discuss resource access and allocation, and receive advice on how the CSDE can support our schools. These organizations include the Connecticut Association of Public School Superintendents, the Connecticut Association of Boards of Education, and the Connecticut Association of Schools, which represents school principals and vice principals. The CSDE also routinely engages with our teachers' unions as well as associations representing school nurses, counselors, social workers, and psychologists, paraeducators, and child nutrition program directors. This collaborative approach is necessary in building effective policy and positively supports the whole child.

## Initiatives and Programs Supporting the Social, Emotional, and Mental Health Needs of Students and Staff

I am privileged to live in a state where education receives robust bipartisan support from the legislature. Last session, Connecticut lawmakers passed the most comprehensive mental health bills in the state's history—including grants for schools to hire staff to support student well-being, bolstering the Governor's homevisiting initiative, increasing summer programs' capacity to support the mental health of their campers, and more.

The pandemic brought keen attention to the necessity of addressing the social, emotional, and mental health needs of our students and school staff. While Connecticut has a longstanding history with this work, COVID–19 significantly increased the demand for mental health services and supports—both in the number of students needing support as well as the severity and complexity of those needs.

Connecticut has prioritized the allocation of human and financial resources toward addressing the comprehensive health needs of our students, encompassing their emotional, mental, physical, and behavioral well-being. Throughout the pandemic, the state implemented a range of interventions and policies that not only catered to immediate challenges but also considered prevention strategies and long-term support. By prioritizing the whole child, Connecticut has paved the way for promising practices that can serve as valuable examples for other regions across the Nation seeking to enhance their educational systems and ensure the overall well-being of their student populations. The following outline some of our most impactful initiatives and programs:

***1. Statewide Behavioral Health Landscape Scan***

The CSDE commenced a statewide behavioral health landscape scan in September 2020 to provide insight into emerging concerns and trends related to the well-being of students in K–12 schools across Connecticut. This was the first step in providing a systematic collection of data to identify needs and enhance existing efforts related to supporting the mental health and well-being of our students.

***2. Connecticut Behavioral Health Pilot***

State level ESSER funding has afforded the CSDE the opportunity to support resources to fully fund the Connecticut Behavioral Health Pilot. Currently, our Behavioral Health Pilot is underway in seven districts in partnership with community-based behavioral health partners to assess their mental health support needs.

The CSDE identified districts of various demographics—from large urban districts, medium sized suburban districts and small rural districts—to participate in the pilot program to implement targeted supports based on needs identified from the landscape scan and focus group discussions. The specific needs and gaps in service will drive the development and implementation of these systems of care. The pilots will then inform plans to scale these systems statewide for implementation in similarly situated Connecticut districts. Robust needs assessments are being conducted in each district to document the mental health system components that exist within each district and assess the comprehensiveness of those systems. These data are driving the prioritization of quality improvement efforts and will set into motion systems to track improvements throughout implementation.

Specifically, the district-level assessments examined the efficacy of districts' behavioral and mental health systems by analyzing current and existing programming, as well as human and fiscal capital. This process will help to determine the appropriate, scalable interventions, which will depend on the capacity and resources—both internal and community-based—in each community. Solutions may include increased staffing and service provision; opportunities for training, professional development, technical assistance, and coaching; external referral systems of care through partnerships with mental health providers and primary care facilities; and streamlined and shortened referral processes. These combined efforts will ensure students' emotional well-being, which can support consistent school attendance, engagement, and academic success. All relevant school district staff will then receive adequate trainings and demonstrate increased knowledge in both content and referral processes and systems, which will help to reduce both the total number of student visits to local emergency departments for behavioral health crises and reduce the rates of exclusionary discipline and absenteeism.

The early results of the pilot are already evident. Districts have established priorities and identified community partners to support them. One district realized that it needed more universal mental health assessment capacity. They have subsequently created a liaison position between the school and the community provider to identify students needing a higher level of support. Through their assessment, one of our larger districts identified that over 250 out of their 4,000 students reported having attempted suicide. The district quickly developed partnerships with community providers and created a student response team to address pressing mental health needs.

### *3. Grants to Support Mental Health Professionals*

In a bipartisan effort, the Connecticut General Assembly directed $28 million in American Rescue Plan Act (ARPA) funding across three different grants to support mental health professionals in schools. The legislature directed $5 million toward a School Mental Health Workers grant program to assist Connecticut local and regional school districts in hiring and retaining additional school social workers, school psychologists, school counselors, school nurses, and licensed marriage and family therapists. An additional $15 million was directed to support a School Mental Health Specialist grant program to assist school districts in hiring and retaining additional school social workers, school psychologists, trauma specialists, behavior technicians, board certified behavior analysts, school counselors, licensed professional counselors, and licensed marriage and family therapists. Over 70 clinicians have been or will be hired through these grants to support students through three school years. Last, the legislature directed $8 million to a Summer Mental Health grant program to support the delivery of mental health services for students when school is not in session. Funding is available to school districts, operators of youth camps and other summer programs.

These grants, funded entirely through Federal ARPA dollars, are essential for local efforts to adequately address the needs of children and youth. The CSDE understands the critical need to maintain these positions and the vital services they provide for our students, and districts will require new mechanisms and resources to retain these essential staff when the ARPA funding expires. The CSDE is looking at opportunities under Medicaid to sustain this critical investment.

### *4. Summer Enrichment Grant Program*

Connecticut has invested $33 million in ESSER and ARPA funding toward a multi-year Summer Enrichment Grant program, initiated in summer 2021. The program was created in an effort to connect K–12 students whose education may have been negatively impacted by the pandemic with low or no-cost, high-quality enrichment opportunities when they are out of school during the summer months, including at summer camps, childcare centers, and other similar programs, with a priority for those in communities that were disproportionately impacted by the pandemic.

Programs place a strong focus on social-emotional, physical, and mental health; academic acceleration, intellectual growth, and exploration; and student-peer relationships during the summer months. This investment also enables summer camps to hire additional staff such as behavioral specialists or other personnel to serve more students. An evaluation of the 2021 program concluded that the initiative successfully connected more than 108,000 Connecticut students with summertime enrichment opportunities that year. An evaluation of the 2022 program will be released soon.

### *5. After-School Grants*

In 2022, the CSDE released $2.2 million in ESSER funding to support after-school Innovation Grants for underserved communities to address the academic, social, emotional, and mental health needs of students, especially for those who have been disproportionately affected by COVID–19. Innovation Grants enabled smaller towns, districts, and non-profit organizations to create innovative after-school programs. This was an addition to $8.7 million used to expand and enhance Connecticut's existing after-school programs, for a total combined funding of $10.9 million.

The Innovation Grants focused on creating new after-school programs to reach underserved target populations while building districts' capacity through the assistance of local and community partnerships. This grant provided successful applicants with the necessary funding to design and implement new, high-quality after-school programs that address the academic, social, emotional, and mental health needs of students across the state.

### *6. Deveraux Student Strengths Assessment System (DESSA)*

Through ESSER funding, the CSDE implemented the DESSA System. The DESSA is a strength-based observation tool that teachers use to capture how frequently they have observed a student demonstrating positive behaviors (e.g., getting along with others, taking turns, considering different opinions, active listening, etc.) rather than inappropriate behaviors. Focusing on strengths can build students' self-efficacy and help them persevere when they face difficulties and challenges in the classroom and the school environment. This helps teachers better support their students in feeling, confident, successful, engaged in learning and connected to school. Close to half of Connecticut school districts are participating in the DESSA System. Following the first year of implementation, half of students were already demonstrating positive growth in pro-social competence and behavior. Our high school students are invited to participate in the DESSA Student Self-Report (SSR), which engages students in reflecting on their own strengths and empowers them to steer their learning in a way that aligns with their needs. The SSR is a student self-rating that delivers real-time results and immediate strategies to incorporate student voice and choice in learning, which has a significant impact on learner engagement, motivation, and achievement.

Supporting the well-being of our K–12 administrators, educators and staff is also vital for them to be able to ensure student growth and success. This initiative is a pilot program designed to help educators give their best to students while also caring for themselves. It includes a comprehensive set of research-based resources that provide educators with professional development tools, self-assessments, personal development plans, self-directed strategies, and teaching practices.

### *7. Components of Social, Emotional, and Intellectual Habits for Grades K–12*

The CSDE has developed the Components of Social, Emotional, and Intellectual Habits for Grades K–12. This guidance represents the knowledge, skills, and habits that form an essential blueprint for students' well-being and equip every student with the knowledge and skills necessary to succeed in college, careers, and civic life. While attention to core academic subjects remains important, positive habits set the stage for all future learning, promoting intrapersonal, interpersonal, and cognitive competence. This guidance provides grade-specific competencies for districts and schools to integrate into academic content areas so that students will learn and model essential life habits. Some examples of the competencies include: (1) *Acknowledging and welcoming constructive feedback from others that challenges and builds resilience and identifies strengths and areas for growth and* (2) *demonstrating critical thinking skills when solving problems or making decisions, recognizing there may be more than one perspective or solution to the problem.*

### *8. Leveraging Medicaid Reimbursement*

The CSDE's partnership and collaboration regarding leveraging Medicaid reimbursement began with the Connecticut Department of Social Services (CTDSS) prior to the pandemic due to the existing challenges of providing healthcare supports to all students in Connecticut. The current patchwork of Medicaid, private coverage, SAMHSA, local and state educational authority funding makes it very challenging to implement consistent, evidence-based, sustainable and comprehensive systems within schools. Current medical models in which reimbursement is provided based on individual student clinical services do not allow for a systems approach to meeting the needs of all students. Schools and school districts do not have the capacity or expertise to bill as medical providers or manage complex grants, and districts with the greatest needs often have the least capacity in this regard. Eligible students currently receive coverage and care through Medicaid via the Medicaid School Based Child Health Program (administered by the CT DSS). This program allows school districts to seek federal Medicaid reimbursement for many Medicaid-covered services, such as assessment, audiology, clinical diagnostic laboratory, medical, mentalhealth, nursing, occupational therapy, physical therapy, respiratory care, speech/language, and optometric services. Districts may also pursue federal reimbursement for administrative activities which support provided Medicaid health services. Currently 118 of Connecticut's 205 school districts are enrolled in the Medicaid School Based Health Program. Medicaid covers roughly 250,000 young people (ages 5-17) in the state of Connecticut. Prior to the pandemic, the CSDE was in active communication with the CTDSS on how to leverage Medicaid reimbursement for students. With the new Centers for Medicare and Medicaid Services guidelines, CT DSS is actively looking into two options to streamline Medicaid coverage and reimbursement. These are (1) School Based Child Health (the district is the provider and biller) and (2) School Based Health Center (private health care provider embedded in the school). The partnership between the CSDE and CT DSS will actively work to ensure that schools and school districts can leverage these added resources and that a robust plan is in place to ensure the greatest number of students possible are eligible for Medicaid. In addition, the sustainability of funding a robust professional mental health work force within schools is tied to our ability to leverage Medicaid funds for students. As mentioned above, we also see Medicaid as a tool to sustain some of the impactful work enabled by ESSER funds once those funds are no longer available.

***9. Bipartisan Safer Communities Act (BSCA)***

Connecticut received $9.12 million in federal BSCA funding to create a Stronger Connections Grant. These grants are competitive subgrants that SEAs can provide to high-needs LEAs to fund a broad range of activities including school-based mental health services, early identification of mental health issues, substance use prevention, trauma-informed care, and appropriate referrals to support services, which may be provided by school-based mental health service providers or in partnership with a public or private mental and behavioral health providers.

Our Request for Proposals (RFP) will be released this month and will reflect feedback provided from our many stakeholders. It must be noted that this timeline to release the Bipartisan Safer Communities Act RFP is purposeful following the awarding of the robust $28 million in School Mental Health Grants mentioned above. This allows for the CSDE, as well as school districts, to be strategic in first planning for the use of existing ESSER funding to support student mental health and then determining the gaps in resources that can be supported by the School Mental Health Grants. This will ensure that BSCA funds will be strategically utilized to support the most pressing needs.

***10. School Based Health Centers***

Connecticut's School-Based Health Centers (SBHCs) are comprehensive primary health care facilities licensed as outpatient clinics or hospital satellites. SBHCs are intentionally located in schools where students have historically experienced health care access disparities and are often publicly insured, underinsured, or uninsured. Multi-disciplinary teams of pediatric and adolescent health specialists staff the health centers, including nurse practitioners, physician assistants, social workers, physicians and in some cases, dentists and dental hygienists. SBHCs provide all levels of care for students including medical services and mental health services. Connecticut currently funds 90 SBHCs and efforts are underway to expand that number in areas and schools not currently served by an existing SBHC or other health care center.

***11. Mobile Crisis Intervention Services***

Mobile Crisis Intervention Services is an initiative developed and administered by the Connecticut Department of Children and Families (CT DCF), the state's child welfare and behavioral health agency. Accessible by simply calling 2–1–1, or 9–8–8, Mobile Crisis providers deliver a range of crisis response and stabilization services to children, youth, their families and caregivers. Mobile Crisis providers are experts in meeting the complex needs of students experiencing psychological or behavioral issues. Districts in Connecticut are required to contract with community-based Mobile Crisis providers to respond to schools and families when students are in crisis. As a result of the pandemic, Connecticut invested an additional $8.6 million in ARPA funding for an annual total of $19 million to ensure access 24 hours per day, 7 days per week, 365 days per year. In the event of a psychiatric emergency, a trained screener will, within 15 minutes, facilitate direct contact with a licensed Mobile Crisis staff member or other emergency service as necessary. The trained screener will connect the caller real-time with a clinician during the call and the clinician can respond in person to the caller's location within 45 minutes if needed.

## Initiatives to Support Healthcare Workforce Development

As stated, Connecticut is not immune to shortages of mental and behavioral health staff. As a result, a concerted cross-agency effort to recruit and retain a quality behavioral and mental health workforce is underway in Connecticut.

***1. Connecticut Office of Workforce Strategies (CT OWS) Initiatives***

The Connecticut Office of Workforce Strategy (CT OWS) has several workforce initiatives related to healthcare career pathways. While these programs are not focused specifically on school-based practitioners, they are geared toward increasing the number of clinical workers in the state. The education and training provided these programs will increase the supply of clinical healthcare workers entering schools as school-based practitioners. Many of these projects have stemmed from inter-agency collaborative efforts, including between the CSDE, CT State Colleges and Universities (CSCU), and CT OWS.

(a) One such program is the CT Health Horizons, which CT OWS launched with $35 million in state ARPA funds. The goal of this program is to increase the number of graduates from the nursing and social work program (prioritizing the MSW degree, which is the precursor to becoming a Licensed Clinical Social Worker, the most in-demand position in behavioral health), with a focus on diversifying the workforce. Grants will soon be available to address three areas: (1) Tuition Support to incentivize low-income and minority students to enter accelerated and cost-effective nursing and social work programs, (2) Increase faculty to expand seat capacity and train an influx of nursing and social work students, and (3) Promote employer-driven innovation programs to support entrance into high-demand careers in nursing and social work. Grants were provided to independent colleges and universities that coordinated efforts to increase access to accelerated nursing and mental health programs. Students are enrolling in programs that start fall semester 2023.

(b) In addition, CT OWS has invested $11.6 million in two CareerConneCT grants focusing on health care training. The Academy for Human Service Training (AHST) is a 15-week comprehensive classroom and hands-on training opportunity for roles in Community and Social Services/Human Services; Case Managers, Direct Support Professionals, Psychiatric Aides, Recovery Assistants, etc. The Health CareerX Academy is designed to support the scaling of the Southwest Healthcare Career Academy statewide to train individuals in entry-level healthcare roles.

(c) An OWS legislatively mandated report is recommending a plan to work with high schools across the state to develop and strengthen pathways that encourage students to pursue careers in healthcare.

### *2. Connecticut Department of Public Health (CT DPH) Initiatives*

Similar to the CT OWS, the CT DPH has recognized the pressing need to bolster its mental health workforce to effectively address the growing demand for mental health services. In response to this imperative, the state has embarked on a series of robust public health initiatives aimed at increasing the number of mental health professionals.

a. In 2022, CT DPH joined the Psychology Interjurisdictional Compact (PSYPACT®) designed to facilitate the practice of tele-psychology and the temporary in-person, face-to-face practice of psychology across state boundaries. The Interstate Medical Licensure Compact is an agreement among participating U.S. states and territories to work together to significantly streamline the licensing process for physicians who want to practice in multiple states. It offers a voluntary, expedited pathway to licensure for physicians who qualify.
b. In 2022, the Connecticut General Assembly passed two public acts providing DPH resources to strengthen the mental and behavioral healthcare workforce in Connecticut, to include:
    I. PA 22–81 encourages pediatric offices to integrate behavioral health into their practices. This is accomplished through a new grant program to provide pediatric offices with a 50 percent match for costs associated with paying the salaries of licensed social workers providing counseling and other services to children receiving primary health care from such providers.
    II. PA 22–47 increases the number of child and adolescent psychiatrists available in the state to provide services to school-aged children. This is accomplished by the establishment of child and adolescent psychiatrist grant program to provide incentive grants to employers for recruiting, hiring, and retaining child and adolescent psychiatrists.

## Focus on Attendance and Engagement

With any discussion on mental and behavioral health supports, it is critical to include the importance of student attendance and engagement in school. Attendance is a precursor to engagement which is a precursor to learning. When students regularly attend school, they have access to not only in-person relationships with their peers but also to critical social and emotional supports. Therefore, the CSDE has placed a significant focus on improving attendance. Two practices the CSDE implemented to decrease chronic absenteeism include:

***1. Increased Data Collection***

Beginning with the 2020–21 school year, the CSDE rolled out two new data collections—weekly collection of learning models (e.g., in-person, hybrid, or remote) and enrollment, as well as expanding the collection of student attendance from yearly to monthly, to allow us to make data-informed decisions in real time to focus resources on student engagement and participation.

***2. The Learner Engagement and Attendance Program (LEAP)***

The state's response to this data collection was the Governor's Learner Engagement and Attendance Program, or LEAP, which was announced in April 2021. Underway in 15 high-needs districts, LEAP is the CSDE's research-based, relational home visiting model proven to increase student attendance and family engagement. Home visitors establish relationships with families and students and connect them with school and community resources, including behavioral health resources as needed.

As of December 2021, nearly 7,000 students across the 15 LEAP school districts had received more than 12,000 contacts from home visitor staff to encourage and support increased student attendance in school. Thanks to financial commitments of our legislature, this program will continue.

LEAP, by design, is supportive and creates trusting, relationship-based partnerships with parents. This helps parents resolve barriers to attendance and other life stressors. The Center for Connecticut Education Research Collaboration's (CCERC) evaluation of the LEAP program found that home visitors and families noted eight main benefits of LEAP including:

- Improved family school relationships
- Increased student attendance
- Increased student achievement
- Increased feelings of belonging
- Increased access to resources for families
- Increased expectations of accountability
- Greater gratitude and appreciation

CCERC conducted the largest, most robust study ever completed of a home visit program. The research shows that when implemented with fidelity, the LEAP model has a positive impact on students and families.

The results of the quantitative analysis indicated the following findings:

- Visits that were made in-person had more impact than virtual visits or phone calls.
- One month after the initial home visit, participating students showed a 4 percentage point increase in attendance.
- Six months after the visit showed a 10 percentage point increase in attendance among pre-K to grade 5.
- Six months after the visit showed a 20 percentage point increase in attendance among grades 6–12.

## Evaluating Effectiveness and Sustainability

Scientifically researching and evaluating the effectiveness of the referenced initiatives, programs and investments is at the heart of our strategy in Connecticut. ESSER funds were used to establish the first-of-its-kind research collaborative we call the Connecticut COVID–19 Education Research Collaborative (CCERC). CCERC is a research partnership between the CSDE and public and private institutions of higher education across Connecticut that works collaboratively on program evaluations. Given the value of the research collaboration beyond COVID–19 research efforts, it was recently rebranded as the Center for Connecticut Education Research Collaboration (CCERC), keeping the same acronym, and continuing this partnership well after the COVID–19 pandemic.

The rebranded CCERC's mission is to address pressing issues in the state's public schools through high quality evaluation and research that leverages the expertise of researchers from different institutions possessing varied methodological expertise and content knowledge. District and school leaders across our state are critical partners in this work. Many of the projects require an in-depth review of local policies and practices, especially when there have been large investments in the area of study. These important evaluation studies require district cooperation with researchers.

In addition to evaluation studies released on LEAP, summer enrichment, and remote learning, nine additional projects are underway and include the behavioral health pilot, identifying effective and equitable socio-emotional supports for students and educators, equity in academic recovery, and more.

CCERC demonstrates the CSDE's commitment to programmatic accountability and sustainability, building evidence on the effectiveness of its interventions and knowing what works. As the end of the ESSER funding approaches, Connecticut will have the strength of results to fund and sustain what works.

## Policy Recommendations

As we gather here today to address pressing youth mental health challenges, I would like to draw your attention to a set of policy recommendations below that I believe warrants your consideration.

***1. Allocate Resources for State and Local Evidence-Based Program Evaluation***

Program evaluation initiatives such as CCERC provide an objective and evidence-based assessment of the efficacy of educational programs, allowing policymakers, educators, and administrators to make informed decisions. These evaluations help identify strengths and weaknesses in funded programs/initiatives, measure impact on student outcomes, and pinpoint areas for improvement. By understanding what works and what does not, states and school districts can better direct resources to strategies that have a proven track record of success, ultimately benefiting students, educators and communities. As Congress considers reauthorizing the Education Sciences Reform Act, I encourage you to help states build capacity to evaluate program effectiveness and support effective uses of limited resources.

***2. Provide Funding for the Continuation of Prevention and Intervention Initiatives***

By the end of 2024, states and school districts will have fully invested the Federal education funding that Congress provided under three relief packages to mitigate COVID–19 and address its lasting impacts upon student achievement and well-being. In 2024, the end of this funding will significantly limit schools' ability to access the resources and supports students and communities need to recover from the ongoing effects of the pandemic. Moving forward, we are committed to effective uses of more limited funds but also encourage Congress to make additional investments in K–12 education to ensure that we can continue to meet the needs of students and families.

***3. Support Educators' Focus on Student Physical Health***

Student physical health is a critical factor in youth development and overall health and needs to be part of the package of supports for students. Childhood obesity is again on the rise along with increased sedentary habits in our Nation's youth. Diminished physical health, especially in underserved populations is a doorway to other issues and concerns, including mental and behavioral health, potentially leading to negative impacts on overall health and well-being. Programs and services to support physical fitness and wellness, as well as expansion of the Federal child nutrition programs for all students, are foundational to lifelong health and success.

***4. Incentivize Collaboration between Federal Agencies***

Federal agencies need to coordinate to leverage different entry points to mental health support so that, regardless of the agency that has a high touch with a family, any one of them are able to provide entry into supports for children and students experiencing trauma and struggling with access to services and care. Such collaboration is critical to address the Social Determinants of Mental Health. Augmenting traditional behavioral health services with additional health-enhancing supports and positive youth development opportunities has the power to develop well-rounded students with the knowledge, skills and confidence to support their lifelong wellness and success. Such opportunities include: focused investments targeting protective factors; providing for basic needs such as stable housing; supporting comprehensive wraparound supports for emerging adults; providing innovative education opportunities outside of school that focus on building skills and confidence; providing opportunities for employment or training; and, providing access to mentors with lived experience in behavioral health, juvenile justice, and child welfare systems.

As Connecticut's Commissioner of Education, I am greatly appreciative for the invitation to be part of this national discourse to share what Connecticut has done to support youth mental health and to describe potentially scalable initiatives to inform Federal investments and policies. Addressing non-academic barriers to learning will serve to improve educational attainment. Your willingness to model transparent bipartisan national discourse such as this will lead to enhanced access to needed services and ultimately improved academic supports and outcomes for our young people, and I appreciate these efforts. I am part of a strong, nationwide network of state commissioners working together with the Council of Chief State School Officers, and I can guarantee you no two stories are alike. What I can surely guarantee you is that we all collectively wake up every morning with our students and their families, educators, and school staff at the forefront of our minds, because it is when our schools are supported our students achieve more, our communities achieve more, and together—we all achieve more.

We must use this moment to think holistically across all levels of government about the continuum of supports necessary for our students and nation to thrive.

Finally, none of the practices and initiatives that I bring from our great state would be possible without the leadership of our Governor, our sister agencies, the excellent staff at the CSDE, our State Board of Education, our school district superintendents, administrators, educators and staff, our policymakers, and the many education partners in our state. That truly is the Connecticut Difference!

Chair Sanders, Ranking Member Cassidy, and HELP Committee Members, thank you once again for the opportunity to share Connecticut's story with you today.

## [Summary Statement of Charlene M. Russell-Tucker]

The social isolation and stress of the COVID–19 Pandemic exacerbated existing mental health challenges facing our youth and also exposed gaps in the behavioral and mental health care system. This is evident from the results of the Connecticut School Health Survey, which indicated that feelings of sadness and hopelessness in high school students reached a new high in the fall of 2021. The Connecticut Department of Education (CSDE) built on existing systems and leveraged new funding to address this critical need in our students.

### Stakeholder Involvement and Collaboration

Stakeholder engagement is a pillar of Connecticut's response to addressing mental health concerns in students. The Commissioner's Roundtable for Family and Community Engagement in Education represents a diverse constituent group of education stakeholders representing school and district staff, advocacy organizations, parents and guardians, community members, and students, to advise the Commissioner of Education regarding policy and programmatic priorities. Voice4Change, the first statewide student participatory budgeting initiative in the country, gave students a direct say in how a small portion of state set-aside ESSER funding should be spent across Connecticut schools. Students overwhelmingly voted for projects that supported student and staff mental health. The AccelerateCT Education Taskforce was launched in 2021 to develop a statewide education recovery and acceleration framework and programming for students across the state beginning with enhanced learning and enrichment opportunities, which included a focus on social, emotional, and mental well-being. Engaging associations representing school superintendents, principals, teachers, nurses, counselors, social workers and others are also part of Connecticut's play book for success.

## Supporting the Social, Emotional, and Mental Health Needs of Students and Staff

Connecticut created programs and rolled out grants to strategically build the infrastructure to support schools and students. Efforts include: $183 million district ESSER funding prioritized for mental health; $28 million in school mental health personnel grants; $35 million after-school and summer enrichment grants; the school behavioral health pilot program; expansion of Mobile Crisis Intervention Services; School Based Health Center expansion plans; guidance and systems to support positive growth in pro-social competence and behavior in students.

## Initiatives to Support Healthcare Workforce Development

Key initiatives spearheaded by the CSDE's partnerships with other state agencies include workforce grants and training programs for mental health professionals to increasing the number of social workers and psychologists for school-aged children including $35 million to support students in nursing and social work programs, and funding incentive programs for employers of clinicians to strengthen the mental and behavioral healthcare workforce.

## Focus on Attendance and Engagement

The CSDE understands the power and importance of real-time evaluation data. Increasing the collection of attendance data from yearly to monthly allowed the CSDE to address root causes of chronic absence and disengagement in real time. These data points led to the development of the Governor's Learner Engagement and Attendance Program (LEAP). LEAP is the CSDE's research-based, relational home visiting model proven to significantly increase student attendance and family engagement.

## Evaluating Effectiveness and Sustainability

A commitment to evaluation is at the heart of our strategy in Connecticut. Data-driven decisionmaking is key to informed and effective policymaking. To that end, the CSDE invested a portion of our ESSER funds to establish the first-of-its-kind, research collaborative called the Connecticut COVID–19 Education Research Collaborative (CCERC). Recently rebranded as the Center for Connecticut Education Research Collaboration, CCERC is a research partnership between the CSDE and institutions of higher education across Connecticut. This research center allows the CSDE to leverage the strong collaboration that exists in our state to scientifically research and evaluate the effectiveness of our initiatives and investments.

## Policy Recommendations

The policy recommendations in this testimony for consideration to support youth mental health include: allocate resources for state and local evidence-based program evaluation; provide funding for the continuation of prevention and intervention initiatives; support a focus on student physical health; and incentivize collaboration between Federal agencies.

* * *

The CHAIR. Thank you very much. We are going to jump over Dr. Garcia for a second. We are to go to Dr. Joy Osofsky, who will be introduced by Senator Cassidy.

Senator CASSIDY. It is a joy to introduce Dr. Joy Osofsky. She is the head of pediatric mental health at LSU Medical School, a developmental psychologist, and a national leader in early childhood development. I have learned a lot from Dr. Osofsky.

She is who taught me that you can actually begin picking up separation disorder from day zero. It was just amazing to me. And she was very influential in what Chris Murphy and I did, at least my part of the mental health reform bill of 2016, so I owe a lot to her.

She has expertise in trauma informed care, helped many Louisiana families recover from Hurricane Katrina, and apply that expertise during the COVID–19 pandemic. She received numerous awards and recognition for her work. Dr. Osofsky, thank you for being here.

## Statement of Joy Osofsky, Professor of Pediatrics, Psychiatry, and Public Health, Head of Division of Pediatric Mental Health, Louisiana State University Health Sciences Center, New Orleans, LA

Dr. OSOFSKY. Thank you very much, Senator Cassidy, for the invitation, and Senator Sanders. I very much appreciate being here.

One of the things that I want to say in introducing my testimony is how important the opportunity has been for me, actually together with my husband who is a psychiatrist, to be able to consult with Senator Cassidy on mental health issues, to identify and support community and state agencies that work individually and collaboratively in supporting the mental health needs of children and families, including cross-state efforts.

We started this in 2016. We have been pleased to support his efforts to increase mental health support in schools and in communities. And we didn't talk earlier as much about communities, and I think we need to integrate that in the conversation we have now.

Bipartisan Safer Communities Act and Support Act would expand community based behavioral health services and access to mental health care services in schools and communities in both rural and urban areas. And we know in rural areas, it is much harder to access mental health services in general.

The Act would provide funding also for the National Child Traumatic Stress Network to improve trauma informed training, treatment, and services for children, adolescents, and families who have experienced trauma. I have been fortunate enough to work with the National Child Traumatic Stress Network being funded since 2003, to develop mental health collaboration with schools and communities.

Our latest effort, and I think one that is really very much reflective of the direction of the National Child Traumatic Stress Network is going, has been to not just work in one community, but develop regional coalitions so that we spread the work that we do and the efforts that each of us make in working with children who have been traumatized in different ways and experienced trauma, to be able to share that knowledge with other communities.

For example, and I actually happened to be quite fortunate during the COVID pandemic, we had a center within the National Child Traumatic Stress Network that just ended, a terrorism and disaster coalition for child and family resilience.

Through that coalition, we built regional relationships across states, one in the Gulf South, where we already had relationships due to the disasters, Hurricane Katrina and the Gulf oil spill, but then in the Northeast region of the United States, across five states.

The regional coalitions are composed of people from all different backgrounds, state agencies, education agencies, stakeholders in the community, people who are involved in policy, we have some politicians involved, so that we were able to share information across the different groups for much better preparedness, as we share information, response, and then recovery when a disaster of any type occurs.

Not just a natural or technological disaster, but also a terrorist attack or a shooting that has occurred in a community, or a shooting that has occurred in schools, that we can share information and have immediate response to those situations. I really feel about the work of the National Child Traumatic Stress Network speaks to some of the issues that have already come up in terms of integrating across community innovative ways to provide mental health services in ways that would be quite acceptable.

The other thing that I want to bring up that has not been discussed is the importance of how to support resilience—how to support resilience in children, and how to support resilience in families. Certainly, we have seen families being pressed immeasurably during the COVID pandemic. What I call it is an indefinite information.

Everything changed all the time, indefinite uncertainty. We didn't know what was going to happen from 1 day to the next. How can a family come together and how can a school system or a community come together when you don't know how things are going to change from day to day? And the issue came off of how to communicate, and I think that is why there has been so much excess use of social media as a way to connect.

We were told we couldn't be around people, so how can children relate to their friends? And how can one have a sense of family, if you can't see people and relate to them? So, I think that it is really very important for us to think about how to establish connections across families and connections across communities.

One of them, I will give you—I see I am just about out of time. I was going to give you a brief example how we brought together families and children after Hurricane Katrina on some of the cruise ships that housed people who did not have housing. And how we work together, including mental health, as a way of just being there.

That is something that we have to think about. Also, it is supporting parents to be able just be there and listen to their children and give support to parents to be able to do that. Thank you very much.

[The prepared statement of Dr. Osofsky follows:]

## Prepared Statement of Joy Osofsky

Since 2016, we have had the opportunity to work with Senator Cassidy to identify and support community and state agencies that can work individually and collaboratively in supporting the mental health needs of children and families including cross-state efforts. We have been pleased to support his efforts to increase mental health support in schools and communities. The Bipartisan Safe Communities Act and SUPPORT Act would expand community based behavioral health services and access to mental health care services in schools and communities in both rural and urban areas. This Act would also provide funding for the National Child Traumatic Stress Network to improve trauma informed training, treatment, and services for children, adolescents, and families who have experienced trauma.

### Effects of Trauma on Youth

Youth are exposed to trauma in many ways, for example, experiencing abuse and neglect, exposure to domestic violence, substance use, and community violence. Youth are also exposed to natural and technological disasters and, in the past 3 years, to the COVID–19 pandemic with its many effects on children and families, including parental and caregiver loss. There is much evidence that exposure to trauma affects development in different ways. For very young children, exposure to abuse and neglect can impact on their brain development. For all children, their cognitive, social, and emotional development can be affected by abuse and neglect (Center for the Developing Child at Harvard, 2023). Many studies have shown that children who are exposed to adverse life experiences (ACEs) early in their lives are at significant risk for developing serious and long-term problems, both medical and psychological, later in development. Trauma-informed and trauma-responsive interventions and evidence-based mental health treatments have been developed to help youth who have been exposed to trauma. It is crucial to recognize that recovery from trauma and development of resilience with meaningful, consistent relationships which means that parent and caregiver availability and support, in addition to mental health services, will help children and adolescents recovery from trauma exposure and also support resilience (Masten, 2021). The COVID–19 pandemic has contributed to increased risk of mental health problems for several reasons. Children of all ages, including adolescents, are likely to develop well with consistency in their schedules, positive relationships with a parent or caregiver in a supportive environment, and, as they grow older, consistent peer relationships. Few of these positive supports for youth development were in place during the COVID –19 pandemic.

## The Mental Health Impact of Natural and Technological Disasters on Youth Compared to the COVID–19 Pandemic

While the psychological and social impact of the COVID–19 pandemic shares some similarities to natural and technological disasters, there are also major differences that need to be considered related to the mental health impact on youth, having contributed significantly to the increase in anxiety, depression, and other mental health disorders. Unlike the COVID–19 pandemic, natural disasters commonly impact on designated regions of a city, community, state, or country, allowing those not impacted to be available to help with recovery. A second difference is that it is often possible to predict, with some variations, the duration of natural and technological disasters; however, with the COVID–19 pandemic, there has been much uncertainty about the duration and, therefore, the recovery process. Third, and perhaps most important, is that recovery from natural and technological disasters is helped to a great extent by supportive in-person relationships that have been unavailable during COVID–19. Psychological and social well-being has been affected significantly by "stay at home" orders, social distancing, and other safety precautions needed to contain the pandemic that preclude social relationships. Further, the psychological and social impact is influenced by fears of becoming sick as well as having to cope with friends and family being sick and dying mostly alone from COVID–19. Youth have reported that they often worried about going to school when they opened being fearful of bringing COVID back to a parent or other caregiver in the family. Recent data has shown that intrafamilial spread is often due to apparently well children. The number of fatalities from COVID–19 also has taken a toll on psychological well-being. Following Hurricane Katrina, Louisiana experienced an estimated 1,700–2,200 fatalities. In contrast, as of May 2020, there were already more than 2,281 fatalities in Louisiana from COVID–19 (NOLA.com, 2020) and in 2023, a total of 18,835 deaths which was 1 in 247 residents. The death rate for the African American population is 2.65 times the rate for all other groups. As with many major disasters, socioeconomic difficulties and preexisting health conditions are contributing to racial disparities in COVID–19. The mental health repercussions following disasters like Hurricane Katrina have been significant with both adults and children reporting high incidences of depression, anxiety, posttraumatic stress disorder, and substance abuse that went down slowly over time with growing family and community stability. This outcome has not been the case with COVID–19. Rather there have been reports of increases in anxiety, depression, substance use, and an exacerbation of previous mental health problems. Early in the pandemic, crisis counseling (Psychological First Aid), as is offered with disasters, was provided remotely. However, generally, there were limited clinical services and outreach support for individuals and families dealing with the stresses of temporary or permanent layoffs, decline in income, having to provide remote learning for children, and worries about illness and possible death. Mental health support also emphasizes the importance of establishing new routines and schedules for daily life including a schedule for youth to get up in the morning, have breakfast and go to school. During COVID, both youth and families experienced continual uncertainty about school, work, virtual schooling, homework, meals, self-care for parents, and time with children not only for virtual schoolwork, but also for positive play or conversation. The new routines also needed to include virtual ways to maintain friendships and family relationships using telephone or social media if available. While systematic reporting has been hampered with Stay-at-Home orders, concerns were raised, but not fully substantiated, about possible increases in child abuse and domestic violence with perpetrators and victims living in close quarters. Additional stress was contributed by family members becoming ill with COVID and not being able to be with loved ones when they were severely ill or dying from the virus. Further, youth experienced death of a parent, grandparent, or caregiver being taken to the hospital or leaving in an ambulance when sick with COVID never to return. For all children, this experience has been traumatic and, for younger children, confusing and difficult for them to understand. Clinically, we have heard many reports of young children continuing to stand at the window of their homes waiting for a parent to return. And with such losses, the remaining caregivers have had to find ways to support the children while also grieving themselves. The issue of inequities with COVID– 19 is striking. In Louisiana, African Americans represent 32.7 percent of the population but account for 70 percent of the deaths from COVID–19. These figures for Louisiana have been repeated across the United States with a much higher incidence of illness and death from COVID for Black/African Americans, Latino, Native Americans, Alaska Natives, Pacific Islanders among the many groups heavily impacted. This figure and inequities are likely related to having less access to care. Further, limited health care, which has contributed to a higher percentage of underlying conditions such as heart disease, hypertension, diabetes, and respiratory problems, places these individuals at higher risk if they become sick with COVID–19. The only conclusion to be drawn is that the COVID–19 pandemic is an unmitigated disaster in many ways comparable but worse than traditionally defined disasters such as hurricanes, earthquakes, tornadoes, and fires. Natural and technological disasters disrupt the essential consistencies in children's environments that are important for positive development. However, in most cases, substitute support can be established relatively quickly. However, the COVID–19 pandemic was different requiring a prolonged lockdown and social distancing requirements that should have been called physical distancing for safety so that social interactions that are so important for youth development would continue to occur, even if done virtually. Many young children could not really understand what happened and why their lives had changed from going to day care, preschool, or school to being isolated at home. For youth and adolescents of health care providers, they were often confused about why could they not see or hug their mother or father when they came home from work. Why could they not see or visit their grandparents who played such an important part in their lives? Also, the role of parents and caregivers in supporting their children is very important. If a parent is available to listen to their child, it can be extremely helpful even before mental health support may be available. A study done by Sesame Workshop during the pandemic that asked children to answer questions about their experiences during COVID, found that most children said that their parents would take care of them and keep them safe and secure.

Youth and parents were continually living with "indefinite uncertainty" with schools, including preschools, being closed and then opened and closed again if there was spread of COVID. Further, the pandemic exposed inequities as for many families, virtual schooling was not possible with parents needing to work and limited access to internet and the technology needed for virtual schooling. This constantly changing environment interfered for children and adolescents with many of the important components for positive development including consistent peer relationships. The Rapid Assessment of Pandemic Impact on Development Early Childhood Survey, that was designed to collect essential information from households and families of young children during COVID, indicated that the level of emotional distress in households for both parents and children was related to the number of material hardships encountered. Further, they found that financial and material hardships contribute to caregiver distress that impacts on child distress. Virtual schooling with little support may have added to the stress for both youth and parents contributing to mental health symptoms.

Youth mental health has been impacted by the "indefinite uncertainty" as a result of the pandemic with inconsistencies in schedules, feelings of isolation and anxiety with schools being closed, and an inability to be with friends. While virtual communication was possible for many youth, having to depend totally on this type of interaction may have also contributed to feelings of isolation and anxiety. Given that ideally for positive youth development, the use of social media, both content shared with friends and time spent, should be monitored by parents. During the pandemic, both children and parents depended more on virtual communication to interact with friends and family members. While some use of social media is reasonable for development. Unfortunately many youth and also their parents became more dependent on this method of communication and sharing during the pandemic. On the one hand, youth likely felt less isolated using social media; however, it could also have led to their feeling more isolated if they saw others interacting more with peers than they were doing. The main point is that use of social media for youth of any age should be monitored carefully by parents or caregivers which was made more difficult during COVID when this became a main way for youth to communicate and to receive education.

## Integrating Mental Health Support in School and Community Settings

Following Hurricane Katrina, we had the opportunity to develop an innovative community-academic partnership program in a temporary building with school personnel, all of whom had lost their homes and now their schools, the former principals and teachers collaborated with our mental health team to encourage high school students to take a leadership role in recovery by helping older citizens and younger children come back to school and the community. The youth in the "Young Leadership Program" who were mainly higher risk adolescents felt responsibility for leadership in the recovery giving them a sense of purpose and also helped other students and their community—giving them a sense of purpose. Other youth leadership programs were being planned for high-risk students when the COVID–19 pandemic closed schools.

From extensive school and community-based experiences in providing mental health supports following Hurricane Katrina and the Deepwater Horizon Oil Spill, our team learned about the importance of delivering mental health supports and services in collaboration with schools and community groups. In several of the rural parishes where few mental health supports are available, we also collaborated with community clinics to bring more mental health support for youth. Further, and not unexpectedly, we also learned about the importance of providing trauma-informed training for school personnel including teachers, counselors, nurses, other school staff, and administrators most of whom were also impacted personally by the disasters. To be supportive of students who experience trauma, it is important for school personnel to understand the impact of trauma and how it may be affecting the students. In this relationship-based approach, the students can feel understood and heal from trauma. The training and support for schools also includes information about vicarious traumatization and compassion fatigue in trying to support children who have also experienced trauma. The situation has been similar with the COVID– 19 pandemic from survey research with teachers, childcare providers, and administrators who have experienced due to illness and loss in their families, the pressures of doing virtual schooling, and their concerns related to re-opening schools and possible illness. Many of the teachers reported being concerned that it would be difficult for them to provide the support that the youth needed while also teaching them. Emphasis on these recommendations also comes from a recent experience shared by a psychologist who worked closely with us during our NCTSN grants supporting students in school settings. He shared with me that he walked into the school where he provides services and learned that two students had been shot and killed they day before. There was no supportive work done for the students or the teachers whether or not they knew the boys as all attended the same school. There are strategies that have been established to support schools, students, teachers, and staff when a student has been traumatically injured. It was hard for us to imagine the feelings at the school with no intervention and supportive work being done. Trauma-informed interventions and support should be in place for all students, teachers, staff, and families when needed.

To deliver mental health services most effectively in school settings, collaboration with school personnel is important especially with counselors and nurses whom the youth see if they are having problems. Unfortunately, there are many schools across the country that have no school counselors. In the work of our team after natural disasters, we learned the importance of school personnel being "trauma-informed," in order to recognize that behaviors like anxiety, irritability, or symptoms like stomach aches may reflect the child or adolescent's anxiety related to exposure to trauma. After Hurricane Katrina and the Deepwater Horizon Oil Spill, our team worked collaboratively with schools to obtain parental consent, which is required for mental health services for youth, to provide services at the school setting. It also provides an opportunity to also meet and work with the parents.

## Providing Mental Health Support in Collaboration with Community Groups

Not only partnering with schools in delivery of mental health services, but also collaborating with community groups where children may come for recreation or after school activities may be a place to identify increased anxiety or depression in youth and provide support. Trauma-informed community programs can play an important role in identifying and helping with mental health and substance use problems earlier. We have had experience with a successful community program in New Orleans, Son of a Saint, started 11 years ago by an innovative young man who lost his father, a New Orleans Saints player, due to natural causes when he was 3 years old. While his mother was very devoted, he found the teenage years difficult without having a father and was determined after he finished his education to start a program for adolescents. Boys ages 10–12, who had lost their fathers to violence or incarceration. Ninety percent of the youth are minorities and 80 percent are Black. While there are some mental health services provided for the program, most of the support is done by mentors who are well trained to provide ongoing support for the youth and adolescents, including the important encouragement of a consistent relationship. Since the beginning of the program, all have graduated high school, many have gone on to college, and none have had problems with the law.

## References

Center for the Developinng Child at Harvard—https:// developingchild.harvard.edu/.

Fisher, et al. (2023) Rapid Survey-https://rapidsurvey3years.com/.

Kaiser Family Foundation (2022) Recent trends in mental health and substance use concerns among adolescentshttps://www.kff.org/coronavirus-covid-19/issue- brief/recent-trends-in-mental-health-and-substance-use-concerns-among-adolescents/.

Masten, A. (2021) Resilience of children in disasters: A multisystemic perspective.

International Journal of Psychology, 56, 1–11. DOI:10.1002/ijop.12737.

Osofsky, J.D., Osofsky, H.D., Mamon, L.Y. (2020). Psychological and social impact of COVID–19. Psychological Trauma: Theory, Research, Practice, and Policy. Advance online publication. http://dx.doi.org/10.1037/tra0000656.

Osofsky, J.D. and Osofsky, H.J. (2020). Hurricane Katrina and the Gulf Oil Spill: Lessons Learned about Short and Long-term Effects. International Journal of Psychology,DOI: 10.1002/ijop.12729.

Osofsky, H., Osofsky, J., Hansel, T., Lawrason, Speier, A. (2018) Youth Leadership Program https://muse.jhu.edu/article/692848/pdf.

Sesame Workshop https://sesameworkshop.org/our-work/impact-areas/covid-response/.

## [Summary Statement of Joy Osofsky]

Since 2016, we have had the opportunity to work with Senator Cassidy to identify and support community and state agencies that can work individually and collaboratively in supporting the mental health needs of children and families including cross-state efforts. We have been pleased to continue to support his efforts to increase mental health support in schools and communities in urban and rural areas to help youth and families.

In my written testimony, I review and provide some important references for this work:

1. The Effects of Trauma on Youth including ways to support resilience following trauma exposure. Children of all ages, including those exposed to trauma, are likely to develop well with consistency in their schedules, positive relationships with a parent or caregiver in a supportive environment.
2. Mental health impact of natural and technological disasters on youth compared to the COVID–19 pandemic.
3. Natural disasters are often more predictable and are time limited. The COVID–19 pandemic has been marked by indefinite uncertainty. Recovery from disasters is helped by supportive in-person relationships. Mental health support following natural disasters is helped by supportive in-person relationships. Mental health support following natural disasters can be provided in schools and community settings.
4. With COVID–19, in order to limit spread of the virus, lockdowns and social distancing was imposed with no in-person contact. Schools that are important for recovery following disasters were closed during the pandemic with much stress imposed on families, particularly those with fewer resources having to work and do virtual schooling. Family stress after natural disasters is helped with community support. With COVID–19, increased financial and other family stress due to lockdown contributed to child stress. Both parents and youth depend on social media to maintain contact with family, friends and peers. Difficult to set suggested limits on use of social media with

COVID–19. Inequities were apparent with both natural disasters and the pandemic. Inequities were even more pronounced with serious illness from COVID–19.

5. Integrating Mental Health Support in Schools and Community Settings. Mental health services in collaboration with schools worked well in providing support for youth of all ages. Trauma-informed training and support in preparation for or following disasters for teachers, administrators, and other school staff to help them be more sensitive to students, especially given vicarious trauma and compassion fatigue.
6. Providing mental health collaboration with community groups and school collaborations will be very helpful in supporting youth mental health following the COVID–19 pandemic. Additional initiatives in school and community settings following disasters were helpful for high-risk youth with an illustrative example provided.

The CHAIR. Thank you. Our next witness is Dr. Joshua Garcia. Dr. Garcia is the Superintendent of the Tacoma, Washington School District. He previously served as Deputy Superintendent, Assistant Superintendent, High School Principal, Assistant Principal, Athletic Director, and Teacher. Other than that, not much. All right.

[Laughter.]

The CHAIR. Thanks very much for being with us, Dr. Garcia.

## Statement of Joshua Garcia, Superintendent, Tacoma Public Schools, Tacoma, WA

Dr. GARCIA. Chairman Sanders, Ranking Member Cassidy, and Members of the Committee, I am a proud Superintendent of the Tacoma school district and honored to share the viewpoint of superintendents for this important hearing focused on mental health of our Nation's youth, and to speak with you about what we have observed, what we have been doing, and what we might do together to curb the youth mental health crisis in America.

Tacoma is fully committed to each of our students being safe, engaged, supported, healthy, and challenged. We recognize mental health impacts us all. Mental health includes our emotional, psychological, and social well-being. It affects how we think and act. It helps us determine how we handle stress, relate to others, and make healthy choices.

During a highly critical phase of development, the lack of support and comprehensive approaches are significantly impacting our students' ability to grow socially, emotionally, and their academic development. Tacoma Public Schools, more than 28,000 students represent 170 tribes and ethnicities.

Over 2,000 of our students qualify as homeless. Over 55 percent of our students qualify as low income. And over 15 percent qualify for special education students. In the 2011 and 2012 school year, each of our high schools was labeled as a dropout factory. We were in a dire state, and we needed a new approach.

We started the Tacoma Whole Child Initiative, an intentional action plan that recognizes students are learning 24 hours a day, 7 days a week. Fast forward to 2022, 90.2 percent of our students graduate in 4 years. 86.7 percent of our high schools take college level classes. This year alone, over 12,000 participants in kindergarten through eighth grade have engaged in after school activity, and a record number of high school students are participating in paid job experience.

Tacoma has been able to make big strides to improve outcomes, but we know the challenges our students are facing are only growing. In the last year, our students, Tony, Angel, Brielle, Isiah, Marco, DJ, Wyatt, Xavier, Larry, and Iyana have been shot in our community. Our students have to survive human trafficking, battle homelessness, drug abuse, physical and mental abuse, and social media harassment and bullying.

Although these may not be new challenges to us as a nation, the speed of the incidences and the traumatic stress are only increasing. Like you and I, students are being bombarded with images, news events, daily experiences of trauma, and hate and stress.

Unlike us, they are doing this without fully developed brains, coping skills, or access to preventative and therapeutic services. In 2021, 13,239 of our 10th graders in our states made a plan for suicide. As you heard, Washington State is not unique. Our students are facing tremendous challenges and schools can't do this work alone.

Through the Tacoma Whole Child Initiative, we have moved away from episodic events to sustainable practices across our buildings and our community. They are focused on three elements, prevention strategies, response strategies, and therapeutic services. Our prevention strategies.

Each of our schools develop an intentional plan to support social emotional learning. They contextualize each plan at each school site. Our students are engaged in physical and mental wellness supports during the day and in the afterschool ecosystem. We do this with the Beyond the Bell and Club B, which uses a shared business model, common mental health supports, community assets, and align funding with over 70 partners.

Our system of positive behavioral supports ensure students understand schoolwide expectation, fostering stability and reinforcing healthy mental health habits. We also provide a safe space for our students to build belonging during evening and non-school hours. Our responsive strategies.

We have invested in professional development focused on trauma sensitive practice. We support and train facilitate restorative practice that bring voice with intentional healing and understanding And we also provide tiered supports, focusing on target intensive support for students at risk. Using ESSER and U.S. Department of Education grants, we were able to invest in therapeutic supports.

During a robust prevention and strategy, TPS is not able to alone meet the needs. To meet this challenge, we are implementing an ambitious plan to increase the ratio of students to mental health providers. Here are a few things I encourage us to think about doing together. Expand on the bipartisan Safe Communities Act. I know budget decisions are tough, but with the message students are telling us, we just—we have to listen to.

Pay for health care services with health care dollars to ensure Medicaid access. Incentivize the health care industry to formalize partners with schools, prioritizing youth first. Build on categorical funding opportunities.

Increase flexibility with the support for the Carl Perkins and Department of Labor grants to build hope. Require states to match your investment. Has Tacoma done everything we could? Not yet. Tacoma is learning, responding, and making a difference.

We have evidence. We know that through engagement, tiered supports, and shared strategies, our students are being more successful dealing with their individual emotions and stresses, developing their social awareness, and working academically at all times.

Finally, America's schools and individual communities can't do this alone. We must work in partnership, and we know that it is not easy. There are egos, turf battles, and frustrations. However, we are truly better together.

We may not be united on everything, but our future is with us now, and we must be united in our commitment to serving youth first. Thank you.

[The prepared statement of Dr. Garcia follows:]

## Prepared Statement of Joshua Garcia

Good morning, Chairman Sanders, Ranking Member Cassidy and Members of the Committee.

My name is Josh Garcia, and I am the proud Superintendent of the Tacoma School District. I am honored to share the viewpoint of school superintendents for this important hearing focused on the mental health of our Nation's youth and to speak with you today what we have observed, what we have been doing in Tacoma Public Schools and what we might do together to support the youth mental health crisis in America.

What do we want for every child in America? A simple question that has a complex and nuanced response. As one school district, we're thinking and working to take action every day. We are fully committed to each of our kids being safe, engaged, supported, healthy and challenged. We recognize mental health impacts us all, students, staff, and community. Mental health includes our emotional, psychological, and social well-being. It affects how we think, feel, and act. It also helps determine how we handle stress, relate to others, and make healthy choices. The need for this hearing is more critical than ever.

As we know, the human brain is developing during the K–12 experience. At the most impactful phase in human development, the lack of support and comprehensive approaches are significantly impacting our students' ability to grow their social, emotional, and academic development.

### 1. Tacoma

For those that don't know our beautiful community, Tacoma WA is an urban port city that is diverse. Our Tacoma Public Schools represent more than 28,000 students representing over 170 tribes and ethnicities. Over 2,000 of our students qualify as homeless, over 55 percent qualify as low income, and over 15 percent receive special education services.

In the 2011–2012 school year, each of our high schools was labeled as drop out factory by *U.S. News and World Report*. We were in a dire state, and we needed a new approach. We started the Tacoma Whole Child Initiative, which is an intentional action plan that recognizes that students are learning 24 hours a day, 7 days a week. It's a recognition that focusing all our community energy on solely transforming the student experience during schools is a bad model, when schools only have students one-third of the time. We knew we had to transform schools and leverage the other two-thirds of the time to truly make gains and provide the supports necessary to reach our desired academic and mental health goals.

Fast Forward to 2022, 90.2 percent of our students graduate in 4 years. 86.7 percent of high school students take college level classes. We have record numbers of students engaged in extra-curricular activities and athletics. This year alone over 12,000 participants in K–8 have been engaged in after school activities, STEM, fitness, arts and more. A record number of High School students are participating in paid job experiences through work-based learning and Jobs 253. Tacoma has been able to make big strides to improve student outcomes. But we know that the challenges our students are facing are only growing. Our kids are in pain—in our own homes, neighborhoods, cities, states and in our own Nation. We need a united response.

## 2. Mental Health Youth Crisis

Everyday our students face the challenges that are ripping our great nation apart. In the last year, 10 of our students—Tony, Angel, Brielle, Isiah, Marco, DJ, Wyatt, Xavier, Larry, and Iyana—have been shot, our students have had to attempt to survive human trafficking, battle homelessness, drug abuse, physical and mental abuse, and social media harassment and bullying. If we pause and read the news, we will see that our students are like many American youth in the trauma they face daily. Although these may not be new challenges for us as a Nation, the speed of the incidents and the traumatic stress are more intense than ever.

Like you and I, our students are relentlessly being bombarded with images, news events and daily experiences of trauma and stress. Unlike you and I, they are doing this without fully developed brains, coping skills and access to preventive and therapeutic services. This repeated attack on the human brain is putting our youth on high alert, which brings us all here today.

In 2021, 72 percent of our 10th graders reported feeling anxious, nervous or on edge regularly (68 percent across the state) and 60 percent reported not being able to stop worrying (55 percent across the state).

17 percent of our 10th graders made a suicide plan in the last year compared to 15.6 percent across the state. This translates into 13,239 students in our state making a plan to commit suicide.

Unfortunately, it is hard to imagine that 10th grade kids in Washington are unique. That same data would show the number is higher in 8th grade (16.2 percent of 85, 819) = 13,902.

## 3. How Tacoma Faces These Challenges Head on

The challenges our students and schools face are tremendous, and schools can't do this work alone! Communities, states, and our great nation need sustainable action plans that are functional, continuous, and comprehensive. We must all acknowledge our responsibility without blame. Through the Tacoma Whole Child Initiative, we have moved away from episodic events to sustainable practices across our school buildings. Our sustainable practices related to supporting whole child to improve student outcomes are focused on three elements: prevention strategies, response strategies, and therapeutic supports.

### *Prevention Strategies*

In Tacoma we have an intentional plan to support social emotional learning defined at the local level: each of our schools has developed their own social emotional learning plan and publishes it annually to ensure feedback from families and community stakeholders.

We also make sure our students are engaged in solid physical and mental wellness supports during the school day as well as in the afterschool ecosystem. Locally we do this with Beyond the Bell and Club Beyond which serves over 12,000 participants using a shared business model, common mental health supports, accessing community assets and aligned funding with over 70 partners. Through our shared signature strategies, we make sure students are greeted warmly, which builds a sense of belonging, and we focus on relationship building through strategies like, "circles" (building community, empathy and equitable story telling) and "emotion checks" (fostering self-regulation and understanding of others).

Our system of positive behavioral supports ensures students understand—school wide expectations to foster stability, encourage positive expectations and outcomes and reinforce healthy mental health habits.

We also provide a safe place for students to build belonging during the evening; Tacoma has launched 12 summer sites across town where teens can belong, break bread, and have equitable access to safe environments.

***Responsive Strategies***

We have invested in professional development focused on trauma sensitive practices.

We support, train, and facilitate restorative practices that bring voice with the intention of healing and understanding for all participants.

We also provide tiered supports—focusing on targeted support for some students (check in, check out) and intensive supports (students at risk of harming self or others).

***Therapeutic Supports***

Using Federal ESSER funding and U.S. Department of Education grants we were able to invest in therapeutic supports. We have learned that we must build partnerships and be honest about what our schools can and can't do for our students. We have 10 healthcare partners that are providing site based mental health supports to our students to keep them engaged in school and learning alongside their peers.

***How Can We Move Forward Together***

Expanding on the lessons we have learned and successes we have had in Tacoma to date, I would encourage Congress to do the following:

1. Continue to expand on your work with Bipartisan Safer Communities Act. I know that budget decisions are difficult and there is never enough. However, it would be foolish for us all to ignore the signs are youth are sending us. If we don't invest now, our costs will be 10 times what they are now in the future. In particular, the School-Based Mental Health Services Grant and the Mental Health Service Professional Demonstration (MHSP) grants will help districts train and retain desperately needed school mental health professionals.
2. Pay for healthcare services with healthcare dollars by ensuring every district can bill Medicaid for the healthcare services delivered to Medicaid eligible students, so we can focus our local education funding on other supportive programs and services.
3. Incentivize the Health Care Industry to have formalized partnership with public schools to serve youth with Mental Health Supports. We need to bring therapeutic services to our youth and continue to find ways to support growth in the workforce.

4. Build on categorical funding opportunities like Title IV of ESEA and consider new targeted support specifically for mental health programs and services and require states to match Federal investments. This will allow smaller communities to have sustainable resources for their students.
5. Provide flexibility through the Carl Perkins Grant and Department of Labor Grants to support paid youth job experiences and required financial literacy, building a sense a hope for the future.

***Gratitude***

Has Tacoma done everything we could, far from it! Tacoma is trying, learning, responding, and making a difference, we have evidence. We know that through engagement, tiered supports, and shared strategies, our students are being more successful dealing with their individual emotions and stresses, developing their social awareness and its impact on others. They are making responsible decisions for their future and building relationship skills. We are seeing students give back, feel seen, fostering their own sense of belonging, and working academically at all time high levels.

America's public schools and our beautifully unique communities can't respond to the mental health needs in isolation. In Tacoma, we work in partnership and that is not easy, there are egos, turf battles and frustrations. However, we recognize that we are better together, that we may not be united on everything, but our future is with us now and we must be united in our commitment to serving youth first. Personally, and professionally, I am grateful for your willingness to do more and better. I know that out of the 27,141 Washington students who reported the made a plan to commit suicide, 751 of those students are in our city. I challenge us all to know how many youth are in crisis in our own communities.

Thank you!

## References

Data Dashboard—Healthy Youth Survey (askhys.net)
Report Card—Washington State Report Card (ospi.k12.wa.us)

## [Summary Statement of Joshua Garcia]

Tacoma is an urban port city that is diverse, with more than 28,000 students representing over 170 tribes and ethnicities. Over 2,000 of our students qualify as homeless, over 55 percent qualify as low income, and over 15 percent receive special education services. In the 2011–2012 school year, each of our high schools was labeled as drop out factory by *U.S. News and World Report*. We were in a dire state, and we needed a new approach. We started the Tacoma Whole Child Initiative, an intentional action plan that recognizes that students are learning 24 hours a day, 7 days a week. Fast Forward to 2022, 90 percent of our students graduate in 4 years and 87 percent of high school students take college level classes. But we know that the challenges our students are facing are only growing. Our kids are in pain and we need a united response. Everyday our students face the challenges that are ripping our great nation apart. In the last year, 10 of our students have been shot, our students have had to attempt to survive human trafficking, battle homelessness, drug, physical, and mental abuse, and social media harassment and bullying. In 2021, 72 percent of our 10th graders reported feeling anxious, nervous or on edge regularly and 60 percent reported not being able to stop worrying. 17 percent of our 10th graders made a suicide plan in the last year. This translates into 13,239 students in our State making a plan to commit suicide.

Our sustainable practices related to supporting whole child to improve student outcomes are focused on three elements: prevention strategies, response strategies, and therapeutic supports. In Tacoma each of our schools has developed their own social emotional learning plan and publishes it annually to ensure feedback from families and community stakeholders. Our system of positive behavioral supports ensures students understand—school wide expectations to foster stability, encourage positive expectations and outcomes and reinforce healthy mental health habits. We also provide a safe place for students to build belonging during the evening with 12 summer sites where teens can belong, break bread, and have equitable access to safe environments. We have invested in professional development focused on trauma sensitive and restorative practices that bring voice with the intention of healing and understanding.

Expanding on the lessons we have learned and successes we have had in Tacoma to date, I would encourage Congress to (1) continue to expand on your work with Bipartisan Safer Communities Act. In particular, the School-Based Mental Health Services Grant and the Mental Health Service Professional Demonstration grants; (2) ensure every district can bill Medicaid for the healthcare services delivered; (3) incentivize the Health Care Industry to have formalized partnership with public schools to serve youth; (4) increase funding for Title IV of ESEA; and (5) Provide flexibility through the Carl Perkins Grant and Department of Labor Grants to support paid youth job experiences and required financial literacy.

We know that through engagement, tiered supports, and shared strategies, our students are being more successful dealing with their individual emotions and stresses, developing their social awareness and its impact on others. They are making responsible decisions for their future and building relationship skills. We are seeing students give back, feel seen, fostering their own sense of belonging, and working academically at all time high levels. America's public schools and our beautifully unique communities can't respond to the mental health needs in isolation. In Tacoma, we work in partnership and that is not easy. However, we recognize that we are better together, that we may not be united on everything, but our future is with us now and we must be united in our commitment to serving youth first.

* * *

The CHAIR. Thank you very much. Let me begin the questioning. Mrs. Russell-Tucker, you mentioned the importance of afterschool and summer programs.

I think one of the things we all agree on is that we are going to have to do a lot of treatment, but on the other hand, we are going to have to give young people a lot of positive community based activity.

Can you talk a little bit about the impact that increased funding for summer and afterschool programs has had in Connecticut?

Ms. RUSSELL-TUCKER. Thank you, Senator. Really important for—I appreciate that question, because it is such an important piece of the work that we have been doing. Under ARP ESSER fund, or ESSER funding, that we received $11 million for some enrichment, and we immediately put that to work. And our state stepped up and added more funding for the subsequent summers.

We are now up to $33 million of state investment around summer enrichment. We are able, in that space—the first summer was to really try to get students back together, back with their peers, back in that environment, allowing them to work with sometimes behavioral—behavior therapists in that space while they are having a really good time with each other, right.

It is enrichment, which is so important. And so, we have been able now, we have also evaluated the impact of that reimbursement. As I mentioned in my testimony of our 108,000 students we served that first summer, we are now into summer No. 3, and we are evaluating it rigorously to make sure we know what is happening and so that we can——

The CHAIR. Let me guess that you would like Congress to continue that kind of funding. Is that a good guess?

Ms. RUSSELL-TUCKER. [continuing]. Exactly. Fund what works, right. That is one way of thinking about sustainability. Same is true for our after school program that we also we see funding to support.

The CHAIR. We significantly expanded those programs in the American Rescue Plan.

Ms. RUSSELL-TUCKER. Yes, absolutely. And so, it is important that we are funding what works, and that is why I am so proud that we are evaluating the impact of those investments.

The CHAIR. Okay. Dr. Garcia, I want you to pick up on that. Again, we want to treat the millions of young people who are struggling, but we also want to challenge them. We want to bring them together.

We want to have proactive activities. It sounds to me like in Tacoma, you are challenging young people. You are trying to provide job opportunities, among other things. Talk about the importance of treating young people with respect and allowing them to use their energies in productive ways.

Dr. GARCIA. Thank you, Senator. I think it is important that each community has the opportunity to define what respect, responsible, and safe looks like, and that is what our social emotional learning plans do. They bring voice, student voice to that conversation. They bring staff voice to that conversation. And they bring family voice. Each of our plans is published, so——

The CHAIR. Young people are involved in the development of those plans?

Dr. GARCIA. Absolutely. Absolutely. And they define what it looks like in each location, right. Respect looks a little differently in a classroom than it does in a lunchroom, right. There are different settings. It looks different than in your neighborhood.

We have to build community through a common language, and that is important. We bring respect, and how does that look in the afterschool world? How do we hear their voice and what are the activities that they want to participate in?

It is very much an intentional effort to bring community together to define that, but those common words are across all the town.

The CHAIR. I am gathering that the empowerment of young people, giving them a voice in the community, has a positive impact on mental health, among other things.

Dr. GARCIA. We bring voices in several ways, and we also hear from students. Students have asked me, they have said, Josh, stop asking us our opinions and bringing others to ask our opinions if the adults aren't going to do anything.

That is a really important message. So, we bring voice through empathy interviews. We bring data around positive interactions. We have student voice at our board meetings. We—students will vote with their feet, if you will.

The increased activities in extracurricular activities, not what the adults want to offer, but what do they want to participate in. They have also told us they don't want to be engaged in the business model. They want to know the activity of that. We survey their interest regularly.

The CHAIR. Okay. Let me ask Dr. Osofsky a question. You use the term indefinite uncertainty. What impact you walk through the streets of Washington this morning, you breathe the air, which is a result of terrible fires in Canada. Young people worry about climate change.

We have heard discussions, Senator Kaine mentioned, on school, gun violence in the school. Kids worry about gun violence. Families all over the country are struggling economically. Louisiana, Vermont.

What impact does all of that and more have in indefinite uncertainty about worrying what the future is going to look for these young people, whether there will be a decent future, from an environmental point of view, from an economic point of view, from a violence free point of view? What impact is that having on the lives of young people?

Dr. OSOFSKY. I really appreciate you are asking that question because this is something that I struggle with and a lot of us struggle with, us in the mental health world. What children need, of all ages growing up, is they need to have schedules. They need to have routines. They need to know what is expected.

For example, having a schedule of knowing they get up in the morning and they go to school, and who is going to pick them up at school, or where they are going to go and what their activity might be. And what happened, unfortunately, with the COVID pandemic is that changed continually.

One of the things that we recommended is set a new schedule, have the children involved with setting the schedule so there is something predictable for them. But it went on for a very long time in that way. We also tried to support the parents, too, because parents were having—didn't have a schedule either.

Instead of getting up, and if they went to work, going to work and doing whatever, they were having to balance that with educating their children virtually, if they were fortunate to have the internet and the equipment that is needed to do that. And every day that changed as well for them.

The other thing that is very important for the young people is their peers at every age. For the younger children, being able to play with them and get to know them. For the older children, we know that it gets more complicated in adolescence and that kind of thing, which as I mentioned, contributes to some of the extensive use of social media.

It is very, very important now that schools are open again for there to be that kind of schedule and things that parents can count on and children can count on to be able to move forward. I also wanted to make a comment on the involvement of youth.

We found that to be extremely helpful after there was so much destruction with Hurricane Katrina, that there were a lot of teenagers who were on the streets because there was nothing there for them to do with themselves. They couldn't—there were no activities. So, we involved them with recovery.

The teachers, who also didn't have classrooms and schools, they involved with recovery, so that the teenagers, instead of being in trouble, were able to contribute in positive ways.

The CHAIR. Thank you very much. My time is long expired. Senator Braun, or Senator Cassidy? Senator Cassidy.

Senator CASSIDY. Dr. Osofsky, in some schools, they are limiting information sharing between parents and teachers, effectively cutting parents out of their child's life. What does your research say about the role of parents when students are going through traumatic experiences?

Dr. OSOFSKY. That is such an important issue that you bring up, Senator Cassidy, because we know the important role that parents play for children, to be there, for them to listen, to advise them, and to be very much a part of their life.

One of the studies that was done during COVID by Sesame Workshop sent out information to families, different backgrounds, racial groups, and asked them to have their children talk about what is important to them during COVID and what is going to help them. And the No. 1 issue was their parents.

Their parents were the hero. The parent was going to keep them safe, and that was so important to them. And also, from a mental health point of view, if parents are available, can be emotionally available, like say to not just be there and listen to the children, and be involved with their activities, that is going to be very important.

They will know when things are happening sometimes before the school will know, but obviously that collaboration is very important. But parents play a key role in mental health, in supporting the mental health of their children.

Senator CASSIDY. In the bipartisan Safer Communities Act, there are significant dollars put forward for tele-mental health. Does that work equally well for adolescents? Is there a role for that to be used in school health settings?

Dr. OSOFSKY. We found tele-mental health to be very helpful and it does work well generally for adolescents. They kind of like that. They are more used to being on the screen than others are, and it is a way to stay in contact.

We are very pleased that they allowed a lot of mental health work to be done using telehealth during the pandemic because it was a way that we were able to stay in touch and help people. For younger children, it can be a little bit challenging.

They may want to go press a button or something like that, but we found it to be very successful in working with teenagers related to telehealth, and I hope that opportunity will continue as a way to reach them.

Senator CASSIDY. I keep asking questions I don't know the answer to, but hearing you speak today, it suddenly occurred to me that the people that decided to lock down our economy, who had the noble goal of limiting death but of course ended up increasing isolation, did they actually have children, psychiatrists, psychologists involved in their deliberations to do a cost benefit ratio, if you will, a risk benefit ratio of if we lock down, we are going to have X amount happen because of isolation, as much as that was foreseeable? Do you know that process? I don't, I am asking.

Dr. OSOFSKY. Yes. I don't know for sure about that process either. Certainly, we were communicating, a number of us, and talking about it. And I recall almost every time I did an interview, I specifically recall an interview with an NPR reporter who had two children at home, and he took 15 minutes before he did the interview to talk to me about how can I support my children under the circumstance.

They can't see their grandparents. The holiday was coming. It was a very important part of their lives. So, the tele—telecommunication was really helpful. But I am not sure, Senator Cassidy, whether they did consult——

Senator CASSIDY. But what I am hearing from you is actually, it wasn't an imponderable. It was actually predictable that when the children were isolated, that they would have some of the problems that we now see. Is that a fair statement?

Dr. OSOFSKY. I think it is. I think in families, it is very clear in families where they have more resources, for example, where they could work remotely, where they could get help, where they could set up separate learning areas for a few kids. Where they consist in kids that wouldn't have to be afraid of COVID.

I know many families with resources who were able to do that. But for families with fewer resources, it was going to set up an ongoing problem, including learning over time and catching up where many of these children had problems to begin with.

Senator CASSIDY. Last, when I FaceTime with my 8 year old grandson, almost nine, he has got like 3 minutes for me, then he's gone. I say that because you mentioning that tele-mental health actually works.

But as the younger child, they want to hit a button. At what point does it begin to work? Because we will be asked to support these programs in schools of various ages. At what point does it begin to work, and at what point—or is it just a little boy who has got ADD? Like a squirrel, squirrel, squirrel.

Dr. OSOFSKY. Yes, I think certainly with what we call latency in children. Children about 8 years old and older, as we found with the earlier—that they were able to pay attention better when we did something—

Senator CASSIDY. Boys, girls difference or the same?

Dr. OSOFSKY. Sorry—?

Senator CASSIDY. Boy and girl——

Dr. OSOFSKY. Oh, I didn't—we didn't see differences between boys and girls, but we found the earlier work, at that age and older, seemed to be going pretty well. But on the other hand, we provided mental health services for younger children, but again, that was in person. I think it is the really little ones.

As you know, we work with very young children like under the age of five that may have more difficulty with that. But again, if the parent is with them and working with them, and it is really a combination. It is not just the mental health person dealing with a three or 4 year old, it is working with the parent together.

A dyadic work, and then the parent learns how to support the child. We are finding now in mental health in general, even in person, but certainly virtual, that involving parents, even with teenagers, with older children, is very important as a way to support them.

Senator CASSIDY. Thank you.

The CHAIR. Thank you.

Senator Markey.

Senator MARKEY. Thank you, Mr. Chairman, before I begin my questions, I want to address and make a comment about the health of trans youth, reiterating some of what Senator Baldwin mentioned earlier.

In the past 6 months, state legislators have passed 75 bills discriminating against LGBTQ Americans and blocking access to gender affirming care. Drag shows have been attacked, hospitals providing gender affirming care are receiving bomb threats, and local clinics are installing security systems.

Human Rights Campaign declared a national state of emergency for LGBTQ Americans, and the discriminatory actions and statements by elected officials at every level of Government are fueling the fire and making the youth mental health crisis worse. Passing bills into law is a tough process.

What is easy is giving people the freedom to be themselves. What is easy is not using hate fueled rhetoric on trans kids to score cheap political points. And we need to do this, especially during pride week, to identify this as a huge problem in our Country. So, I want to turn to other issues that obviously the Surgeon General was addressing. But you are on the front lines. One in three teenage girls contemplated suicide last year. One in ten teenage girls attempted suicide last year.

One in five LGBTQ youth attempted suicide last year—one in five LGBTQ youth attempted suicide last year. So, this is a real crisis, and we know that it is totally exacerbated by big tech and the role that they are playing in the lives of these children in our Country, because it is just unregulated in terms of what it can do to teenagers in our society. No protections, no safeguards.

They collect an avalanche of personal information, and they use it up to send back an endless stream of toxic content into the minds of young people in our society. And the results are clear. More money for big tech, more pain for kids and teenagers in our Country. And we know that it is Instagram. We know that it is— we know that it is Facebook. We know that it is TikTok.

We have to take action to pass a comprehensive law. We know that it is Disney. We know that it is Paramount. They are collecting information and sending it right back in a form that advances the financial interests of these companies. So, my question to you is, Ranking Member Cassidy and I have introduced a piece of legislation that would create an online privacy bill of rights for teenagers in America.

There is a law on the books right now for 12 and under, but there is no law for a 13 year old girl with bulimia or anorexia from being targeted by these companies with information that actually worsen the situation. So here is what the legislation would do. Just would love to get your comments on it.

One, the bill would ban targeted ads to children and teens. Two, it would establish a youth marketing and privacy division at the Federal Trade Commission. And three, it would limit the collection of children and teens' personal information.

It would actually say to parents, you have a right to say to the companies, erase this stuff that you have gathered about my child. Do you think that is necessary? Would you support legislation to accomplish that goal, so that the parents and the kids have protections against big tech?

Ms. RUSSELL-TUCKER. Well, thank you, Senator, for the background and information that you have just shared. And it is so important, I think, critically, recognizing the impacts of all of this on our youth, that we are really paying close attention.

I really believe hearing the voices, so having youth voices as a part of what is proposed, which is what we try to do in Connecticut. Hear from all the voices, including our families. Inform ultimately the impact, right, of the proposal being made. And so, we will really be looking at that very closely to get a sense of all that is being proposed, but anything that we can do——

Senator MARKEY. But in general, do you believe that teens and children need an online privacy bill of rights?

Ms. RUSSELL-TUCKER. No, I believe that.

Senator MARKEY. Thank you. Yes, sir.

Dr. GARCIA. Thank you, Senator. Yes, I do. I also was struck by the comments earlier this morning, and I don't know if we are using the tools to our advantage. The data would tell us that when kids are talking about suicide, that we could inform them right there online and require companies to give them suicide information. If they are struggling with food, we could require those companies to push that information to them as well to curb that support as well.

Senator MARKEY. What about upfront just putting the preventative action in place?

Dr. GARCIA. Yes, Senator.

Senator MARKEY. That way the kids and the parents have a bill of rights so that the kid isn't targeted, that exacerbates the situation, so that they do become excessively depressed and contemplate suicide. Do we need those protections put in place?

Dr. GARCIA. I have three teenagers and I would say yes, please.

Senator MARKEY. Okay, yes. And doctor?

Dr. OSOFSKY. Yes, I would agree with my with two other panelists here. One of the things I was thinking about, but it doesn't in any way negate what I just said that I agree with that. We also know that for many of these youth, that is how they make relationships, too. And so, if there was a way that we would be able to help support them in some way, at the same time that we are protecting them, I think it would be very important.

Senator MARKEY. Yes, I would say that we are in a crisis. We hear it today, we know that big tech plays a big role in creating this amongst kids. So, we are urgently in need of passing comprehensive legislation in my opinion.

AI that we are discussing right now is just algorithms on steroids. But we already have algorithms on steroids by big companies who target children in our Country. We have to put the protections in place.

If we can't do that, we are never going to be able to deal with the consequences for AI on steroids. If we can't protect children, we are not going to be able to protect our society. Thank you, Mr. Chairman.

The CHAIR. Thank you.

Senator Braun.

Senator BRAUN. Thank you, Mr. Chairman. Senator Kaine asked Dr. Osofsky about parents' role. I am going to turn to Mrs. Russell Tucker. I served on a school board many years ago, didn't have the issues I think that we now contend with. It is a lot different now than then. Parents were always the primary stakeholder on almost any issue.

Generally, it ended up being a disciplinary one, not what we deal with currently. In your testimony, you list in terms of on the mental health issue, the stakeholders, the Office of the Governor, and the State Board of Education, state agencies, educators, administrators, families, students, advocates, policymakers, local health officials, and more.

I tried to tease out of Secretary Cardona on who the main stakeholders should be in our own kids' education and could not get parents out of his mouth the first time. After the Virginia election and it was made an issue there, he did begrudgingly say that parents should be a stakeholder, not the primary.

When we are talking about mental health, there is a list of a lot of, and I believe sometimes that village doesn't need to be consulted, but I would think that in any of these issues, the parents ought to be the primary and everything else ancillary.

By the way, you stated that. Would you agree with parents being the primary, all these other ancillary, or do you have a different way of saying what you are meaning what you said there?

Ms. RUSSELL-TUCKER. Thank you, Senator. And I have long, if you saw from my testimony, as you mentioned, recognized the value and importance of parent voice in everything that we do in education. It is really important that they are at the table.

They are a stakeholder. And the family engagement roundtable that I mentioned is doing just that. As a matter of fact, they have worked together through their voices to define what family engagement means in Connecticut.

They truly are very important. And every time we have a chance to do any program, any policy, that their voices are actually are there at the table so we can understand, hear from them, and hear their perspectives. Because it really—so they are key stakeholders——

Senator BRAUN. Are they consulted first in any navigation through a mental health issue in terms of getting with them first, are they just part of the group?

Ms. RUSSELL-TUCKER. They are very much important about the health of their children. And so, I know for a lot of the initiatives that we have in the state, they are consulted and provide consent for services that is being provided. And so, in that case of health, I think it is very important that they are very much key and there to make decisions, to help to make decisions around their children.

Senator BRAUN. Thank you. And Dr. Garcia, briefly on that topic.

Dr. GARCIA. Yes. They are very much a part of the process. At certain ages in Washington State, students can access services without family consent.

Senator BRAUN. Would you say they are the primary, not just part of it?

Dr. GARCIA. I don't think it is a simple answer because I have experiences as families are in different spots. And so there is a recognition that I have, is that some families are not in a place where they are able to be at the table for work, social issues, a variety of things. And so, as a school system, it is not a luxury of one——

Senator BRAUN. But whenever possible and able to, you would probably consider them the primary.

Dr. GARCIA. We engage them. Yes.

Senator BRAUN. Another question, over the years, we have spent billions on the issue, and I would like each panelist, we have got about a minute and a half left here, do you think we have implemented what we have already put in the law and the money that we have devoted to it properly?

Do you think that has been done in a way that would justify more? Do we need to do better at that? And where does the state fit in terms of maybe being able to do that better? We will start with Mrs. Russell Tucker. Give it about 30, 40 seconds, and move on down the panel.

Ms. RUSSELL-TUCKER. Really important that we are continually evaluating so we know what works. We implement, but we must know the results and the impact. And so, at the state level, we have done that. You can see that in my testimony in making sure that we are indeed doing that. So, we can tell you what works, so we can actually talk about sustainability.

Senator BRAUN. Yes or no, have the Federal programs and everything we have sent your way, do you think we have implemented that as good as it needs to be?

Ms. RUSSELL-TUCKER. I think there is always room for improvement.

Senator BRAUN. Thank you. And Dr. Garcia.

Dr. GARCIA. In my testimony, I ask that you work with states to require them to match your investments. My rural colleagues—let me know that categorical funding, direct streams are important, and competing for grants are oftentimes problematic alone. And so, I would encourage us to think about how we can do direct spend through categorical investments to build on sustainability.

Dr. OSOFSKY. Yes, I believe very strongly that the investment, at least one program that I am involved with, and that is the National Child Traumatic Stress Network, has been extremely helpful because we focus on trauma.

We have been talking about trauma. How to help children. And there has also been creative ways to spread what we have learned and also address the issues that we are concerned about with children. So that money has been very well spent.

Senator BRAUN. Thank you.

The CHAIR. Thank you, Senator Braun. That concludes our hearing today. And I want to thank all three of our witnesses for their excellent presentations. For any Senators who wish to ask additional questions, questions for the record will be due in 10 business days, June 23rd at 5.00 p.m.

Finally, I ask unanimous consent to enter into the record five statements from stakeholders outlining their youth mental health priorities, and that will take place.

[The following information can be found on page 80 in Additional Material:]

The CHAIR. The Committee stands adjourned. Thanks.

## Additional Material

American Occupational Therapy Association,
AOTA.ORG.
*June 8, 2023,*

Hon. BERNIE SANDERS, *Chairman*,
Hon. BILL CASSIDY, *Ranking Member*,
*U.S. Senate Committee on Health, Education, Labor, and Pensions,*
*428 Dirksen Senate Office Building,*
*Washington, DC.*

RE: Why Are So Many American Youth in a Mental Health Crisis? Exploring Causes and Solutions

Dear Chairman Sanders and Ranking Member Cassidy:

The American Occupational Therapy Association (AOTA) greatly appreciates the Senate Health, Education, Labor, and Pensions Committee's hearing on the youth mental health crisis. We are pleased to provide testimony and resources in support of this hearing.

## Background

AOTA is the national professional association representing the interests of more than 244,500 occupational therapists, occupational therapy assistants, and students of occupational therapy across the Nation. The practice of occupational therapy is science-driven, evidence-based, and enables people of all ages to live life to its fullest by promoting health and minimizing the functional effects of illness, injury, and disability.

Occupational therapy (OT) is a vital component of a complete mental health team to address the youth mental health crisis. Roughly one third of the profession are already working with children in a range of settings, such as schools, pediatric outpatient clinics, and hospitals. OT practitioners focus on an individual's ability to engage in day-to-day activities to maximize independence, function, and performance. They are trained to identify how factors such as the environment, cognition, and sensory processing support or hinder recovery and participation.

## A History and Scope in Mental Health

The profession was founded in public psychiatric hospitals over a century ago, based on the observation that a person's ability to engage in their desired roles, routines, and activities, could dramatically affect their mental health and overall well-being. Today, occupational therapy practitioners still focus on an individual's ability to engage in day-to-day activities.

For decades, OT was a core part of the interdisciplinary mental health services. With the call for deinstitutionalization of individuals with mental illness, which culminated in the 1963 Community Mental Health Act, occupational therapists and occupational therapy assistants began working in community mental health. However, the role of occupational therapy in working with those with behavioral health disorders has declined, despite OT's focus on the promotion of functional skills and independence.

One of the barriers to providing the services they are trained to provide, is a lack of clear and complete understanding of the profession and what they are allowed to provide by law. This barrier has created the misconception OT mental health services aren't eligible for reimbursement. However, statute in all 50 states and the District of Columbia, the explicitly allows OT practitioners to provide interventions and procedures for the development, remediation, or compensation of cognitive, psychosocial, or psychological deficits.

Occupational therapists have been included in imperative legislation to combat workforce shortages in mental and behavioral health, addressing chronic pain, and expansion of community mental health services. The Federal Government recognizes occupational therapy as a valued part of the behavioral health workforce. Occupational therapy services provided to a beneficiary with a mental health diagnosis have long been reimbursable under Medicare.

Occupational therapy is included under the staffing suggestions for Certified Community Behavioral Health Centers, a Medicaid demonstration program. In 2016 occupational therapy education programs were made eligible to receive Behavioral Health Workforce Educations Training Grants, and since 2018, the Health Resources Service Administration (HRSA) has included occupational therapy among the professions making up the behavioral health workforce.

### School and Community-Based Settings

AOTA believes the schools are the most effective setting to provide basic and universal mental health support. Children spend a vast majority of their time outside of the home in schools, where they have access to a range of specialized instructional support personnel (SISP) who work in mental health, such as occupational therapists, psychologists, social workers, and counselors.

Academic success is critical, but schools must be equipped to address children's social, emotional, and behavioral needs in order to make it possible for them to learn in the classroom. These needs and their educational progress cannot be minimized or separated. This emphasized by research that demonstrates the relationship between improved mental health and improved outcomes for students. Occupational therapy uses activity or occupation-based interventions to enable students to achieve their potential by increasing their functional skills for better participation in school and later in adult life, as well as to minimize the effects of disabilities.

As part of a larger treatment plan, occupational therapy practitioners help persons with schizophrenia, bipolar disorder, and major clinical depression, regain, build, or maintain skills that are essential to independent functioning, health, and well-being. In particular, occupational therapy practitioners are able to assist individuals with the cognitive impairments commonly associated with serious mental disorders that impact independent function, and compromise speech, memory, attention, and executive decision-making of all kinds.

### Indiana: The National Model

The State of Indiana should be the national model for coverage of mental health OT services. In September 2021, the Indiana Health Coverage Programs (IHCP) issued a *bulletin* clarifying coverage of occupational therapy services for eligible IHCP persons. The IHCP supported including occupational therapists on a substance use disorder (SUD) or behavioral health treatment team when the occupational therapists provide services within their scope of state licensure.

In addition, the IHCP guidance specifies that when occupational therapy is delivered to patients with mental illnesses or addiction treatment disorders, the scope of occupational therapy includes "services that are provided to promote health and wellness, prevent disability, preserve functional capabilities, prevent barriers for occupational performance from occurring, and enable or improve performance in everyday activities." The agency noted that the scope of occupational therapy practice allows for the provision of psychosocial interventions, and the IHCP supported including occupational therapy in the treatment plan of members receiving mental health care and addiction treatment services.

### Conclusion

As is well known, there is a documented shortage of mental health professionals in America with at least 152 million Americans living in a mental health professional shortage area. While occupational therapy practitioners continue to provide services in multiple mental and behavioral health settings, such as acute care hospitals and Certified Community Behavioral

Health Centers, they remain an underutilized part of this workforce. The profession is already well positioned to support efforts to address the youth mental health crisis. In early 2023, two occupational therapy programs received funding to strengthen the mental health workforce pipeline from the Department of Education's Mental Health Service Professional Grant Program.

AOTA strongly urges the Committee to build on past successes broadening OT's visibility with regards to mental health services and prioritize methods to promote the inclusion of occupational therapy in future policy discussions.

Thank you for the opportunity to provide these comments. AOTA stands ready to provide any additional information you need and to collaborate on any efforts in this area. Please contact Abe Saffer if you have questions or need additional information.

Sincerely,

ABE SAFFER,
*MPM American Occupational Therapy Association.*

## Prepared Statement of the Child and Adolescent Mental Health Coalition

On behalf of our organizations, which are leading members of the Child and Adolescent Mental Health Coalition (CAMH),[41] we commend the Senate Health, Education, Labor, and Pensions Committee for holding a hearing on youth mental health. We thank you for your bipartisan commitment to addressing the youth mental health crisis and look forward to working with you to ensure that Congress crafts legislation that addresses the full continuum of child and adolescent mental health needs.

In October 2021, the American Academy of Pediatrics, the American Academy of Child and Adolescent Psychiatry, and the Children's Hospital Association declared a *national emergency* in child and adolescent mental health. Since then, important work has been done to address the mental and behavioral health needs of the Nation's youth, but it is not enough. Suicide is the second leading cause of death for youth ages 10–18 in the United States.[42] In 2021, 42 percent of high school students reported feeling persistently sad or hopeless, and 29 percent reported experiencing poor mental health.[43] Additionally, 20.1 percent of youth ages 12–17 had a major depressive episode in the past year, compared to only 15.7 percent of youth

---

[41] CAMH is a coalition of organizations dedicated to promoting the mental health and well-being of infants, children, adolescents, and young adults. Our organizations reflect a diversity of viewpoints and expertise, ranging from clinical providers to school-based services to suicide prevention organizations and others. As a coalition, we seek to advance a robust mental health safety net, inclusive of programs, supportive payment models, and infrastructure, that provide the full continuum of mental health care, in a manner that facilitates easy and prompt access to services. Our coalition has prepared a set of core principles, *available here*. Our full coalition consists of over 30 organizations; entities specifically endorsing this statement are specified at the conclusion of this statement.

[42] National Vital Statistics System. Leading Causes of Death, United States. Centers for Disease Control and Prevention; 2020 *https://wisqars.cdc.gov/data/lcd/home*.

[43] Youth Risk Behavior Survey Data Summary & Trends Report, 2011–2021. Centers for Disease Control and Prevention; 2023. *https://www.cdc.gov/healthyyouth/data/yrbs/yrbs-data-summary-and-trends.htm*.

in 2019.[44] We urge Congress to make new dedicated investments that are designed to support a full range pediatric mental and behavioral health services and to grow the pediatric mental health workforce to deliver this essential care, across settings.

The experiences and needs of children and adolescents are different from those of adults, and the system and funding must be designed to address their needs across the continuum of mental health care services, from promotion and prevention to early identification, intervention and treatment, to care for children and youth in crisis. To support this continuum of care, new dedicated investments in pediatric health care services and infrastructure are vital, including to grow the pediatric behavioral health workforce. It is clear that current Federal programs and investments are not sufficient, as currently structured and funded, to alleviate the national emergency in children's mental health and to ensure that children's mental health needs are prioritized, identified, and addressed with timely, high-quality care.

By some estimates, as many as 19 percent of children have mental health symptoms that impair their functioning without meeting criteria for a disorder. Programs and funding that are limited to children with serious emotional disturbance (SED) miss a key opportunity to support early prevention and early intervention. Our organizations were pleased to see a prevention set-aside within the Community Mental Health Services Block Grant for early identification and early intervention in the *Mental Health Reform Authorization Act of 2022*. A similar provision to allow Community Mental Health Services Block Grant funds to be used for prevention and early intervention passed the House in H.R. 7666, Restoring Hope for Mental Health and Well-Being Act of 2022. We were disappointed that these provisions which would enable the Community Mental Health Services Block Grant to better meet children's needs did not become law last Congress. Children urgently need access to prevention and early intervention services to improve outcomes and prevent worsening conditions.

The Community Mental Health Services Block Grant is SAMHSA's primary investment in community mental health services, yet children's mental health needs continue to be insufficiently met by this program. A set aside for prevention and early intervention would allow states to fund programs that provide help upstream to people who have not been diagnosed with SED or Serious Mental Illness (SMI). Research shows that early intervention and prevention activities can mitigate, or in some cases, prevent the incidence of mental health conditions. With a prevention and early intervention set-aside in place, the block grant would allow flexibility for states to determine what prevention and early intervention programs are needed in their communities and fund those initiatives. This can include mental health literacy programs, outreach programs, and integrated services in primary care and school settings that reach underserved communities.

We strongly support a 5 percent set aside for the Community Mental Health Services Block Grant targeted for prevention and early intervention to begin addressing these needs not currently met with these funds. We encourage a greater emphasis on addressing the mental health needs of children, including young children and children who do not have a diagnosis or who have a mental health condition that is not considered an SED. Congress must make

---

[44] Substance Abuse and Mental Health Services Administration. Key Substance Use and Mental Health Indicators in the United States: Results from the 2019 National Survey on Drug Use and Health. US Department of Health and Human Services; 2020. *https://www.samhsa.gov/ data/report/2019-nsduh-annual-national-report*; Substance Abuse and Mental Health Services Administration. Key Substance Use and Mental Health Indicators in the United States: Results from the 2021 National Survey on Drug Use and Health. US Department of Health and Human Services; 2023. *https://www.samhsa.gov/data/report/2021-nsduh-annual-national-report*.

targeted investments in expanding the availability of a full spectrum of mental health care for children and the critical infrastructure to support these services. While this set aside is a good first step, it is unlikely to be enough to facilitate the expansion needed to meet children's mental health needs across settings and across the continuum of mental health service levels.

CAMH has identified nine priority areas and offers the following policy solutions that, if enacted, will help to increase access to quality pediatric mental health care. For more information, please see the *CAMH Principles*:

Prevention, Early Identification, and Early Intervention

- Roughly half of lifetime cases of mental illness begin by age 14 and almost three-quarters begin by age 24.[45]
- Congress should ensure new and existing Federal investments in mental health are tailored to include prevention and early intervention services.

School-Based Mental Health

- School-based mental health services help ensure children receive screenings and care.
- Congress should increase resources and financing mechanisms available to schools for mental health services.

Integration of Mental and Behavioral Health into Pediatric Primary Care

- Primary care is where most families access care and where identification, initial assessment, and care of mental health conditions in children often occur.
- Congress should support models of co-location or integration of mental health providers in all pediatric primary care settings.

Child and Adolescent Mental and Behavioral Health Workforce

- There is a dire shortage of practitioners specializing in mental and behavioral health to care for infants, children, adolescents, and young adults.
- A nationwide cross-sector strategy to expand the supply, diversity, and distribution of the behavioral health workforce, along with appropriate payment for pediatric mental health services, must be developed and implemented.

Insurance Coverage and Payment

- Even when covered by Medicaid, CHIP, or private insurance, children's access to timely, quality mental health care is often limited by high costs.
- Barriers to care like carve-outs, same day billing restrictions, inadequate payment rates for mental and behavioral health services, and lack of payment for emerging conditions that do not yet have a diagnosis should be addressed.

Mental Health Parity

- There is a persistent need to improve oversight and compliance with the requirements of the Paul Wellstone and Pete Domenici Mental Health Parity and Addiction Equity Act (MHPAEA).
- Congress should expand MHPAEA to children in Medicaid fee-for-service arrangements and ensure meaningful compliance and enforcement.

---

[45] Kessler RC, Berglund P, Demler O et al. Lifetime prevalence and age-of-onset distributions of DSM-IV disorders in the National Comorbidity Survey Replication. Arch Gen Psychiatry; 2005; 62(6):593–602. Doi:10.1001/archpsyc.62.6.593.

Telehealth

- Telehealth utilization has surged in the past few years, offering an efficient way to support youth in rural, underserved, and low-income communities who continue to face the most barriers to care.
- Congress should ensure that telehealth continues to be a part of a comprehensive set of care options available to children with mental and behavioral health needs.

Infants, Children, and Adolescents in Crisis

- Providers are witnessing an alarming number of children and adolescents in behavioral health crisis, with emergency departments seeing increases in suicidal ideation and self-harm.
- Congress should designate funding specifically intended to target youth crisis care needs, including consistent and sufficient funding for 988 and to support access to step-down programs.

Justice-Involved Youth

- The prevalence of mental health disorders among justice-involved youth ranges from 50 percent–75 percent.
- Congress should invest in incarceration diversion programs, including specialized mental health and substance use programs.

We thank the Senate Health, Education, Labor, and Pensions Committee for your continued attention to child and adolescent mental health and the critical roles of child serving professionals within both education and health care. More action is needed now to end the national emergency in child and adolescent mental health and ensure children and families can access the mental health services and support they need.

American Academy of Pediatrics. American Academy of Child and Adolesecent Psichiatry. American Foundation for Suicide Prevention. Children's Hospital Association.

* * *

NATIONAL EDUCATION ASSOCIATION,
Washington, DC,
*June 7, 2023.*

U.S. Senate,
*Committee on Health, Education, Labor, and Pensions,*
*428 Dirksen Senate Office Building,*
*Washington, DC.*

Dear Senator:

On behalf of our 3 million members and the 50 million students they serve, we would like to submit the following comments for the record of tomorrow's hearing, "Why Are So Many American Youth in a Mental Health Crisis? Exploring Causes and Solutions." This is a vital topic as students and families emerge from the COVID–19 pandemic. We embrace public dialog on mental healthcare for our Nation's students.

Our youth are in crisis. According to the Centers for Disease Control and Prevention (CDC), more than a third (37 percent) of high school students reported experiencing poor mental health during the pandemic, and 44 percent reported feeling persistently sad or hopeless during the past year. In addition, more than 1 in 5 students (22 percent) seriously considered attempting suicide and 1 in 10 (10 percent) attempted suicide. Suicide attempts occurred more often among Black students than students from other groups, and increased among Black and White students from 2011 to 2021.

We are pleased that Congress responded to this crisis through the Bipartisan Safer Communities Act, creating and funding two programs that begin to address these needs. We urge continued support for the:

- *Mental Health Service Professional Demonstration Grant Program* that provides competitive grants to support a strong pipeline into the mental health profession, including innovative partnerships to prepare qualified school-based mental health service providers for employment in schools.
- *School-Based Mental Health (SBMH) Services Grant Program* that provides competitive grants to states and school districts to increase the number of qualified mental health service providers delivering school-based mental health services to students in local educational agencies with demonstrated need.

In addition, we urge continued support for the *Full-Service Community Schools Program* that meets the unique needs of the locations they serve by engaging with parents, students, and the community. Through this grant program, student and family needs are assessed, and programs developed and opportunities created in partnership with students, families, and community members to meet those needs. A critical aspect of these opportunities is the ability to help youth and their families access mental health services and supports.

We know that the programs cited above are not the only programs to address the mental health and overall health of students, and that we must continue to partner to address the crisis facing young people today. NEA and its members stand ready to work with you to do so.

We thank you for holding this hearing and giving us the opportunity to submit these comments.

Sincerely,
Marc Egan,
*Director of Government Relations.*

## Prepared Statement of the American Association of Child and Adolescent Psychiatry

On behalf of the American Association of Child and Adolescent Psychiatry (AACAP), we thank the Committee for hosting this hearing and for the opportunity to submit testimony on why so many American youth are in a mental health crisis and to offer AACAP's recommendations on causes we should consider and solutions that can make a difference.

AACAP represents over 10,000 child and adolescent psychiatrists and trainees all of whom grasp the gravity of our Nation's pediatric mental health crisis and continue to respond to it. Our members work in every child-facing system of care: in urban and rural communities and from hospitals to schools.

AACAP, along with the American Academy of Pediatrics and the Children's Hospital Association, have declared a national state of emergency in children's mental health.[46] While there are many factors that contribute to poor access to pediatric behavioral health care, we emphasize the impact the insufficient behavioral health workforce has had and continues to have on access to care and note the importance of ensuring equity, diversity, and inclusion. Along these lines, we recommend policy solutions toward addressing this crisis.

## Background

There has been a silent pediatric mental health pandemic building for decades, disproportionately impacting minoritized groups including racial, ethnic, and gender diverse youth, and those living in poverty. The social disruptions and fear and grief caused by the COVID–19 pandemic turned the world upside down for all children, especially those vulnerable to mental illness and substance use disorders.

Rates of childhood mental health concerns and suicide rose steadily between 2010 and 2020 and by 2018, suicide was the second leading cause of death for youth ages 10–24. The pandemic intensified this crisis: across the country we have witnessed dramatic increases in Emergency Department visits for all mental health emergencies, including suspected suicide attempts.

The pandemic struck at the safety and stability of families. According to the National Institutes of Health, more than 140,000 children in the United States lost a primary and/or secondary caregiver, with youth of color disproportionately impacted. Child and adolescent psychiatrists are caring for young people with soaring rates of depression, anxiety, trauma, loneliness, and suicidality. We must identify strategies to meet these challenges through state, local and national approaches to improve access to care. We must work as a community to address mental health awareness, prevention, and treatment.

The Declaration of a National State of Emergency in Children's Mental Health outlined the following shared recommendations for how we address the crisis we face (in no order of priority):

Increase Federal funding dedicated to ensuring all families and children, from infancy through adolescence, can access evidence-based mental health screening, diagnosis, and treatment to appropriately address their mental health needs, with particular emphasis on meeting the needs of under-resourced populations.

Address regulatory challenges to improve access to technology to assure continued availability of telemedicine to provide mental health care to all populations.

- Increase implementation and sustainable funding of effective models of school-based mental health care, including clinical strategies and models for payment.

---

[46] Pediatricians, CAPs, and Children's Hospitals Declare National Emergency (*aacap.org*).

- Accelerate adoption of effective and financially sustainable models of integrated mental health care in primary care pediatrics, including clinical strategies and models for payment.
- Strengthen emerging efforts to reduce the risk of suicide in children and adolescents through prevention programs in schools, primary care, and community settings.
- Address the ongoing challenges of the acute care needs of children and adolescents, including shortage of beds and emergency room boarding by expanding access to step-down programs from inpatient units, short-stay stabilization units, and community-based response teams.
- Fully fund comprehensive, community-based systems of care that connect families in need of behavioral health services and support for their child with evidence-based interventions in their home, community, or school.
- Promote and pay for trauma-informed care services that support relational health and family resilience.
- Accelerate strategies to address longstanding workforce challenges in child mental health, including innovative training programs, loan repayment, and intensified efforts to recruit underrepresented populations into mental health professions as well as attention to the impact that the public health crisis has had on the well-being of health professionals.
- Advance policies that ensure compliance with and enforcement of mental health parity laws.

## Policy Actions for Committee Consideration

### *Access to Specialty Care and the Child and Adolescent Psychiatry Workforce*

To increase access, we can extend the reach of the child and adolescent psychiatry workforce by supporting primary care providers and school-based providers in identifying, assessing, and stabilizing children with pediatric behavioral health disorders and then escalating to specialty behavioral healthcare when a patient's needs require a higher level of care.

### 1. Support Child Psychiatry Consultation Programs

Pediatric Mental Healthcare Access (PMHCA) consultation programs, run through the Maternal and Child Health Bureau (MCHB) at the Health Resources and Services Administration (HRSA), school-based mental health care, and integrated behavioral health and primary care models, connect patients to behavioral health care.

These consultation programs, commonly called child psychiatry access programs (CPAPs), have been implemented in most states across the country, and are funded through HRSA grants, state funding, or institutional funding, or a combination of these funding resources, yet some states with large rural and underserved areas have not yet developed such programs.[47] Pediatricians utilize CPAPs in their state to consult with child and adolescent psychiatrists about treatment options for the children and youth they see who may need mental and

[47] Map—NNCPAP National Network of Child Psychiatry Access Programs.

behavioral health care. Research has shown that the use of CPAPs significantly improves outcomes for the patients who receive integrated medical and behavioral health care through this model compared to treatment as usual.[48] AACAP encourages the Committee to support replication of the CPAP program in every state.

AACAP is grateful for recent congressional investments in these programs and urges the Committee to continue to support these resources and promote state and provider adoption to ensure these models are sustainable. We must meet children where they are and eliminate additional barriers.

**2. Support Integrated Care Arrangements**

Integrating behavioral healthcare, including child and adolescent psychiatry, into primary care practices facilitates primary care provider's in accessing real time, immediate support for behavioral and mental health issues that present during patient visits. AACAP encourages the Committee to support integrated care arrangements, like the collaborative care model, that support pediatric practice engagement with child and adolescent psychiatrists.

**3. Build a Pipeline of Child and Adolescent Psychiatrists**

Before the COVID–19 pandemic, the workforce shortage of child and adolescent psychiatrists was significant, and this shortage continues. As physician subspecialists who conduct 4 years of medical school, complete a medical residency in psychiatry and complete a residency fellowship in child and adolescent psychiatry, the training is extensive and costly. AACAP recommends the following strategies for supporting a pipeline of child and adolescent psychiatrists:

- Support targeted student loan repayment programs—S. 462, the "Mental Health Professionals Workforce Shortage Loan Repayment Act of 2023," sponsored by Committee Members Senators Tina Smith, Lisa Murkowski, and Maggie Hassan, would repay up to $250,000 in eligible student loan debt for mental health professionals who work in mental health professional shortage areas.
- Support efforts to defer student loan payments on an interest-free basis during training—S. 704, the "Resident Education Deferred Interest (REDI) Act," would allow borrowers to qualify for interest-free deferment on their student loans while serving in a medical residency program.

**4. Advocate for Mental Health Parity—Coverage and Payment**

We must support mental health parity to ensure mental health is on equal footing with physical health and surgical care. Lack of medical coverage and poor reimbursement for mental health care are disincentives to recruiting medical students into child and adolescent psychiatry and building robust psychiatric services for children. Lack of parity contributes to limited in-network psychiatry access, longer wait times for children and youth, and higher expenses for patients who are often forced to go out of their insurance networks to find any care. Full parity in insurance coverage and reimbursement rates for mental health and substance use treatment

---

[48] Integrated Medical-Behavioral Care Compared With Usual Primary Care for Child and Adolescent Behavioral Health: A Meta-analysis—PubMed (*nih.gov*).

across insurance plans would support children's access to high quality and timely mental health care.

The *Paul Wellstone and Pete Domenici Mental Health Parity and Addiction Equity Act of 2008* (MHPAEA) aims to ensure that insurance coverage for mental health and addiction treatment is no more restrictive than insurance coverage for other medical care. This goal needs to be realized to tackle mental health access issues. AACAP appreciates the authorization of state parity assistance grants in the *2023 Consolidated Appropriations Act*, as well as the sunsetting of the non-government health plan opt-out of MHPAEA. AACAP respectfully asks Congress to fund the state parity assistance grants.

AACAP urges the Committee to support granting the Department of Labor authority to levy civil monetary penalties on ERISA plans found out of compliance with MHPAEA. In addition, the Committee should encourage more technical assistance to state regulators to ensure health plans are complying with MHPAEA.

AACAP also recommends that insurance regulators require health plans to use nationally recognized service intensity technological tools developed by professional medical organizations in making medical necessity determinations. With respect to children and adolescents, service intensity instruments such as the Child and Adolescent Service Intensity Instrument[49] and the Early Childhood Service Intensity Instrument,[50] are standardized assessment tools that provide determinations of the appropriate level of mental, behavioral, substance use, or other service needed by a particular child or adolescent and his or her family.

**5. Build a Behavioral Health Workforce That Represents Communities Being Served**

The current pediatric mental health care system does not sufficiently serve the needs of all of our communities. The COVID–19 pandemic amplified pre-existing mental health disparities in minoritized children and adolescents, including gaps in access to high quality mental health care. To truly bridge the gap in all children's access to mental health and substance use disorder care, we need a behavioral health workforce that understands and identifies with their patient's experiences, language, and background. We can do this by investing in the recruitment, training, and broader distribution of a more diverse and representative workforce through the workforce programs supported by HRSA and the Substance Abuse and Mental Health Services Administration (SAMHSA). Physicians who speak the same language as their patients and can identify with their patient's life experiences are best equipped to overcome stigma and gain the trust of their providers. AACAP encourage Congress to support programs that improve health equity by training a racially and ethnically diverse pediatric behavioral health workforce through scholarship, tuition assistance, and professional development opportunities.

We hope to work with the Committee to advance these priorities to improve existing programs and create new models to address the series crisis in children's mental health care.

---

[49] CASII (aacap.org).

[50] ECSII (aacap.org).

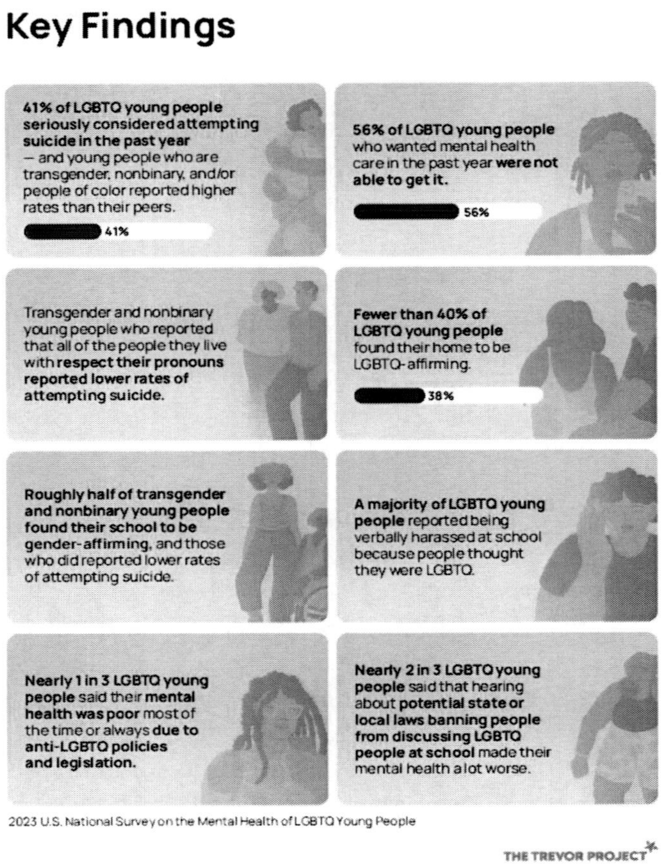


* * *

Congress of the United States,
Washington, DC,
May 9, 2023.

The Hon. Lawrence Tabak,
*Acting Director, National Institutes of Health,*
*9000 Rockville Pike,*
*Bethesda, MD.*

Dear Dr. Tabak:

We write today with grave concerns regarding a study funded by the National Institutes of Health (NIH) in which two young people tragically died by suicide.

The study, titled "Psychosocial Functioning in Transgender Youth after 2 Years of Hormones," evaluated the psychosocial effects of cross-sex hormones on "transgender and nonbinary youth."[51] In this study, researchers examined young people between the ages of 12

---

[51] *https://doi.org/10.1056/nejmoa2206297.*

and 20 who identify as transgender and were given cross-sex hormones. Of the 315 subjects, 240 were minors.[52]

Notably, the four clinics and some of the researchers who conducted this experiment are outspoken advocates for conducting gender transition interventions on children. In a video it later removed from its YouTube channel, Boston Children's Hospital, one of the clinics involved, went as far as to claim that children can know their gender identity "from the womb."[53] Johanna Olson, a co-author of this paper, told CNN in 2014, "We're definitely in the middle of a gender revolution and it's exciting."[54] This same researcher later received a Federal grant for a study in which she altered protocol to allow children as young as 8 years old to receive cross-sex hormones.[55]

During this study, two young people died by suicide and 11 reported suicidal ideation.[56] Rather than shutting the study down after such serious adverse events, the researchers published their paper, concluding that the study was a success because cross-sex hormones had altered subjects' physical appearance and improved psychosocial functioning.[57] However, the researchers admitted that they were not able to properly establish causality between the administration of cross-sex hormones and improved psychosocial functioning because their study lacked a control group.[58]

Despite glaring shortfalls, this government-funded research is already being used to further the fallacy that chemically transitioning children is safe and effective.[59] It is alarming that vulnerable young people died by suicide while participating in a taxpayer-funded study that will almost certainly inflict devastating physical harm on those who participated. Twenty-four participants in this study received cross-sex hormones after puberty suppression or "in early puberty" and are likely sterile as a result.[60] Further, participants are now at increased risk for cardiovascular disease, blood clotting, and a host of other complications.[61]

Research shows that gender dysphoria in minors often resolves as they progress through puberty—completely undermining the idea that children should have their bodies permanently altered to match their changing identities.[62] Despite overwhelming evidence that chemically transitioning children is not safe, the NIH plans to give more than $10.6 million to experiment on children and adolescents through 2026.[63] We are deeply concerned about your agency's use of taxpayer dollars to advance experiments on children who will be irreversibly harmed by radical gender ideology.

---

52 Ibid.

53 *https://first-heritage-foundation.s3.amazonaws.com/live-files/2023/01/230130-DNHNEJM-Response.pdf.*

54 *https://www.cnn.com/2014/06/27/living/transgender-youth-pride-march/index.html.*

55 *https://docs.wixstatic.com/ugd/3f4f51-a929d049f7fb46c7a72c4c86ba43869a.pdf.*

56 *https://doi.org/10.1056/nejmoa2206297.*

57 Ibid.

58 Ibid.

59 *https://www.nbcnews.com/nbc-out/out-health-and-wellness/hormone-therapy-improves-mental-health-trans gender-youths-new-study-fi-rcna66306*; *https://abcnews.go.com/Health/gender-affirming-care-trans-youth-improves-mental-health/story?id=96510337*; *https://www.washingtonpost.com/business/trans-teens-benefit-from-gender-affirming-care/2023/01/20/955f807c-98bd-11ed-a173-61e055ec24ef-story.html.*

60 *https://doi.org/10.2147/AHMT.S110859.*

61 *https://pubmed.ncbi.nlm.nih.gov/36238954/.*

62 *https://www.dovepress.com/getfile.php?fileID=40774.*

63 *http://gendersanity.org/documents/NIH-funding-from-progress-report-12-15-21.pdf.*

We request your full and complete response to each question below no later than June 9, 2023. Please provide a separate response to each question, rather than a narrative response.

1. Were the individuals who tragically died by suicide while participating in this study minors?
2. At which study sites did the two participants who died by suicide receive treatment? On what date did the researchers from these sites inform researchers at other participating sites that a study participant had died by suicide?
3. Please list the steps that were taken to halt and review the study after the first and second deaths and the dates on which these actions occurred.
   a. If a review took place, please provide the outcome of that review.
4. Were the other participants, as well as their parents, notified that two participants died by suicide? If so, who provided this notification?
5. Were participants and their parents given the opportunity to reconsider their consent and withdraw from this research in light of the suicides?
6. What steps were taken to provide ongoing monitoring of other children participating in the study to ensure they were not at risk for suicidal ideation?
7. Have study participants been evaluated to assess sterility or impaired fertility as a result of receiving cross-sex hormones? If so, how many participants are now sterile or suffering from impaired fertility?
8. Will a follow-up occur to evaluate the long-term physiological state of the subjects? If so, please provide an expected date for this follow-up.
9. The study notes that "6 participants withdrew from the study." Please provide the ages and Tanner stages at which these participants withdrew and their reasons for withdrawing.
10. Please provide all closed-meeting minutes from the NIH regarding the approval of funding for this study.
11. Please provide all closed-meeting minutes from the NIH, researcher Johanna L. Olson, the Children's Hospital of Los Angeles, and any relevant review boards regarding the approval of children as young as 8 years old to receive cross-sex hormones in the study titled "The Impact of Early Medical Treatment in Transgender Youth," redacting any information that personally identifies study participants if applicable.
12. Please provide all information that participants and their parents received specifically regarding sterility or risks of impaired fertility resulting from the use of cross-sex hormones, redacting any information that personally identifies study participants if applicable.
13. Does the NIH still commit to funding Project Number R01 HD082554 through 2026? If so, please provide justification for continuing this funding and detail what additional steps will be taken to prevent such serious adverse events going forward.
14. Please detail any ongoing or proposed NIH funding for studies involving transgender or nonbinary identified minors.

Thank you for your attention to this important matter.
Sincerely,

Josh Brecheen
*Member of Congress*

Ted Budd
*U.S. Senator*

Marco Rubio
*U.S. Senator*

Rand Paul, M.D.
*U.S. Senator*

James Lankford
*U.S. Senator*

Michael S. Lee
*U.S. Senator*

Mary Miller
*Member of Congress*

Randy Weber
*Member of Congress*

Lauren Boebert
*Member of Congress*

Chip Roy
*Member of Congress*

Andy Biggs
*Member of Congress*

Ronny L. Jackson, M.D.
*Member of Congress*

Eli Crane
*Member of Congress*

Jeff Duncan
*Member of Congress*

Michael Cloud
*Member of Congress*

## No One Knows How Many L.G.B.T.Q. Americans Die by Suicide

Death investigators in Utah are among a handful of groups trying to learn how many gay and transgender people die by suicide in the United States.

By Azeen Ghorayshi
June 1, 2023

Cory Russo, the chief death investigator in Utah, is used to asking strangers questions at the most excruciating moments of their lives. When she shows up at the scene of a suicide, a homicide or another type of unexpected death, her job is to interview the grievers about how the deceased had lived.

How old were they? What was their race? Did they have a job? Had they ever been hospitalized for psychiatric issues? How had they been feeling that morning?

Over the past couple of years, she has added new questions to the list: What was their sexual orientation? What was their gender identity?

Ms. Russo, who works in the Office of the Medical Examiner in Salt Lake City, is one of the relative few death investigators across the country who are routinely collecting such data, even though sexuality or gender identity can be relevant to the circumstances surrounding a person's death.

She recalled the recent suicide of a young man who died in the house of older adults. During her interviews, Ms. Russo learned that the man had been living with them for a year, ever since his family had kicked him out of their house because he was gay. He had struggled with emotional upheaval and addiction.

"It was heartbreaking to hear," said Ms. Russo, a lesbian who has lost loved ones to suicide. "In that case, it was very relevant to understand that piece."

Studies of L.G.B.T.Q. people show they have high rates of suicidal thoughts and suicide attempts, factors that greatly increase the risk of suicide.

But because most death investigators do not collect data on sexuality or gender identity, no one knows how many gay and transgender people die by suicide each year in the United States. The information vacuum makes it difficult to tailor suicide prevention efforts to meet the needs of the people most at risk, and to measure how well the programs work, researchers said.

The absence of data is especially unfortunate now, they said, when assumptions about suicide rates among L.G.B.T.Q. groups are frequently thrust into high-stakes political debates. Some L.G.B.T.Q. advocates have warned that bans on gender-affirming care for transgender minors will lead to more suicides, for example, while some Republican lawmakers have claimed that deaths by suicide are rare.

Utah, which like many mountain states has a high rate of suicide mortality, has been at the forefront of efforts to collect such data since 2017, when its State Legislature passed a law mandating detailed investigations of suicides.

The lawmakers were "frustrated with being asked to respond to the suicide crisis in our state with a blindfold on," said Michael Staley, a sociologist who was hired to lead the data-collection effort in the Utah medical examiner's office. "It's a five-alarm fire."

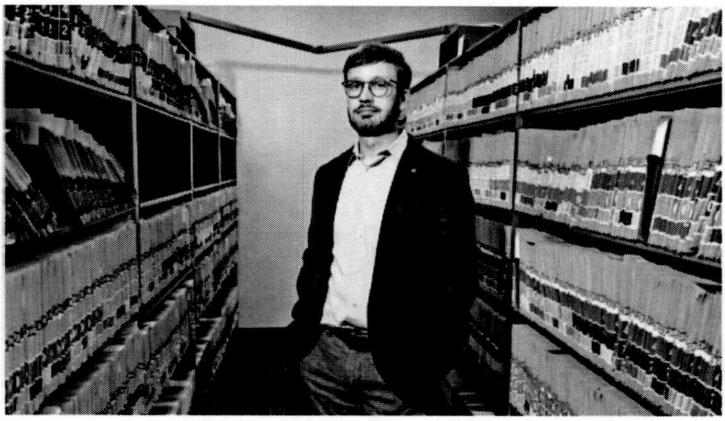

*Michael Staley, a sociologist who works in the Salt Lake City Medical Examiner's Office, conducts "psychological autopsies" in the months after a death by suicide or drug overdose. Kim Raff for The New York Times*

In the months after investigators like Ms. Russo show up at the scene of a death, Dr. Staley's team of six people conducts "psychological autopsies," contacting family members of everyone in the state who dies by suicide or drug overdose for detailed information about the lives of the deceased.

Such data — which includes information on sexual relationships and gender, as well as housing, mental health, drug problems and social media use — can be used to help understand the complex array of factors that contribute to people's decisions to end their lives, Dr. Staley said. He plans to release a report later this year describing interviews with the families of those who died by suicide in Utah over the last five years.

For children and adolescents who die by suicide, the team interviews not just parents and guardians, but also several close friends. In some cases, Dr. Staley recalled, friends knew about the deceased's struggles with sexuality, gender or drug use that the parents did not.

These conversations can be exceedingly difficult. John Blosnich, head of a research initiative called the L.G.B.T. Mortality Project at the University of Southern California, has done ride-alongs to observe and train death investigators on the importance of collecting data on gender and sexuality. His training also helps investigators navigate distress or stigma about the questions from the deceased's friends and relatives.

"They're talking with families who are in shock, who are infuriated, who at times are catatonic because of their loss," Dr. Blosnich said.

So far, Dr. Blosnich has trained investigators in Utah, Nevada, Colorado, New York and California, where a 2021 state law started a pilot program to collect data on sexual orientation and gender identity. In a recent study of 114 investigators in three states, Dr. Blosnich reported that only about 41 percent had directly asked about a deceased person's sexual orientation, and just 25 percent had asked about gender identity, before going through the training.

Medical examiners send reports of homicides and suicides to the Centers for Disease Control and Prevention, which maintains a database of violent deaths with extensive demographic, medical and social information, including toxicology tests, mental health diagnoses and even stories of financial and family hardships. But a study of more than 10,000 suicides among young adults reported to the C.D.C. database found that only 20 percent included information on the deceased's sexuality or gender identity.

Another agency in the health department, the Office of the National Coordinator for Health Information Technology, is trying to set new standards that would require any hospital that receives federal money to ask its patients about their sexuality and gender identity.

Death investigators are "limited by the fact that they can't ask the person the question," said John Auerbach, who worked on standardizing questions about sexuality and gender at the C.D.C. from 2021 to 2022. If doctors were routinely talking to their patients about sexuality and gender identity, that information could help answer other public health questions as well, such as those regarding the relative risk of cancer or diabetes in the L.G.B.T.Q. community, Dr. Auerbach said.

But that approach has its limits. Patients may not feel comfortable disclosing that information to their doctors. And those who don't interact with the health care system may be at especially high risk of suicide.

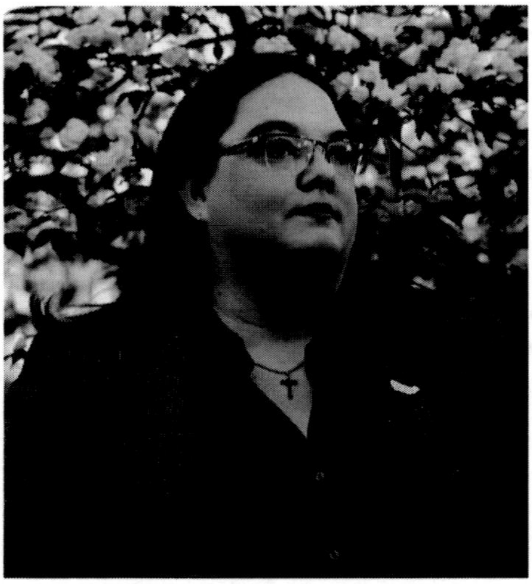

*"Lacking in data, it is all too easy to dismiss us," said Casey Pick, director of law and policy at the Trevor Project. Shuran Huang for The New York Times*

L.G.B.T.Q. advocates said that obtaining that data had become more urgent in the past couple of years, as states across the country have imposed restrictions on many aspects of life for gay and transgender people.

"Lacking in data, it is all too easy to dismiss us," said Casey Pick, director of law and policy at the Trevor Project, a nonprofit organization focused on suicide prevention among L.G.B.T.Q. young people that has lobbied at the state and federal levels to begin collecting that data.

"I have heard it too many times: Lawmakers and public witnesses in hearings suggest that the L.G.B.T.Q. community is crying wolf on suicide because we don't have this data to point to," Ms. Pick said.

It's also important to acknowledge the unknowns, Dr. Staley said. Although studies have reported a high rate of suicidal thoughts and suicide attempts among lesbian, gay and transgender people, that doesn't necessarily mean a high rate of suicides. He noted that although women have a higher rate of suicide attempts than men do, men have a much higher rate of dying by suicide, partly because they have more access to guns.

And Dr. Staley, who is gay, cautioned against political narratives that "normalize suicide as part of the queer experience."

"I would argue that if anything, this life experience sets us up to be resilient," he said. "Our fate is not sealed. Our story is not written."

If *you are having thoughts of suicide, call or text* 988 *to reach the* 988 *Suicide and Crisis Lifeline or go to SpeakingOfSuicide.com/resources for a list of additional resources.*

*Azeen Ghorayshi* covers the intersection of sex, gender and science for The Times.

A version of this article appears in print on , Section A, Page 16 of the New York edition with the headline: Utah Is Driving Push to Fill Void on L.G.B.T.Q. Suicide Data

[Whereupon, at 12:26 p.m., the hearing was adjourned.]

# Chapter 2

# Promoting Mental Health and Well-Being in Schools: An Action Guide for School and District Leaders*


## Centers for Disease Control and Prevention


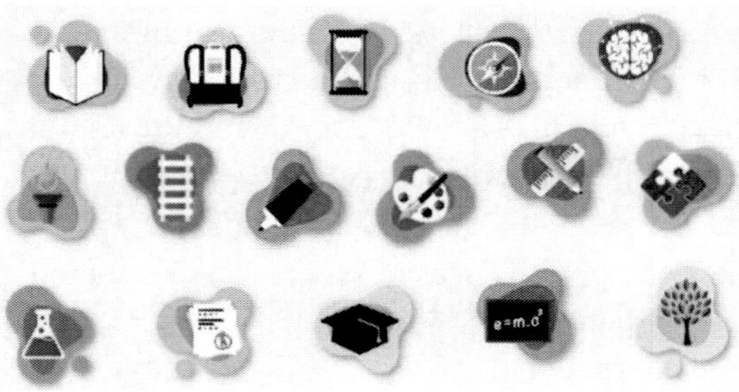


### Acronyms and Abbreviations

| | |
|---|---|
| ACT | acceptance and commitment therapy |
| CASEL | Collaborative for Academic, Social, and Emotional Learning |
| K–12 | kindergarten through 12th grade |
| LGBTQIA+ | lesbian, gay, bisexual, transgender, queer or questioning, intersex, asexual, and other sexual minority identities |
| MTSS | multitiered systems of support |


### Acknowledgments

This action guide is based on research about school-based comprehensive mental health promotion programming and intervention services that contribute to improved student mental health. It was developed by the Centers for Disease Control and Prevention's (CDC) Division


* This is an edited, reformatted and augmented version of Division of Adolescent and School Health (DASH), National Center for Chronic Disease Prevention and Health Promotion (NCCDPHP), Centers for Disease Control and Prevention (CDC), dated December 2023.


In: Understanding Youth Mental Health
Editor: Michael A. Post
ISBN: 979-8-89530-700-7

of Adolescent and School Health and RTI International (Contract # GS00F354CA, order number 75D30121F12871).

## Contributors

Autumn Barnes, RTI International
Adina Cooper, PhD, Centers for Disease Control and Prevention
Marci Hertz, MPH, Centers for Disease Control and Prevention
Kesha Hudson, PhD, RTI International
Sarah Lee, PhD, Centers for Disease Control and Prevention
Sandra Leonard, RN, FNP, DNP, Centers for Disease Control and Prevention
Bailee Peralto, RTI International
Mary Schauer, MSPH, Centers for Disease Control and Prevention
Katy Suellentrop, MPH, RTI International
Jorge Verlenden, PhD, Centers for Disease Control and Prevention
Natalie Wilkins, PhD, Centers for Disease Control and Prevention
Camara Wooten, RTI International
Anna Yaros, PhD, RTI International

## External Reviewers

We appreciate the hard work of the many individuals and organizations who shared their knowledge and helped inform our understanding of school-based strategies that support mental health. We extend our gratitude to the National Center for School Mental Health, in particular, Sharon Hoover and Nancy Lever, for helpful feedback, support, and encouragement for this resource. We especially thank focus group participants, who provided key evidence for this report, and the following 17 subject matter experts, who participated in the listening sessions and provided feedback during the development of the package:

Olga Acosta Price, The George Washington University
Riana Elyse Anderson, Stanford University
Melinda Baldwin, Substance Abuse and Mental Health Services Administration (SAMHSA)
Renee Bradley, U.S. Department of Education
Catherine Bradshaw, University of Virginia
Jessie Coffey, Nebraska Department of Education
Sean Darling-Hammond, University of California, Los Angeles
Dorothy Espelage, University of North Carolina at Chapel Hill
Jamie Freeny, Mental Health America of Greater Houston
Anne Gregory, Rutgers University
Jakatae Jessup, Shelby County Public Schools (Tennessee)
Brittani Kindle, Chicago Public Schools
Kurt Michael, The Jed Foundation (JED)
Jason Okonofua, University of California, Berkley

Farzana Tabitha Saleem, Stanford University
Joyce Sebian, Federal/National School Mental Health Partnership
Trish Shaffer, Washoe County Public School System (Nevada)

## Introduction

This action guide was designed for school administrators in kindergarten through 12th grade schools (K-12), including principals and leaders of school-based student support teams, to identify evidence-based strategies, approaches, and practices that can positively influence students' mental health.

Mental health is important for everyone, and includes our emotional, psychological, and social well-being [6, 7]. It affects how we think, feel, and act as well as how we handle stress, relate to others, and make choices. For children and youth, mental health also includes reaching developmental and emotional milestones, and learning skills to cope with challenges and function well at home, school, and in their communities. Mental health is a component of behavioral health, which also includes choices or actions that affect overall wellness.

Schools play an important role in promoting the behavioral and mental health and well-being of students through education, prevention, and early intervention efforts [8-10].

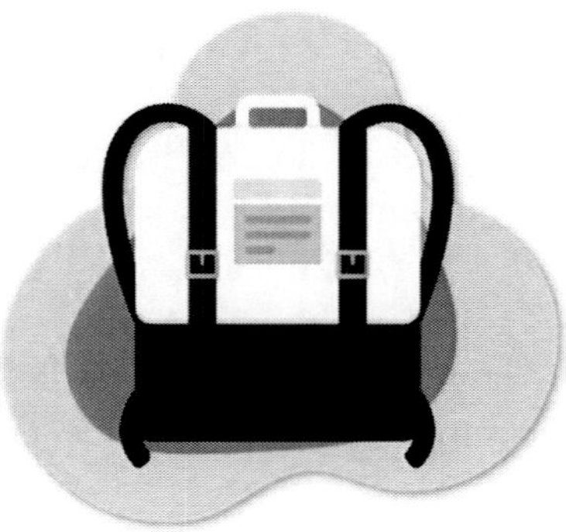

Schools have the potential to establish safe and supportive environments that connect students to caring adults and encourage positive peer relationships. Many schools also play an important role in linking students and families to behavioral and mental health services, especially for students living in low-income settings.

The work schools do to promote student mental health and well-being helps them achieve their educational mission. Poor mental health can interfere with students' ability to learn and can affect classroom behavior, school engagement, and peer relationships [11].

This action guide describes six in-school *strategies* that broadly promote and support mental health and well-being. The strategies in this guide are not intended to replace the individual behavioral and mental health treatment services that are critical to the children and young people who need them. For each strategy in this action guide, *approaches* or specific ways to use the strategy are provided, and a summary of evidence-based policies, programs, and practices that illustrate each approach is included. Tips to support successful and equitable implementation of strategies are described, with considerations for how to ensure all students are benefitting from mental health promotion and well-being efforts.

Recent data shows adolescent mental health is getting worse and has brought national attention to the important role schools play in promoting mental health and well-being.

- In 2021, 42% of high school students reported having felt so sad or hopeless for at least two weeks in the past year that they couldn't engage in their regular activities, and 22% of high school students reported that they had seriously considered suicide [1].
- The data for female students, lesbian, gay, bisexual, queer or questioning students, and students who have experienced racism in school shows they are even more likely to experience poor mental health [1, 3].
- When youth experience poor mental health, they are also at increased risk of school absence and dropout, risky sexual behavior, and illicit substance use [4, 5].

The strategies and approaches included in this action guide are based on findings from a review of peer-reviewed research literature. The equity and implementation considerations were informed by focus groups and listening sessions with students, parents/caregivers, school-based mental health staff (e.g., counselors, social workers, and psychologists), other school staff (e.g., teachers, nurses, administrators), and experts in school-based mental health and well-being from nongovernmental organizations (NGOs), universities, and federal, state, and local educational agencies. For more information on how the evidence in this action guide was assessed see Appendix A.

Strategies included in this action guide do not represent all school-based strategies that are important for promoting student well-being, such as school nutrition and physical activity programming. For more information about additional school-based health promotion strategies, see Healthy Schools | CDC.

**Table 1.** Action guide strategies and approaches

| Strategy | Approach |
|---|---|
| Increase Students' Mental Health Literacy | • Deliver classroom-based mental health education curricula<br>• Implement peer modeling programs |
| Promote Mindfulness | • Deliver classroom-based mindfulness education<br>• Dedicate time for students to independently practice mindfulness<br>• Offer small group mindfulness activities |
| Promote Social, Emotional, and Behavioral Learning | • Provide classroom instruction focused on building social skills and emotional development<br>• Offer targeted education focused on teaching social skills and emotional development |
| Enhance Connectedness Among Students, Staff, and Families | • Provide relationship-building programs |
| Provide Psychosocial Skills Training and Cognitive Behavioral Interventions | • Promote acceptance and commitment to change<br>• Provide cognitive behavioral interventions<br>• Engage students in coping skills training groups |
| Support School Staff Well-Being | • Offer mindfulness-based training programs<br>• Provide therapeutic resources |

There are also additional strategies, approaches, policies, programs, and practices that have an impact on bullying, externalizing behaviors (e.g., aggression, disruptive behavior, attention problems), substance use, chronic absenteeism, and physical health promotion, which are not included in this action guide. Additional evidence-based resources for addressing these other important aspects to student well-being may be found in the following program registries and resources:

- Blueprints for Healthy Youth Development
- The California Evidence-Based Clearinghouse for Child Welfare
- CDC Division of Violence Prevention's Resources for Action
- Collaborative for Academic, Social, and Emotional Learning (CASEL)
- Programs That Work, from the Promising Practices Network on Children, Families and Communities
- What Works Clearinghouse

## Things to Keep in Mind When Implementing Strategies to Promote Mental Health and Well-Being in Schools

When implementing strategies related to school-based promotion of mental health and well-being, it is important to consider existing educational practices that may guide decision-making in the school district. It is also important to consider the school and community context, including availability of resources, needs of students, and capacity of staff. This section outlines several of the things to keep in mind when planning and implementing the school-based mental health and well-being approaches outlined in this action guide.

### *Multitiered Systems of Support*

Multitiered systems of support (MTSS) is a framework used by many schools and districts to coordinate systems and services to address students' academic, behavioral, mental health, and social and emotional needs. The MTSS framework uses a public health approach to promote student well-being by identifying three "Tiers" of prevention to support the needs of the entire school population.

- *Tier 1* programs, practices, and policies are often called "universal" or "primary" prevention programs. These are typically implemented schoolwide and meant to benefit the entire student body. Programs implemented by classroom teachers are frequently Tier 1 (universal, primary prevention).
- *Tier 2* programs are described as "targeted" or "secondary" prevention programs. These programs are typically appropriate for students who might benefit from additional supports, skill development, or early intervention to address concerns. Tier 2 (targeted, secondary prevention) programs are often delivered in a small group setting by professionals with specialized training such as school counselors or other school behavioral or mental health professionals.
- *Tier 3* programs are generally individualized and are often described as "indicated" or "tertiary" prevention programs. Tier 3 programs might involve frequent sessions of

longer duration, and often address specific and sometimes more severe behavioral and mental health concerns that a student may be experiencing. Student involvement in Tier 3 programs typically requires parental consent and student assent and is sometimes described in individualized education programs (IEPs). Tier 3 programs are generally provided by certified or licensed professionals qualified to conduct the specific program or intervention.

The strategies in this action guide can align with schools' existing MTSS to enhance the student support efforts schools have already established.

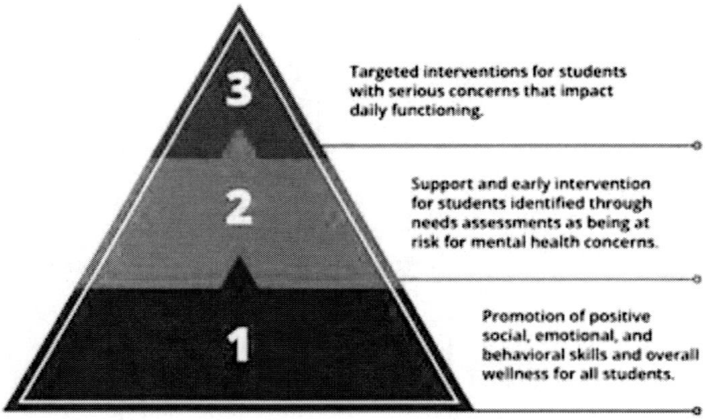


Note: A variety of MTSS models are available to schools. This resource uses the MTSS to describe the general framework, not a specific model.

**Figure 1.** Multitiered Systems of Support.

### *Using Comprehensive Assessment Tools*

Using data to understand and improve both students' and adults' competencies, behaviors, performance, and accountability [12] is critical for assessing need, understanding how students and staff are implementing new programs, policies, and practices, and assessing what effect these practices are having on mental health and well-being. Using student data to make decisions about supports that students need is a central component of MTSS, and school-based screening of students to learn about their social, emotional, behavioral, and mental health concerns is a way to better understand student needs. Screening can also help with linking students to needed services.

- *Social skills and emotional development assessment tools,* for example, might be used to help schools understand their climate and opportunities for improving curricula over time.
  These assessments can also be helpful to teachers as they support skill development in students and tailor curricula to classroom needs [13].
- *Other screening tools* specifically ask about students' mental health needs. Before implementing screening initiatives in a school or district, it is important to decide how students' answers will be used to benefit them. Ethical responsibilities include protecting students' privacy and linking them to mental health supports. For example, if screening uncovers a high need for mental health treatment (which falls into

"tertiary" or Tier 3 services), administrators should determine if those services are available through the school or in the local community. Professional organizations such as the National Association of School Psychologists offer guidance for schools as they consider the adoption of screening in schools. For a more detailed discussion of mental health screening, see the following resources:

- School Mental Health Quality Guide—Screening: https://www.schoolmentalhealth.org/media/som/microsites/ncsmh/documents/quality-guides/Screening.pdf
- The School Counselor and Universal Screening: https://www.schoolcounselor.org/Standards-Positions/Position-Statements/ASCA-Position-Statements/The-School-Counselor-and-Universal-Screening
- Guidance for Trauma Screening in Schools: https://www.ksdetasn.org/resources/1270
- Best Practices in Universal Screening: https://smhcollaborative.org/wp-content/uploads/2019/11/universalscreening.pdf

### *Access to Mental Health Promotion and Treatment*

Students may have difficulty accessing mental health services in their communities because of barriers such as provider shortages, insufficient or no insurance, and transportation. Schools can help their students overcome these barriers by doing the following:

- *Helping link students and families to providers* offering mental health services via telehealth. This is one way schools can help address students' transportation challenges, saving time and costs [14]. In rural communities, telehealth can bridge long distances between providers and those who need services. Schools can also provide access to reliable broadband internet that can support video conferencing for telehealth.
- *Using multiple funding streams and different payment structures* for Tier 3 mental health services based in schools.
- *Embedding mental health supports in school-based health centers (SBHCs)*—SBHCs can partner with community providers to help students meet their mental health needs without having to travel to an additional location [15].

### *Role of All School Staff in Supporting Student Well-Being and Mental Health*

School administrators, teachers, school nurses, and school-based mental health staff all play important roles in supporting the mental health and well-being of students. Implementing new programs or making changes to existing programs requires coordination and collaboration across the school. Consider the responsibilities of staff and how they will work together and with families and other community partners to support implementation. Some key things that can help with staff coordination and collaboration include the following:

- *School-based leaders or champions* who can communicate the purpose of a new mental health and well-being program or practice and may lead plans to integrate it into existing school programs (including academic programming).
- *Consistent administrator buy-in and support* at the district and state level which can send a message of support to teachers and other staff [16].

- *Adequate school-based mental health staffing* (i.e., no more than 500 students per one psychologist; 250 students per one counselor) which is important to consider when selecting new mental health and well-being programs and making changes to established practices and policies [17].
- *Effective and sustained training for staff* aligned with requirements of the programs they will be asked to implement. For example, the Collaborative for Academic, Social, and Emotional Learning (CASEL's) *School Guide* implementation model for supporting social and emotional learning uses leadership teams and ongoing coaching to support implementation [18, 19]. To address training needs and expand the capacity of school personnel, schools might partner with community-based organizations and providers as well as collaborate with local universities and colleges to increase access to resources and training opportunities [20].
- *Partnerships with families, community organizations, and behavioral health providers* which can help ensure mental health and well-being activities meet the most pressing needs of the school community and support program effectiveness and sustainability.
- *Awareness of local, state, and federal policies* which often inform on-the-ground implementation of any program or practice related to mental health and well-being among students.

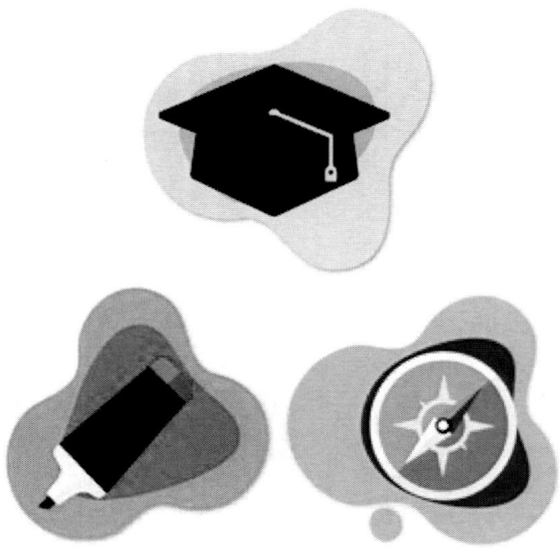

***Diverse Needs of Students***

To effectively and equitably promote mental health and well-being for all students, schools can do the following:

- *Match programs to students' developmental needs.* Many programs are designed for elementary, middle, or high schools and adapted for or tested in other grade ranges. Consider the grades identified by the developer of a program when determining whether it is appropriate to implement.
- *Incorporate culturally and linguistically responsive information* in mental health programming, including input from communities [21].

- *Educate staff on the social, historical, and environmental inequalities* that certain student groups face. For example, inequalities based on race, ethnicity, gender and/or sexual identity [12].
- Support and welcome students, especially those who are at higher risk for *marginalization,* such as students who recently immigrated to the United States, who are living with a disability, or who identify as lesbian, gay, bisexual, transgender, queer or questioning, intersex, or asexual (LGBTQIA+). This can include acknowledging and promoting cultural events, providing multilingual programming, and supporting the creation of student clubs that promote inclusion, such as genders and sexualities alliances (GSAs) [21, 22].
- *Support school attendance by addressing factors that can contribute to absenteeism,* including mental health concerns, exclusionary discipline practices (e.g., suspension), and social or economic factors [23]. Understanding how mental health knowledge and awareness, previous experiences with stigmatizing or discriminatory situations, and cultural norms can contribute to attitudes about mental health and help seeking. Promoting inclusive, nondiscriminatory practices that reduce judgment, blame, stereotypes, and prejudice and that raise awareness of mental health and school-based mental health promotion activities may foster engagement, bolster connections, and reduce barriers to help seeking [17].
- *Review school practices and policies to identify whether they might disadvantage specific groups of students.* For example, consider how a dress code could negatively affect student mental well-being for some students more than others. Items often called out in a dress code, such as hats or hoodies, may have different meaning or value that should be explored with students before the items are banned. Anti-bullying and harassment policies can also better serve the diverse needs of students when sexual orientation, gender identity, and gender expression are specifically listed as protected characteristics in addition to race, ethnicity, national origin, sex, disability, and religion [24].

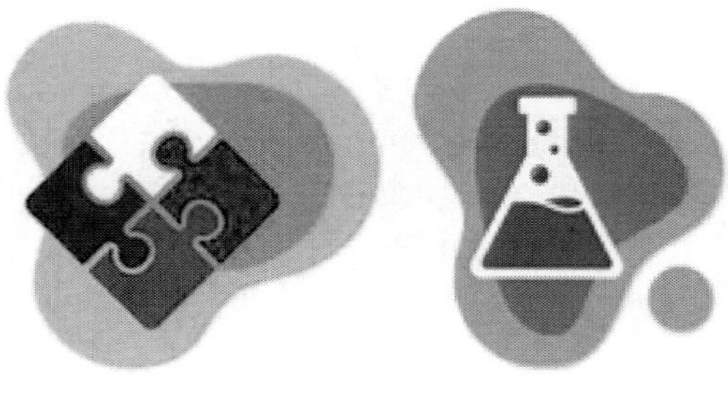

## Strategies for Promoting Mental Health in Schools

This section includes six evidence-based *strategies* for promoting mental health and well-being in schools. For each strategy, specific *approaches* that schools can implement are described, and the evidence of their impact on mental health and well-being is summarized. A list of *example programs* and links to additional resources, considerations for *focusing on equity,* and additional tips for *implementing the approaches* in real-world settings are also provided.

Some general principles around *centering equity* apply across all six strategies. These principles are designed to help schools think about how approaches can result in equitable outcomes for all types of students. Across strategies and approaches, consider the following:

- *Use data* to understand your students and staff. Be aware of the unique groups of students and staff that make up your school—diverse races; ethnicities; gender identities; sexual orientations, mental and physical abilities; income levels; urban, suburban, and rural neighborhoods; religions; household structures; and education levels.
- *Adapt* programs and practices to address the different backgrounds of students in school settings. For example, school-based mental health staff could consider how mental health challenges such as stress might manifest differently for students based on culture or context.
- *Recruit staff* who reflect the unique backgrounds of the students in your school community.

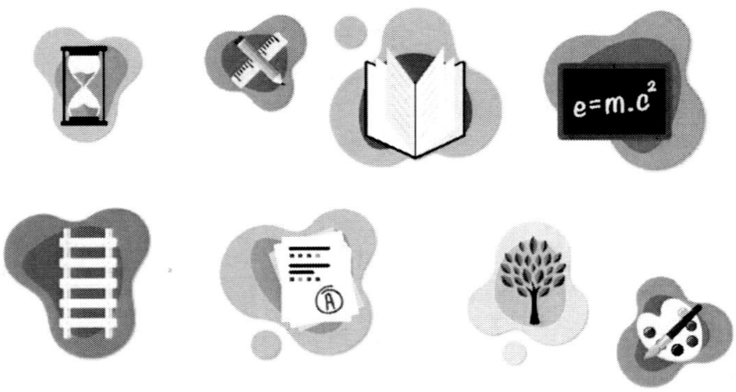


## 1. Increase Students' Mental Health Literacy

Mental health literacy includes having knowledge and understanding of mental health as well as skills that support help-seeking (i.e., reaching out for mental health support when needed). Increasing students' mental health literacy promotes mental health and well-being by helping identify mental health concerns and facilitate access to timely and effective intervention.

Mental health literacy includes increasing knowledge in the following areas: [25, 26]

- How to develop and maintain positive mental health.
- How to reduce stigma around expressing distress or having a mental illness.
- How to effectively engage in help-seeking behaviors (e.g., when and where to obtain help).
- How to identify specific mental health disorders and treatment options.

### *What Can Schools Do?*

Schools can increase students' mental health literacy by delivering classroom-based mental health education curricula and implementing peer-led modeling programs.

## Deliver Classroom-Based Mental Health Education Curricula

*Description of Approach*

Classroom-based mental health education curricula offer a way to increase mental health literacy in schools. Curricula often include interactive, skill-based lessons that incorporate personal testimony from young adults about their mental health journeys, in-class group activities, and homework assignments. Mental health curricula can be delivered in core classes or integrated into comprehensive school health education curricula. Mental health curricula can increase mental health literacy in schools by doing the following:

- Providing information about causes and symptoms of mental illnesses.
- Exploring stigma as it applies to mental illness and explaining how to reduce stigma.
- Emphasizing that mental illnesses are treatable and addressing barriers to seeking treatment.
- Encouraging students to talk with trusted adults and seek treatment.

*Evidence Summary*

Classroom-based mental health education curricula are associated with the following student mental health outcomes:

↑ Mental health knowledge and attitudes [27-32]
↓ Stigma related to mental health [30, 32]
↑ Help-seeking behaviors (i.e., reaching out for mental health support) [29, 31, 32]

*Evidence Description*

Studies have shown that classroom-based mental health education curricula lead to improvements in knowledge, attitudes, and help-seeking behaviors and reductions in stigma among students [27-32]. Middle school and high school students who participated in mental health curricula reported the following:

- Less-negative emotional responses toward people who have a mental illness32 and were more likely to interact with people, including their peers, who have a mental illness [30, 32].
- Improvements in knowledge [27-32] and attitudes toward mental illness that lasted over time [27, 28, 30, 32].

- More help-seeking behaviors (e.g., reaching out for mental health support) and greater optimism about treatment effectiveness [31].
- Fewer worries about sharing personal information with a counselor [32].

One study reported that middle school students who had high levels of mental health symptoms were more likely to seek treatment over the course of the next two years if they had been taught from a mental health curriculum [31].

Learn more about the classroom-based mental health education programs [30, 31] that we reviewed:

- NAMI Ending the Silence (Tier 1).
- Adolescent Depression Awareness Program (Tier 1).
- A School-Based Intervention for Mental Illness Stigma (Tier 1) [30].

## Implement Peer-Led Modeling Programs

*Description of Approach*

Peer-led modeling programs train adolescent peer leaders to model positive attitudes, skills, and behaviors to promote change among students. Programs focused on mental health and well-being teach peer leaders how to promote the development of healthy coping strategies for themselves and their peers. Peer leaders learn about the importance of engaging in healthy activities, having friends who engage in behaviors that benefit or help others, accessing medical and mental health resources, and engaging trusted adults. Through interactive presentations, peer leaders emphasize the importance of identifying resources and strategies for coping with adversity and they share personal narratives about their own experiences. They might also share the names of adults whom they engaged with when experiencing distress and encourage students to identify adults they would trust if they were concerned about the well-being of themselves or a friend [33].

*Evidence Summary*

Peer-led modeling programs are associated with the following student mental health outcomes:

↑ Coping attitudes [33]
↑ Acceptability of seeking help [33]
↑ Perception of adult support [33]

*Evidence Description*

Peer modeling of healthy coping strategies improved high school students' coping attitudes and perceptions of help-seeking behaviors. Improvements were observed in the following things for students:

- Attitudes toward overcoming barriers to engage adults for suicidal youth.
- Attitudes toward seeking help from adults.

- Perceptions about the availability of adult help and peer and family support for seeking help.
- Naming trusted adults.

Importantly, students who reported experiencing suicidal ideation in the past 12 months benefited the most from peer-led presentations that modeled healthy and effective coping behaviors [33].

Learn more about the peer-led modeling program that we reviewed:

- Sources of Strength (Tier 1).

### *Focus on Equity*

*Consider ways to expand the availability of mental health services through partnerships with local, state, and regional organizations as well as community-based groups.* For example, in schools with a large population of Spanish-speaking students, schools can identify clinicians and community organizations who offer supports and services in Spanish. It is also helpful to identify organizations that support students with LGBTQ+identities as well as organizations experienced with supporting the needs of diverse student populations and with providers who reflect the demographics of the students in the school.

*Consider parent, caregiver, and community perceptions of mental health* and how these might affect students' ability and decisions to seek mental health support. If communicating with parents and caregivers, be mindful of the language being used and offer information in a variety of formats. Some parents and caregivers might be comfortable reading materials, whereas others would prefer a conversation with school staff. Consider integrating information about mental health services into other information provided by the school to connect mental health and academics and to normalize information about mental health.

### *Implementation Tips*

Administration-level support is critical for implementing programs, practices, and policies to address mental health literacy. To better support implementation of approaches that increase students' mental health literacy, school administrators can take these actions:

- Identify ways to convey to teachers and staff that administrators understand and support the need for programs, practices, and policies to increase mental health literacy.
- Create consistent guidelines and practices to support any type of mental health training, including mental health literacy training. For example, make sure that school staff know how to support students in distress, how to get help when a student has an immediate need for support, and how to communicate concerns to families.

Use CDC's Health Education Analysis Tool (HECAT) to examine health education curricula, compare strengths and weaknesses of multiple curricula, and develop a scope and sequence for health education that supports mental, emotional, and behavioral health across grade levels. It may also be valuable to consider integrating mental health content into state or district health education standards. The District of Columbia's Health Education Standards provide an example of how this can be accomplished. The National Institute of Mental Health's Resources for Students and Educators also offer a variety of learning resources for students and teachers about mental health and the brain.

> "I feel like the teachers at my school are generally good and aim to promote student well-being, but they don't have the support of the administration behind them, so it can be hard for them to take any real action."
> – Student

## 2. Promote Mindfulness

Mindfulness is a skill that involves intentionally bringing one's attention to the present moment by noticing thoughts and sensations in a nonjudgmental and nonreactive way. Practicing mindfulness can help students manage stress in their everyday lives and regulate their emotions and behaviors.

***What Can Schools Do?***
Schools can promote mindfulness among all students by providing mindfulness education in the classroom and dedicating daily time for independent mindfulness practices. Small-group mindfulness interventions can be provided to students who are experiencing elevated mental health symptoms.

### Deliver Classroom-Based Mindfulness Education

*Description of Approach*
Classroom-based mindfulness education supports students' awareness of the mind-body connection through the following: [34-37]

- Instruction about stress, including the effects of stress on the body and ways to manage stress, develop self-regulation, and build healthy relationships;
- Experiential practice of mindful breathing, meditation, and mindful movement, such as yoga; and
- Group discussion about how to practice mindfulness in everyday situations.

Mindfulness education may take the form of longer lessons in health or wellness education classes [35] or brief sessions that can be incorporated into transitions that occur throughout the school day, such as during morning meetings or advisory periods, after recess, or before the start of a class lesson [34].

*Evidence Summary*
Classroom-based mindfulness education has been associated with the following:

↓ Anxiety [34, 35]
↓ Depressive symptoms [36]
↓ Negative coping behaviors [36]
↑ Positive coping behaviors [37]

*Evidence Description*
Research shows that practicing mindfulness has positive impacts on students' mental health and well-being, including the following:

- Lower ratings of anxiety (by teachers) among elementary-aged girls [34] and fewer self-reported symptoms of anxiety among high school students [35].
- Lower levels of self-reported depressive symptoms and negative coping behaviors (e.g., disengagement, denial, substance abuse, self-blame) among middle school students [36].
- Greater engagement in positive coping behaviors (such as problem-solving, emotion regulation and expression, positive thinking, cognitive restructuring, and acceptance) among middle school students [37].

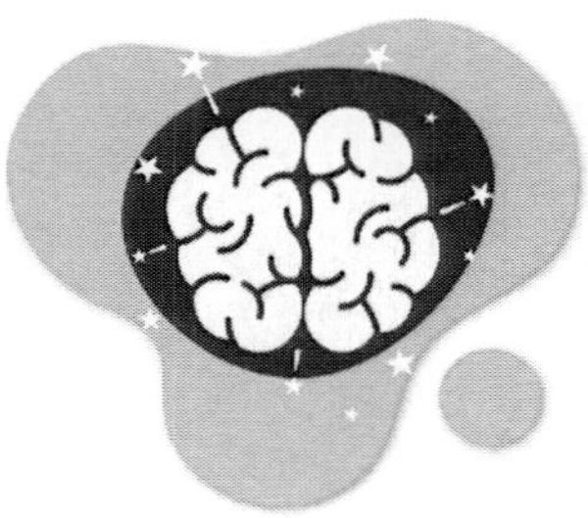

Learn more about the classroom-based mindfulness education programs that we reviewed: [35, 36]

- Master Mind (Tier 1).
- Transformative Life Skills (Tier 1).
- MindUp (Tier 1).

**Dedicate Time for Students to Independently Practice Mindfulness**

*Description of Approach*
Making time for students to independently practice mindfulness daily may also support students' mental health and well-being. Providing students with a few minutes to meditate each day is sufficient for establishing a consistent mindfulness practice.

*Evidence Summary*
Allowing students to independently practice mindfulness has been associated with the following effects:

↓ Anxiety [38]
↑ Resilience [38]

*Evidence Description*
In one study, after learning how to practice meditation, high school students were offered 15 minutes at the beginning and end of the school day to meditate [38]. At the end of the school year, students who were given the opportunity to meditate in the morning and afternoon each school day reported lower anxiety and increased resilience.

**Offer Small Group Mindfulness Activities**

*Description of Approach*
Small groups of students, often led by counselors, learn about and practice mindfulness activities. These interventions aim to promote emotional regulation skills among students experiencing Tier 2 or Tier 3 risk for mental health symptoms. Students learn to understand their thoughts and feelings and develop and practice skills to help them reflect on and manage their emotions in a positive way.

*Evidence Summary*
Students who participated in small-group mindfulness interventions experienced the following changes in self-reported symptoms: [39-41]

↓ Stress [39]
↓ Internalizing behaviors (e.g., feelings of anxiety, withdrawal, and depressive symptoms) [39]
↓ Depressive symptoms [40]

*Evidence Description*
Middle and high school students experiencing mild to moderate depression benefit from small-group mindfulness interventions. Among Latine/Latinx and Asian American middle and high school students experiencing mild to moderate depression, students who participated in small-group mindfulness interventions experienced greater reductions in self-reported stress and internalizing behaviors, including feelings of anxiety, withdrawal, and depressive symptoms compared to students who received no treatment or Interpersonal Therapy - Adolescent Skills Training [39-41]. In one study, researchers reported that the intervention was most beneficial for students who experienced more severe mental health symptoms [39].

Learn more about the small-group mindfulness intervention that we reviewed:

- Learning to BREATHE (Tier 2)

### *Focus on Equity*

**Explore Mindfulness Practice as a Way to Advance Equity**

Mindfulness approaches can help teachers and students develop a more open and inclusive classroom environment [42]. Because mindfulness encourages nonjudgmental observation, it can help individuals in the school reflect on and manage feelings of stress that can result from a disconnect between their identities and that of others in their school or classroom. It can also help teachers reflect on their assumptions and behaviors in ways that are helpful for identifying and reducing bias [43].

**Incorporate Student Voice in the Development of Mindfulness Activities**

Such as by asking students what visualization strategies they like best. Offer students the opportunity to lead mindfulness exercises throughout the school year [42]. It is important to remember that developing a mindfulness practice can help students learn how to cope with stress, but it does not address the factors that cause distress or disruption in students' lives.

Some students may experience events that lead to persistent or highly traumatic distress that may also require additional intervention.

### *Implementation Tips*

To better support the implementation of mindfulness strategies, school administrators can consider doing the following:

- Training teachers and staff throughout the school on the importance of mindfulness, as well as strategies for incorporating it throughout the day.
- Offering mindfulness opportunities for staff and teachers. For example, administrators could give a mindfulness minute for staff at the beginning of each day, or offer mindfulness projects at the district level. These projects could include student-led opportunities to advance mindfulness practice in their schools (e.g., a gratitude wall or wellness conference).

It is important to remember that mindfulness interventions may not be useful for everyone. Teachers, staff, and students should be invited, but not pressured, to incorporate mindfulness strategies into their classrooms or develop an independent mindfulness practice.

## 3. Promote Social, Emotional, and Behavioral Learning

School-based programs can promote social skills and emotional development by focusing on the following: self-management, responsible decisionmaking, relationship skills, social awareness, and self-awareness [44]. These programs have been linked to school climate and positive interpersonal relationships between peers and with teachers. They have also been found to improve specific mental health outcomes such as depressive symptoms and anxiety [45, 46]. Nationally, surveys have observed that there is strong support among school administrators for programs that improve students' social skills and emotional development, as they recognize its significant impact on students' academic performance and mental health outcomes, and its value for promoting positive school climates [12].

### *What Can Schools Do?*

K–12 schools can provide classroom-based programming that includes instruction on social skills and self-regulation for all students. For students at elevated risk of negative mental health outcomes, small-group support might benefit students by providing an opportunity to enhance and practice skills related to social, emotional, and behavioral learning.

### Provide Classroom Instruction Focused on Building Social Skills and Emotional Development

*Description of Approach*

Classroom instruction focused on building social skills and emotional development might cover such topics as the following:

- Recognizing thoughts.
- Understanding feelings.
- Decision-making and problem-solving.
- Healthy relationships.

Programs focused on building social skills and emotional development vary. For example, some programs consist of a single, computer-based session, whereas others include several lessons delivered by a guidance counselor outdoors [47], or a scripted curriculum delivered by classroom teachers twice a week throughout the school year [47-49].

*Evidence Summary*

Programs implemented for all students in either a grade or a classroom (i.e., universal social skill and emotional development programs) were found to have the following effects:

↓ Depressive symptoms [49]
↓ Internalizing behaviors (e.g., feelings of anxiety, withdrawal, and depressive symptoms) [48, 50, 51]
↓ Anxiety [47, 48]
↑ Mental health and well-being [52]
↑ Resilience [53]

*Evidence Description*

Researchers have explored the impact of single-session interventions focused on one skill area, such as growth mindset, as well as longer programs addressing multiple skill areas [47, 51, 53]. For example, a single-session intervention delivered in a rural school with high school students was found to reduce depressive symptoms [49]. A 12 session program implemented in middle schools increased resilience among students. Programs implemented for all students in either a grade or a classroom (i.e., universal social skills and emotional development programs) were found to reduce depressive symptoms, internalizing behaviors, and anxiety and to increase resilience and mental health and well-being among students.

Learn more about the classroom-based skill building programs that we reviewed:

- The PATHs program (Tier 1).
- Project Growing Minds (Tier 1).
- Second Step (Tier 1).
- Speaking to the Potential, Ability, & Resilience Inside Every Kid (SPARK; Tier 1).
- Strong Kids (Tier 1).

**Offer Targeted Education Focused on Teaching Social Skills and Emotional Development**

*Description of Approach*

Targeted education that focuses on social skills and emotional development provides students with small-group or individualized instruction on skills and is tailored to their identified needs. Specific strategies to identify students who might benefit from more specific, small-group instruction might vary depending on age level and rely on teachers' observations along with self-reported feelings and experiences.

*Evidence Summary*

Research has found that targeted education focused on social skills and emotional development had the following effects:

↓ Depressive symptoms [54]
↓ Internalizing behaviors (e.g., feelings of anxiety, withdrawal, and depressive symptoms) [55]
↓ Anxiety [54]

*Evidence Description*

Targeted approaches designed specifically for students at risk for emotional and behavioral disorders were linked to more positive mental health outcomes for these students. When offered as a supplement to universal instruction on social skills and emotional development and integrated into academic subjects, targeted education reduced internalizing behaviors (e.g., feelings of anxiety, withdrawal, and depressive symptoms) among elementary school students

[55]. Similarly, a program focused on processing and responding to interpersonal trauma in relationships decreased anxiety and depression among students [54].

Learn more about the targeted interventions that we reviewed:

- SEL Foundations Curriculum (Tier 2).
- Forgiveness within the Family (Tier 2).

### *Focus on Equity*

*Consider using transformative social and emotional learning to advance equity.* Although promoting equity is not an explicit component of all social, emotional, and behavioral learning, these interventions do offer opportunities to address issues related to equity (e.g., skills for interpersonal relationships) [56]. Transformative social and emotional learning focuses specifically on advancing equity among all students. It incorporates exploration of individual and contextual factors that contribute to inequity (e.g., how issues of race, class, and culture influence society) and focuses on identity, agency, belonging, collaborative problem-solving, and curiosity. Transformative social and emotional learning intentionally addresses structural inequities that students experience in their schools and communities [57]. For example, a transformative social and emotional learning program could provide an opportunity for youth to identify inequities in their communities and develop solutions.

*Consider using screening tools to support students, but examine the tools for potential bias and misuse.* Screening is discussed more specifically in the "Screening to Support MTSS Implementation" section, but it is important to note that in addition to school-based screening for social, emotional, behavioral, and mental health concerns, there are also assessment tools that can be used to identify areas of focus for social and emotional programming. Such screening is a strategy that some schools and districts have used to provide universal and targeted programming for students. However, these tools should be used with care. From an equity perspective, it is critical to look for biases that might be present in screening tools and ask whether these biases influence expectations for different students. It is also important to create a clear plan for using the data, ensure that schools can follow up as needed based on the screening responses, and ensure that the follow-up plan is shared with staff.

### *Implementation Tips*

School administrators can support the implementation of social, emotional, and behavioral learning in schools by doing the following:

- Integrating social skill and emotional development competencies into strategic planning and budgeting, human resources, professional development, and operations, in addition to standard academic programming and initiatives [12]. This includes ensuring that teachers have tools for integrating practices or lessons into their classroom and receive ongoing support during implementation. For example, there are tools to support integration into existing lesson plans and a coaching toolkit that can support implementation efforts.
- Integrating programs at the district level. Outcomes at the district level (e.g., positive climate; buy-in for and commitment to social, emotional, and behavioral learning; clear roles and responsibilities) directly relate to student outcomes (e.g., increased

academic performance, increased mental health wellness, fewer disciplinary actions) [12].

- Monitoring implementation and assessing opportunities for improvement. This could include gathering teacher feedback on the specific curriculum or strategies that the school is using, observing practices and lessons in the classroom, and reviewing data that schools are already collecting, e.g., school climate data [12]. Monitoring and assessment can support continuous quality improvement efforts in implementation.
- Incorporating social and emotional skills-based instruction into academic subjects. For example, one program was implemented as part of a literacy course [55]. Implementation can also take place outside of the classroom. Additional benefits have been observed when social, emotional, and behavioral learning is implemented in an outdoor, natural space [47].
- Integrating programs throughout the school setting. This has been used as a strategy for supporting students and schools as they transition back to in-person instruction after COVID-19-related school building closures. Teachers noted that incorporating social skill and emotional development strategies into classrooms can help support students, but that teachers need appropriate implementation support and professional development to be certain they are implementing strategies with fidelity and in a way that responds to the different needs in their classrooms.

> "They [the school staff] have a system where the teachers almost incorporate it [mental health] in the curriculum. One of my anatomy classes would have us do a self-awareness journal, where we would talk about where we are in the moment.... It was a nice break to have. They would give us resources about ways to handle stress and find people to talk to as well.... That was a new thing they started post-COVID because they realized that it was becoming more of an issue and something that was never talked about previously."
>
> – Student

## 4. Enhance Connectedness among Students, Staff, and Families

School connectedness refers to each student's belief that adults and peers in school care about their learning and about them as individuals. This feeling includes a sense of being cared for, being supported, and belonging at school [58]. Some students, including students of color, students living with disabilities, and students who identify as LGBTQIA+, are at increased risk for experiencing feelings of social isolation or alienation at school [59]. School connectedness can protect and promote students' mental health and well-being.

### *What Can Schools Do?*

Schools can enhance students' feeling of connection to their peers, teachers, and the school community through relationship-building interventions.

## Provide Relationship-Building Programs

### Description of Approach

Relationship-building interventions aim to strengthen connections between students, families, and school communities. These interventions promote positive family–school relationships through frequent two-way communication between parents or caregivers and school staff (e.g., teachers, guidance counselors). The interventions accomplish this by offering (1) group sessions for teachers that focus on how to build strong student-teacher relations and how to collaborate with parents and (2) group or individual sessions for parents that focus on the importance of parental involvement in school and ways to develop collaborative relationships with teachers. Additional supports may include classroom activities to strengthen peer relationships or schoolwide events that raise awareness about various student experiences and needs. Relationship-building interventions can be tailored to meet the unique needs of different student populations.

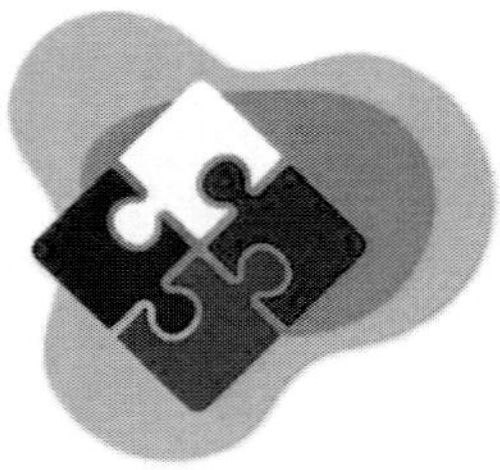

*Evidence Summary*

Relationship-building interventions have been associated with the following:

↓ Internalizing behaviors (e.g., feelings of anxiety, withdrawal, and depressive symptoms) [60, 61].

*Evidence Description*

Research conducted in elementary schools suggests that relationship-building interventions that are tailored to address the unique experiences and challenges facing military-connected children [61] and children with or at risk for disruptive behavior problems [60] lead to reductions in teacher- and parent-reported internalizing behaviors.

Learn about the school connectedness programs that we reviewed:

- Staying Strong with Schools (Tier 1).
- Starting Strong (Tier 3).

### *Focus on Equity*

Approaches to build connection within schools should intentionally include and center students who are at a disproportionate risk for being marginalized and disconnected in school. Girls, youth who report experiencing racism, youth from racial and ethnic minority groups, and youth who identify as LGBTQIA+ often feel less connected at school and experience poor mental health [3, 62].

While racial/ethnic minority students make up over half of the population of students in the U.S. public education system, fewer than two in ten teachers have racial/ethnic minority identities [63]. This is a notable gap since research has found that having school staff who are representative of the racial/ethnic backgrounds of students in the school can increase connectedness within the school and between staff and students [64].

> "What does it mean for a student to be connected and even in the smallest things… like… if a student walks into your classroom, do they see themselves? In the school, do they see themselves? What does that look like? And [you have to be] really being intentional about understanding that intersectionality aspect."
>
> – Focus Group Participant

Other examples of policies and practices that can support connection at school for all students, including students at higher risk for being disconnected include the following:

- Establishing affinity groups for students of color and LGBTQIA+ students (e.g., genders and sexualities alliances).
- Enacting anti-bullying and anti-harassment policies that specifically protect staff and students against gender and sexual identity-based harassment.
- Enacting trauma-informed policies and practices, especially related to disciplinary practices (e.g., restorative practices).

For more information on these policies and practices, see the "Promising Practices" section.

***Implementation Tips***

School administrators can support implementation of connectedness interventions by doing the following:

- Engaging parents and students in the process of identifying and prioritizing relationship-building efforts.
- Supporting professional development for teachers on classroom management approaches that help build relationships with students (for more information about classroom management, see https://www.cdc.gov/healthyyouth/classroom-management/index.htm).
- Making sure that parent engagement activities are being offered at times, locations, and in ways that fit the needs of families.

## 5. Provide Psychosocial Skills Training and Cognitive Behavioral Interventions

Schools can teach specific skills to students to help them cope with their thoughts and behaviors. Cognitive behavioral interventions teach students to identify their own unhelpful thoughts and replace them with alternative thinking strategies. These interventions also often try to get students to engage in positive activities and coping behaviors in their lives, which can improve their moods and other symptoms of mental distress.

Districts and schools can use programs that help students with their thoughts and behaviors (and also improve their well-being and resilience) in one-on-one settings, small groups, and in the classroom. Some of these interventions focus on concepts that are also taught in social skill and emotional development programs, such as self-regulation and decision-making.

### *What Can Schools Do?*

### Promote Acceptance and Commitment to Change

*Description of Approach*

A new category of psychosocial skills training interventions asks students to explore whether their behaviors align with their personal values and, if not, prepares them to make behavior changes. These interventions also promote acceptance of one's current circumstances in ways that are similar to mindfulness. A specific type of therapy, dialectical behavior therapy, incorporates both mindfulness and acceptance and commitment principles.

*Evidence Summary*

Approaches using acceptance and commitment to change show an association with the following effects:

↑ Coping [65]
↓ Depression [66]
↓ Somatic symptoms [66]

*Evidence Description*

One study explored dialectical behavior therapy in a group of students attending an alternative education program and found improvements in somatic symptoms and symptoms of depression [66]. Another study using acceptance-based behavioral therapy in middle schools showed that students increased their use of problem-solving coping strategies [65].

Learn more about the acceptance and commitment program we reviewed:

- Teen Talk (Tier 3)

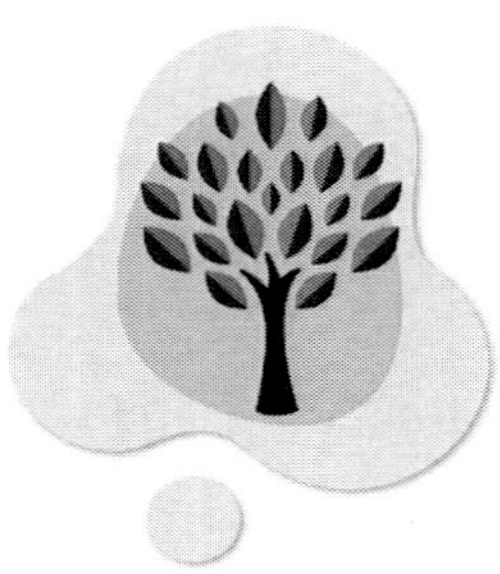

## Provide Cognitive Behavioral Interventions

*Description of Approach*

Cognitive behavioral interventions teach students how to manage their thoughts and behaviors. Cognitive behavioral interventions in schools often include multiple small-group or individual sessions that follow a standardized manual of activities that help students examine their own thoughts and behaviors.

Cognitive behavioral interventions sometimes encourage sharing what students learn about their thoughts and behaviors with others, including parents. Modular cognitive behavioral intervention is one example of this type of intervention in which counselors or therapists focus on a specific topic particularly relevant for a small group of students or one student. Other cognitive behavioral interventions specifically target symptoms of depression, anxiety, or posttraumatic stress.

*Evidence Summary*

Research into cognitive behavioral interventions has shown significant improvements in a range of mental health outcomes in students, including the following:

↓ Internalizing behaviors (e.g., feelings of anxiety, withdrawal, and depressive symptoms) [67-69]

↓ Anxiety, including social anxiety [70-73]

↓ Depression [73-75]

↓ Posttraumatic stress [69, 73, 75, 76]

*Evidence Description*

Research shows that teachers can effectively deliver cognitive behavioral interventions during classroom activities in K–12 schools. In one study, researchers showed that internalizing behaviors (e.g., feelings of anxiety, withdrawal, and depressive symptoms) decreased among elementary and middle school students [68]. High school students who received a cognitive behavioral intervention during a wellness class showed lower levels of depression than students who did not receive the intervention [74]. Modular cognitive behavioral interventions have been shown to help K–12 school students with anxiety and other internalizing behaviors [67, 71, 77, 78].

Small-group and one-on-one cognitive behavioral interventions also have been shown to improve students' ability to cope with trauma and specific anxieties. Several studies of a small-group intervention for elementary and middle school students experiencing anxiety, posttraumatic stress disorder, or both showed improvements in anxiety and posttraumatic stress [69, 73, 75, 76, 79]. Another study tested a cognitive behavioral intervention addressing social anxiety delivered to high schoolers and showed reductions in students' social anxiety [70].

Learn more about the cognitive behavioral interventions we reviewed:

- LARS & LISA (Tier 1).
- Tools for Getting Along Curriculum—Behavior Management Resource Guide (Tier 1).
- Cognitive Behavioral Intervention for Trauma in Schools (CBITS) (Tier 2).

- Footprints (Tier 2).
- Brief Intervention for School Clinicians (Tier 2/3).
- Bounce Back (Tier 3).
- Skills for Academic and Social Success (Tier 3).
- Building Confidence (Tier 3).

### *Engage Students in Coping Skills Training Groups*

#### Description of Approach

Coping skills training groups use principles of cognitive behavioral intervention to teach students skills to help them handle specific struggles and periods of adjustment. Similar to social, emotional, and behavioral learning programs, coping skills training often emphasizes strengthening resilience and learning to practice skills outside of the small group.

*Evidence Summary*

Coping skills training groups have been shown to have the following effects:

↓ Anxiety [80]
↓ Depression [80]
↑ Coping [81]

*Evidence Description*

Coping skills training groups use principles of cognitive behavioral intervention by teaching specific skills for specific struggles and periods of adjustment. Like social skill and emotional development programs, coping skills training often emphasizes strengthening resilience and learning to practice a growth mindset. For example, one study evaluated a coping skills training program for middle schoolers transitioning into high school and showed improvements in both anxiety and depression [80]. Another intervention paired coping skills training with social, emotional, and behavioral learning to help students after a natural disaster and showed improvements in measures of coping with stress [81].

Learn more about the coping skills training group program we reviewed:

- Journey of Hope (Tier 1).
- High School Transition Program (Tier 3).

### *Focus on Equity*

Children who have been exposed to adverse childhood experiences and trauma often receive cognitive behavioral interventions in schools because of their unique mental health needs. It is critical that students who have been exposed to trauma have the opportunity to receive trauma-focused or trauma-informed interventions. These interventions address the unique needs of students who have been exposed to trauma by being sensitive to potential triggers of re-experiencing trauma, being aware of students' fight-or-flight emotional response, and preventing potential outbursts or disruptive behavior caused by extreme emotions (emotional dysregulation). For this reason, some schools have begun implementing whole-school approaches to create trauma-sensitive school climates.

### *Implementation Tips*

Cognitive behavioral interventions and psychosocial skills training occur across a range of tiers of student needs and grade levels. School administrators may do the following:

- Work with school-based mental health staff to find ways for students to practice their new behaviors and coping skills.
- Use the MTSS framework described earlier in this action guide to ensure that students are appropriately screened and matched with classroom, small-group, or individualized interventions depending on their needs.

## 3. Support Staff Well-Being

In a 2022 survey, 73% of K–12 teachers and 85% of principals reported experiencing frequent job-related stress—about twice as high as the average across all work sectors [82]. Compared to other working adults, teachers and principals were also more likely to report burnout and symptoms of depression, and less likely to report feeling resilient. Educators of color, especially Hispanic and Latine/Latinx teachers, were more likely than their White peers to experience symptoms of depression [82]. Poor teacher well-being and mental health is also associated with lower-quality learning environments and poorer academic achievement among students [83].

### *What Can Schools Do?*

Districts and schools may consider incorporating opportunities for teachers and school staff to learn about how supportive practices, such as mindfulness, can be incorporated into daily routines [84-88]. Schools may also make therapeutic resources available to teachers and staff [89].

### Offer Mindfulness-Based Training Programs

*Description of Approach*

Mindfulness-based training programs can help teachers develop skills to effectively manage the demands of teaching and mitigate the physical and psychological impacts of stress. Mindfulness-based programs for teachers and staff are typically group-based and can be delivered over the course of several weeks during planning periods, before or after school [84], or during longer evening or full-day sessions [85, 86]. Across modes of delivery, programs focus on recognizing and understanding one's own emotions and emotional patterns and using mindfulness, meditation, yoga, and breathing exercises to regulate emotions.

*Evidence Summary*

Mindfulness-based training programs have been associated with the following mental health outcomes among teachers and school staff:

↓ Stress [84-86, 88, 90]
↓ Depressive symptoms [85, 86, 88, 90]

↓ Anxiety [85, 86, 88, 90]
↑ Well-being [90]

*Evidence Description*
Positive effects on stress and feelings of depression and anxiety were consistently observed after participation in mindfulness-based professional development programs:

- High school teachers and staff perceived work to be less stressful and reported decreased stress levels overall [84].
- Teachers, including educators of children with special needs, experienced reductions in stress, feelings of anxiety, and depressive symptoms [85, 86].
- School district employees and teachers reported less psychological distress, which included indicators of stress, anxiety, and depression [88, 90] as well as improved overall well-being [90]. One study reported that the program was equally beneficial for school district employees who reported higher anxiety or depressive symptoms before participating in the program and that benefits lasted for 3 months after program participation [90].

Learn about the mindfulness training programs for teachers that we reviewed:

- Healthy Minds Program.
- Cultivating Awareness and Resilience in Education.
- Stress Management and Relaxation Techniques in Education.
- Relaxation Therapy.
- Contemplative/Emotion Training.

**Provide Therapeutic Resources**
Examples include self-help workbooks as a cost-effective option for supporting K–12 teachers' and staff members' mental health.

*Evidence Summary*
Research found therapeutic resources for acceptance and commitment therapy (ACT) had the following effects among teachers and school staff: [89]

↓ Stress
↓ Depressive symptoms
↓ Anxiety

*Evidence Description*

In one study, researchers partnered with a school district to evaluate the effectiveness of a self-help version of ACT that involved reading an ACT workbook and completing exercises. Researchers reported two key findings:

- Reading the workbook and engaging in the exercises prevented the onset of psychological distress for teachers and school district staff who were not experiencing elevated symptoms of anxiety or depression at the start of the intervention. Teachers and staff who were not experiencing elevated symptoms of anxiety and did not receive the self-help workbook were more likely to meet clinical criteria for anxiety and depression at follow-up than were their peers who read the workbook and engaged in the exercises.
- Reading the workbook and engaging in the exercises reduced symptoms of psychological distress among teachers and school district staff experiencing elevated symptoms of stress, anxiety, or depression at the start of the intervention. Teachers and staff who met clinical cutoffs for stress, anxiety, or depression and who read the self-help workbook and engaged in the exercises experienced a greater reduction in symptoms than their peers who did not receive the self-help workbook.

Learn more about the therapeutic resource that we reviewed:

- ACT Bibliotherapy.

***Focus on Equity***

In a recent survey [82], teachers and principals of color were more likely to experience racial discrimination than their White peers. Teachers of color were most often racially discriminated against by other staff, but principals of color were most often racially discriminated against by students' family members. Subsequent analysis then linked that racial discrimination with worse mental health outcomes. This suggests that addressing racial discrimination and promoting inclusivity in schools could have a positive impact on the mental health of teachers and principals of color.

Strategies for reducing racial discrimination and promoting inclusivity include the following:

- Offering culturally relevant mental health and well-being supports that are accessible to staff.
- Building supportive environments within schools by ensuring that efforts to build supportive environments for students include safe spaces for staff (e.g., affinity groups) and activities that provide social support and promote resilience.

***Implementation Tips***

School administrators can support staff well-being approaches by doing the following:

- Asking staff how school practices and policies could be improved to reduce stress.

- Incorporating opportunities to practice mindfulness skills within existing routines. For example, adding a mindfulness minute to start meetings, the school day, or professional development opportunities.
- Engaging school staff in discussions about how to overcome barriers to accessing mental health supports.
- Coordinating teacher and administrator needs with parent–teacher associations or parent–teacher organizations; this provides an opportunity for engaging the community in these efforts. For example, parent–teacher associations could coordinate teacher appreciation activities.
- Depending on the level of support available through school districts, consider allowing school or district mental health and wellness teams to offer some level of support to teachers as well. This might include providing training or support during in-service or professional development days or compiling a robust referral list of mental health providers in the community.

> "School climate is awesome and I'm like, 'Woohoo,' but part of… the reason why is because we're providing psychological supports for the staff."
> — School staff member

Organizational changes can help reduce stress and create consistent opportunities for school staff to engage in positive coping.

- Learn more about how to develop comprehensive plans for teacher and staff well-being using an MTSS approach.
- Organizational changes can help reduce stress and create consistent opportunities for school staff to engage in positive coping. For additional information and resources, see Tips for Promoting School Employee Wellness.

## Promising Practices for Promoting Mental Health and Well-Being in Schools

While the six foundational strategies presented above were supported by a collection of evidence found in rigorous peer-reviewed literature, emerging evidence suggests that approaches for *promoting nurturing and welcoming school environments* may have a positive effect on the mental health and well-being of students and staff but did not have the level of evidence needed to meet criteria for inclusion as a strategy in this Action Guide. These approaches were mentioned by both focus group participants and subject matter experts, and they were found in either the gray literature or peer-reviewed literature that was not rigorous enough to meet criteria for inclusion (e.g., a study without a comparison group; a study that showed impact on outcomes related to mental health, but not mental health directly, etc.). As such, additional research is needed on the effectiveness of the strategies described in this section, but they offer promise for promoting student mental health and well-being. School administrators can consider two primary approaches for promoting welcoming school environments—with the caveat that additional research is needed on their impact on mental health outcomes.

*Restorative practices* can be implemented in schools and are characterized as promoting high levels of warmth and positive relationships between staff and students and high levels of structure and accountability for one's behaviors. Restorative practices often include the following:

- Proactive circles, or community circles, where students are brought together, typically with facilitation by an adult, to set expectations and build relationships among students in a classroom.
- Responsive circles, which are designed to address peer conflict in a school and include the students involved in a specific conflict along with an adult facilitator.
- Restorative conferences, which are held to negotiate a repair after a student's behavior harmed a relationship with another student or staff member.

Restorative practices are most successful when they are used throughout a school building to set expectations for positive relationships and accountability. See the International Institute for Restorative Practices (IIRP) for more information and training on restorative practices in schools.

Many high schools across the United States have implemented restorative practices with promising results, including declines in out-of-school suspension and disproportional exclusionary discipline [91, 92]. In one study in Denver, district suspension rates declined by nearly 47%, with the largest reductions among African American students [92]. Restorative practices are often implemented instead of suspensions or expulsions, which have been shown to affect racial and ethnic minority groups of students at higher rates than ethnic majority groups [93]. Discipline disparities are associated with negative outcomes for Black boys and young men, including lower levels of school connectedness, school engagement, and academic achievement [94]. Restorative practices have shown positive results in reducing exclusionary discipline (e.g., out-of-school suspension [95]), although results from experimentally controlled studies are mixed as to whether or not disparities in discipline for Black students were reduced [96, 97].

### *Genders and Sexualities Alliances*

Schools should consider implementing *internal structures of social support,* such as Genders and Sexualities Alliances, for students who face discrimination.

States with policies that support nondiscrimination of LGBTQIA+ students also have more Gay Straight Alliances (more recently referred to as Genders and Sexualities Alliances) in schools [98]. In addition, emerging research suggests Genders and Sexualities Alliances may be associated with more social support, which buffers against depression and anxiety in LGBTQIA+ youth [99].

## Conclusion

This action guide provides K–12 schools, districts, and administrators with strategies and approaches to promote mental health and well-being in schools based on the most current research evidence, lived experience of students and school staff, and subject matter expert opinions. As mental health concerns for young people have increased in recent years, schools need approaches that are evidence based and feasible. The strategies and approaches presented in this package are best centered in the MTSS that many schools already use to assess and address students' needs. Centering equity in implementation of these strategies and approaches is also critical for prioritizing the unique experiences of students and staff who are disproportionally affected by poor mental health outcomes. School leaders can use this resource to reflect on current practices in their district and schools and explore opportunities for improvement and expansion of strategies to effectively and equitably support student mental health.

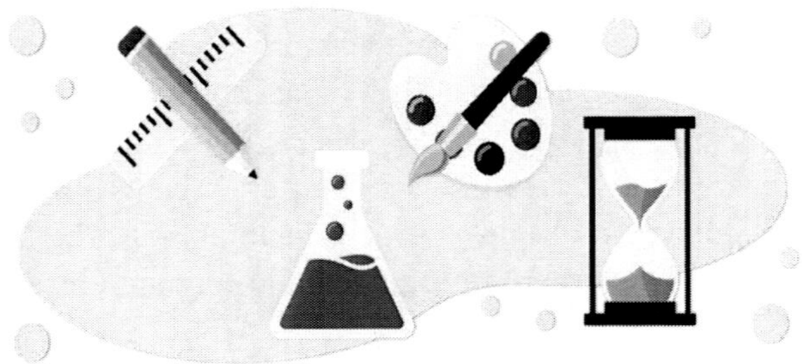

## Appendix A. Assessing the Evidence

### Peer-Reviewed Literature Review

Empirical evidence about programs, policies, and practices was obtained through a review of school mental health-related literature and was included if the following criteria were met:

- Research was peer reviewed.
- Research was conducted in K–12 school settings in the United States with students, teachers, or staff between 2011 and 2021.
- The study was a randomized controlled trial or quasi-experimental study with a statistically controlled comparison group.
- Outcomes related to K–12 students', teachers', or school staff's mental health and well-being were reported (e.g., resilience, coping, depression, anxiety, internalizing problems [often measured as a mix of symptoms including feelings of anxiety, depression, withdrawal, and anhedonia], trauma, stress, suicide).

**Table A.1.** Search strategy

| |
|---|
| Population |
| (kindergarten* OR "elementary school*" OR "middle school*" OR "high school*" OR "K-12" OR (student* AND (child* OR youth* OR adolescent* OR teen* OR "teacher" OR "staff" OR "personnel" OR "nurse" OR "administrator" or "paraprofessional")) OR "school based") |
| AND |
| Mental Health |
| ("mental health" OR "social emotional learning" OR "behavioral problem*" OR "behavior problem*" OR "social problem*" OR "emotional problem*" OR "depression" OR "anxiety" OR "trauma" OR "stress" OR "bullying" OR "verbal aggression" OR "physical aggression" OR "victimization" OR "well-being" OR "coping" OR "emotion*") |

| AND |
|---|
| Supports |
| ("comprehensive school mental health" OR "school mental health service*" OR "school mental health support*" OR "access to care" OR "school psychologist*" OR "school counselor*" OR "school social worker*" OR "family school relationship" OR "school community relationship" OR "school environment" OR "school climate" OR "school infrastructure" OR "multi-tiered systems of support" OR "interconnected system*" OR "framework" OR "Tier 1" OR "Tier 2" OR "Tier 3" OR "cultural responsiveness" OR "culturally responsive" OR "equity" OR "inclusive" OR "inclusion" OR "resilience" OR "training" OR "professional development" OR "employee assistance program/EAP" OR "response to intervention" OR "positive behavioral interventions and support") |

| OR |
|---|
| Population |
| Promotion |
| ("mental health promotion" OR "mental health prevention" OR "mental health intervention*" OR "mental health screening" OR "mental health risk assessment*" OR "teaming" OR "needs assessment" OR "resource mapping" OR "mental health program*" OR "mental health policy" OR "mental health policies" OR "mental health literacy" OR "mental health education" OR "psychoeducation" OR "prevention" OR "policy" OR "intervention") |
| Years |
| 2011–April 12, 2022 |
| Language |
| English |
| Geographic Area |
| U.S. only |
| Population |
| K–12 students or staff |
| Databases |
| PubMed; Web of Science; PsycInfo; ERIC; Embase; CINAHL |

**Table A.2.** Inclusion and exclusion criteria

| Criterion | Include | Exclude |
|---|---|---|
| Populations | K–12 students, teachers, or staff | Populations other than K–12 students, teachers, or staff (e.g., parents, college students) |
| Interventions | Programs; policies; practices implemented in K–12 school settings during the typical school day | Medicine<br>Policies, programs, practices that are implemented outside of K–12 typical school day (e.g., after school) or outside of a school setting |
| Comparisons | Statistically controlled comparison group (e.g., active control condition, usual care, waitlist control). Note: for policies include single group pretest-posttest comparisons | No statistically controlled comparison group (e.g., single group pretest-posttest), except in the case of policies |
| Outcomes | Outcomes that are related to K–12 students' or teachers'/school staff mental health and well-being (e.g., psychosocial outcomes, social-emotional learning, access to care)<br>• mental health/well-being/coping<br>• social-emotional learning<br>• behavioral/social/emotional problem<br>• depression/anxiety<br>• trauma/stress<br>• suicide | Outcomes that are not directly tied to staff or students' social, emotional, and mental well-being (e.g., physical health promotion, academic problems/learning disabilities, substance use, sexual risk behaviors, truancy, homelessness, bullying/verbal aggression/physical aggression/ victimization etc.)* |

**Table A.2.** (Continued)

| Criterion | Include | Exclude |
|---|---|---|
| Study designs | Randomized controlled trials; quasi-experimental designs; systematic reviews; meta-analyses | Case reports, case series; studies that are only descriptive or qualitative; feasibility studies; psychometric studies; cost-only studies (except in the case of policies) |
| Setting | K–12 school settings in the United States | Research conducted in settings other than K–12 schools in countries other than the U.S. |
| Timing | Publications between 2011 and 2021 | Publications before 2011; publications after 2011 based on data collected before 2011 |
| Publication type | Original research | Commentaries, editorials, conference abstracts, study protocols, presentations, dissertations/theses |
| Language | English | Non-English studies |

* Publications that include both mental health outcomes and non–mental health outcomes (e.g., substance use) were included.

A search strategy was developed for the peer-reviewed literature that included search terms and a list of the databases to be searched. The final search was completed in April 2022. The search strategy is summarized in Table A.1.

Inclusion and exclusion criteria related to population, intervention type, comparison group, outcomes, study design, setting, timing, publication, and language were also developed. Whereas some criteria are consistent (i.e., population, setting), others (e.g., comparisons, study design) varied across policies, programs, and practices due to fundamental differences in implementing and evaluating different types of intervention strategies. For example, articles evaluating programs or practices were required to have a statistically controlled comparison group whereas articles evaluating policies were not. Table A.2 lists inclusion and exclusion criteria.

### *Gray Literature Review*

A review of the gray literature (e.g., publications from academic institutions, national organizations and foundations, and federal government resources) was also conducted using the same outcomes and time frame as the peer-reviewed literature search. An online search engine was used to identify sources including government websites and professional organizations' publications. In addition to a key word search, additional searches were conducted to identify gray literature that described the mental health impact of school-based policies, trauma-informed schools, and mental health education.

### *Focus Groups*

Contextual evidence was gathered through focus groups conducted with students, parents/caregivers, school-based mental health staff (e.g., counselors, social workers, and psychologists), other school staff (e.g., teachers, nurses, and administrators), and nongovernmental organization (NGO) representatives. Respondents provided feedback on the availability of programs, policies, and practices to support mental health and well-being in schools, and their perceptions of and suggestions for improved implementation.

***Expert Listening Sessions***

Listening sessions were also conducted with experts in school-based mental health and well-being from NGOs, academia, educational agencies, and federal agencies. They provided additional critical insight around how to frame recommendations, center equity in the recommended approaches, and support implementation of the six strategies described in this action guide.

The example policies, programs, and practices included in this action guide are not intended to be a comprehensive list for each approach but rather to serve as examples that have shown impact on the mental health and well-being of K-12 students and staff based on peer-reviewed literature. It is important to note that programs, policies, and practices that have an impact on outcomes related to mental health and well-being, such as bullying, externalizing behaviors, substance use, chronic absenteeism, physical health promotion, are not included in this action guide. Additional evidence-based resources may be found in existing program registries, such as the following:

- Blueprints for Healthy Youth Development
- The California Evidence-Based Clearinghouse for Child Welfare
- CDC Division of Violence Prevention's Resources for Action
- Collaborative for Academic, Social, and Emotional Learning (CASEL)
- Programs That Work, from the Promising Practices Network on Children, Families and Communities
- What Works Clearinghouse

The strategies included in this action guide also do not represent all school-based strategies that benefit student well-being, such as school nutrition and physical activity programs, which provide important contributions to students' health and well-being. For more information about additional school-based health promotion strategies, see Healthy Schools | CDC.

## References

[1] Centers for Disease Control and Prevention. (2023). *Youth risk behavior survey: Data summary and trends report, 2011-2021.* Retrieved from https://www.cdc.gov/healthyyouth/data/yrbs/pdf/YRBS_Data-Summary-Trends_Report2023_508.pdf.

[2] Pears, K. C., Kim, H. K., & Fisher, P. A. (2012). Effects of a school readiness intervention for children in foster care on oppositional and aggressive behaviors in kindergarten. *Children & Youth Services Review, 34*(12), 2361–2366. https://doi.org/10.1016/j.childyouth.2012.08.015.

[3] Mpofu, J. J., Cooper, A. C., Ashley, C., Geda, S., Harding, R. L., Johns, M. M., Spinks-Franklin, A., Njai, R., Moyse, D., & Underwood, J. M. (2022). Perceived racism and demographic, mental health, and behavioral characteristics among high school students during the COVID-19 pandemic—Adolescent Behaviors and Experiences Survey, United States, January–June 2021. *MMWR Supplements, 71*(3), 22–27. https://doi.org/10.15585/mmwr.su7103a4.

[4] Finning, K., Ukoumunne, O. C., Ford, T., Danielsson-Waters, E., Shaw, L., De Jager, I. R., . . . Moore, D. A. (2019). The association between child and adolescent depression and poor attendance at school: A systematic review and meta-analysis. *Journal of Affective Disorders, 245*, 928-938. https://doi.org/10.1016/ j.jad.2018.11.055.

[5] Conway, K. P., Swendsen, J., Husky, M. M., He, J. P., & Merikangas, K. R. (2016). Association of lifetime mental disorders and subsequent alcohol and illicit drug use: results from the National

Comorbidity Survey– Adolescent Supplement. *Journal of the American Academy of Child and Adolescent Psychiatry, 55*(4), 280-288. https://doi.org/10.1016/j.jaac.2016.01.006.

[6] Centers for Disease Control and Prevention. (Apr 25, 2023). *About mental health*. CDC. Retrieved from https:// www.cdc.gov/mentalhealth/learn/index.htm.

[7] Centers for Disease Control and Prevention. (May 8, 2023). *Physical activity helps prevent chronic diseases*. NCCDPHP. Retrieved from https://www.cdc.gov/chronicdisease/.

[8] National Alliance on Mental Health. *Mental health in schools*. NAMI. Retrieved from https://www.nami.org/ Advocacy/Policy-Priorities/Improving-Health/Mental-Health-in-Schools.

[9] APA Working Group on Children's Mental Health. (2001). *Developing psychology's national agenda for children's mental health: APA's response to the Surgeon General's action agenda for children's mental health* https://www.apa.org/pi/families/resources/national-agenda.pdf.

[10] American School Counseling Association. (2009, 2020). *The school counselor and student mental health*. Retrieved from https://www.schoolcounselor.org/Standards-Positions/Position-Statements/ ASCA-Position-Statements/The-School-Counselor-and-Student-Mental-Health.

[11] National Association of School Psychologists. *The relationship between mental health and academic achievement [Research summary]*. 2020. https://www.nasponline.org/x61337.xml.

[12] Mahoney, J. L., Weissberg, R. P., Greenberg, M. T., Dusenbury, L., Jagers, R. J., Niemi, K., Schlinger, M., Schlund, J., Shriver, T. P., VanAusdal, K., & Yoder, N. (2021). Systemic social and emotional learning: Promoting educational success for all preschool to high school students. *American Psychologist, 76*(7), 1128–1142. https://doi.org/10.1037/amp0000701.

[13] Council of Chief State School Officers, Collaborative for Academic, Social, and Emotional Learning, American Institutes for Research, & al., e. (2021). *SEL MTSS toolkit for state & district leaders*. Retrieved from https://753a0706.flowpaper.com/CCSSOSELMTSSToolkit/#page=1.

[14] Goddard, A., Sullivan, E., Fields, P., & Mackey, S. (2021). The future of telehealth in school-based health centers: Lessons from COVID-19. *Journal of Pediatric Health Care, 35*(3), 304-309. https://doi.org/10.1016/ j.pedhc.2020.11.008.

[15] Reinke, W. M., Stormont, M., Herman, K. C., Puri, R., & Goel, N. (2011). Supporting children's mental health in schools: Teacher perceptions of needs, roles, and barriers. *School Psychology Quarterly, 26*(1), 1-13. https://doi.org/10.1037/a0022714.

[16] Horner, R. H., Sugai, G., & Fixsen, D. L. (2017). Implementing effective educational practices at scales of social importance. *Clinical Child and Family Psychology Review, 20*(1), 25-35. https://doi.org/10.1007/ s10567-017-0224-7.

[17] Habeger, A. D., van Vulpen, K. S., & Simmons, T. F. (2018). Perceptions of rural school mental health services: A focus group study. *Child and Adolescent Mental Health, 30*(1), 1-10. https://doi.org/10.2989/ 17280583.2017.1419250.

[18] Meyers, D. C., Domitrovich, C. E., Dissi, R., Trejo, J., & Greenberg, M. T. (2019). Supporting systemic social and emotional learning with a schoolwide implementation model. *Evaluation and Program Planning, 73*, 53-61. https://doi.org/10.1016/j.evalprogplan.2018.11.005.

[19] Collaborative for Academic, Social, and Emotional Learning (CASEL). (2023). *The CASEL Guide to Schoolwide Social and Emotional Learning*. Retrieved from https://schoolguide.casel.org/.

[20] Borntrager, C., & Lyon, A. R. (2015). Client progress monitoring and feedback in school-based mental health. *Cognitive and Behavioral Practice, 22*(1), 74-86. https://doi.org/10.1016/j.cbpra.2014.03.007.

[21] DeLuca-Acconi, R., Bessaha, M., Velázquez, S. L., & Mendoza, M. R. (2022). How did we get here and where do we go from here?: Supporting undocumented students through a pandemic. *School Psychology, 37*(2), 202-211. https://doi.org/10.1037/spq0000491.

[22] Marx, R. A., & Kettrey, H. H. (2016). Gay-straight alliances are associated with lower levels of school-based victimization of LGBTQ+ youth: A systematic review and meta-analysis. *Journal of Youth and Adolescence, 45*(7), 1269-1282. https://doi.org/10.1007/s10964-016-0501-7.

[23] Bruns, E. J., Duong, M. T., Lyon, A. R., Pullmann, M. D., Cook, C. R., Cheney, D., & McCauley, E. (2016). Fostering SMART partnerships to develop an effective continuum of behavioral health services and supports in schools. *American Journal of Orthopsychiatry, 86*(2), 156-170. https://doi.org/10.1037/ ort0000083.

[24] Kull, R. M., Greytak, E. A., Kosciw, J. G., & Villenas, C. (2016). Effectiveness of school district antibullying policies in improving LGBT youths' school climate. *Psychology of Sexual Orientation and Gender Diversity, 3*(4), 407-415. https://doi.org/10.1037/sgd0000196.

[25] Kutcher, S., Wei, Y., & Coniglio, C. (2016). Mental health literacy: Past, present, and future. *The Canadian Journal of Psychiatry, 61*(3), 154-158. https://doi.org/10.1177/0706743715616609.

[26] Jorm, A. F. (2012). Mental health literacy: Empowering the community to take action for better mental health. *American Psychologist, 67*(3), 231-243. https://doi.org/10.1037/a0025957.

[27] Swartz, K., Musci, R. J., Beaudry, M. B., Heley, K., Miller, L., Alfes, C., . . . Wilcox, H. C. (2017). School-based curriculum to improve depression literacy among US secondary school students: A randomized effectiveness trial. *American Journal of Public Health, 107*(12), 1970-1976. https://doi.org/10.2105/ ajph.2017.304088.

[28] Beaudry, M. B., Swartz, K., Miller, L., Schweizer, B., Glazer, K., & Wilcox, H. (2019). Effectiveness of the adolescent depression awareness program (ADAP) on depression literacy and mental health treatment. *Journal of School Health, 89*(3), 165-172. https://doi.org/10.1111/josh.12725.

[29] Ruble, A. E., Leon, P. J., Gilley-Hensley, L., Hess, S. G., & Swartz, K. L. (2013). Depression knowledge in high school students: Effectiveness of the adolescent depression awareness program. *Journal of Affective Disorders, 150*(3), 1025-1030. https://doi.org/10.1016/j.jad.2013.05.033.

[30] Link, B. G., DuPont-Reyes, M. J., Barkin, K., Villatoro, A. P., Phelan, J. C., & Painter, K. (2020). A school-based intervention for mental illness stigma: A cluster randomized trial. *Pediatrics, 145*(6), 9. https://doi.org/ 10.1542/peds.2019-0780.

[31] Painter, K., Phelan, J. C., DuPont-Reyes, M. J., Barkin, K. F., Villatoro, A. P., & Link, B. G. (2017). Evaluation of antistigma interventions with sixth-grade students: A school-based field experiment. *Psychiatric Services, 68*(4), 345-352. https://doi.org/10.1176/appi.ps.201600052.

[32] DeLuca, J. S., Tang, J., Zoubaa, S., Dial, B., & Yanos, P. T. (2021). Reducing stigma in high school students: A cluster randomized controlled trial of the national alliance on mental illness' ending the silence intervention. *Stigma and Health, 6*(2), 228-242. https://doi.org/10.1037/sah0000235.

[33] Petrova, M., Wyman, P. A., Schmeelk-Cone, K., & Pisani, A. R. (2015). Positive-themed suicide prevention messages delivered by adolescent peer leaders: Proximal impact on classmates' coping attitudes and perceptions of adult support. *Suicide and Life-Threatening Behavior, 45*(6), 651-663. https://doi.org/10.1111/ sltb.12156.

[34] Parker, A. E., Kupersmidt, J. B., Mathis, E. T., Scull, T. M., & Sims, C. (2014). The impact of mindfulness education on elementary school students: Evaluation of the Master Mind program. *Advances in School Mental Health Promotion, 7*(3), 184-204. https://doi.org/10.1080/1754730x. 2014.916497.

[35] Johnstone, J. M., Ribbers, A., Jenkins, D., Atchley, R., Gustafsson, H., Nigg, J. T., . . . Oken, B. (2020). Classroom-based mindfulness training reduces anxiety in adolescents: Acceptability and effectiveness of a cluster-randomized pilot study. *Journal of Restorative Medicine, 10*(1). https://doi.org/10.14200/ jrm.2020.0101.

[36] Sibinga, E. M. S., Webb, L., Ghazarian, S. R., & Ellen, J. M. (2016). School-based mindfulness instruction: An RCT. *Pediatrics, 137*(1), 1-8. https://doi.org/10.1542/peds.2015-2532.

[37] Frank, J. L., Kohler, K., Peal, A., & Bose, B. (2017). Effectiveness of a school-based yoga program on adolescent mental health and school performance: Findings from a randomized controlled trial. *Mindfulness, 8*(3), 544-553. https://doi.org/10.1007/s12671-016-0628-3.

[38] Wendt, S , Hipps, J., Abrams, A., Grant, J., Valosek, L., & Nidich, S. (2015). Practicing transcendental meditation in high schools: Relationship to well-being and academic achievement among students. *Contemporary School Psychology, 19*(4), 312-319. https://doi.org/10.1007/s40688-015-0066-6.

[39] Fung, J., Kim, J. J., Jin, J., Chen, G., Bear, L., & Lau, A. S. (2019). A randomized trial evaluating school-based mindfulness intervention for ethnic minority youth: Exploring mediators and moderators of intervention effects. *Journal of Abnormal Child Psychology, 47*(1), 1-19. https://doi.org/10.1007/ s10802-018-0425-7.

[40] Lau, A. S., Kim, J. J., Nguyen, D. J., Nguyen, H. T., Kodish, T., & Weiss, B. (2020). Effects of preference on outcomes of preventive interventions among ethnically diverse adolescents at-risk of

depression. *Journal of Clinical Child and Adolescent Psychology, 49*(6), 820-836. https://doi.org/10.1080/15374416.2019.1639514.

[41] Fung, J., Guo, S. S., Jin, J., Bear, L., & Lau, A. (2016). A pilot randomized trial evaluating a school-based mindfulness intervention for ethnic minority youth. *Mindfulness, 7*(4), 819-828. https://doi.org/10.1007/ s12671-016-0519-7.

[42] Center for Responsive Schools. (n.d.). *Equity and mindfulness. Culturally responsive mindfulness: Strategies for teachers and students*. Retrieved from https://www.crslearn.org/publication/reflecting-rebuilding-digest-edition/equity-and-mindfulness/

[43] Dray, B. J., & Wisneski, D. B. (2011). Mindful reflection as a process for developing culturally responsive practices. *Teaching Exceptional Children, 44*(1), 28-36. https://doi.org/10.1177/ 004005991104400104.

[44] CASEL. (n.d.). *What Is the CASEL framework? Interactive CASEL wheel* Retrieved from https://casel.org/fundamentals-of-sel/what-is-the-casel-framework/#respon-sible.

[45] CDC. (2022). *Strategies to create a healthy and supportive school environment*. Retrieved from https://www.cdc.gov/ healthyschools/sec_schools.htm.

[46] Cipriano, C., Strambler, M. J., Naples, L., Ha, C., Kirk, M. A., Wood, M. E., . . . Durlak, J. (2023). Stage 2 report: The state of the evidence for social and emotional learning: A contemporary meta-analysis of universal school-based SEL interventions. https://doi.org/10.31219/osf.io/mk35u.

[47] Rian, S. W., & Coll, K. M. (2021). Increased exposure to nature reduces elementary students' anxiety. *Ecopsychology, 13*(4), 257-264. https://doi.org/10.1089/eco.2020.0070.

[48] Calhoun, B., Williams, J., Greenberg, M., Domitrovich, C., Russell, M. A., & Fishbein, D. H. (2020). Social Emotional Learning Program Boosts Early Social and Behavioral Skills in Low-Income Urban Children. *Frontiers in Psychology, 11*, 561196. https://doi.org/10.3389/fpsyg.2020.561196.

[49] Schleider, J. L., Burnette, J. L., Widman, L., Hoyt, C., & Prinstein, M. J. (2020). Randomized trial of a single-session growth mind-set intervention for rural adolescents' internalizing and externalizing problems. *Journal of Clinical Child and Adolescent Psychology, 49*(5), 660-672. https://doi.org/10.1080/15374416.2019.1622123.

[50] Cook, C. R., Frye, M., Slemrod, T., Lyon, A. R., Renshaw, T. L., & Zhang, Y. C. (2015). An Integrated Approach to Universal Prevention: Independent and Combined Effects of PBIS and SEL on Youths' Mental Health. *School Psychology Quarterly, 30*(2), 166-183. https://doi.org/10.1037/spq0000102.

[51] Kramer, T. J., Caldarella, P., Young, K. R., Fischer, L., & Warren, J. S. (2014). Implementing strong kids school-wide to reduce internalizing behaviors and increase prosocial behaviors. *Education and Treatment of Children, 37*(4), 659-680. https://doi.org/10.1353/etc.2014.0031.

[52] Thayer, A. J., Campa, D. M., Weeks, M. R., Buntain-Ricklefs, J., Low, S., Larson, M., & Cook, C. R. (2019). Examining the Differential Effects of a Universal SEL Curriculum on Student Functioning Through the Dual Continua Model of Mental Health. *Journal of Primary Prevention, 40*(4), 405-427. https://doi.org/ 10.1007/s10935-019-00557-0.

[53] Green, A. L., Ferrante, S., Boaz, T. L., Kutash, K., & Wheeldon-Reece, B. (2021). Social and emotional learning during early adolescence: Effectiveness of a classroom-based SEL program for middle school students. *Psychology in the Schools, 58*(6), 1056-1069. https://doi.org/10.1002/pits.22487.

[54] Daunic, A. P., Corbett, N. L., Smith, S. W., Algina, J., Poling, D., Worth, M., . . . Vezzoli, J. (2021). Efficacy of the social-emotional learning foundations curriculum for kindergarten and first grade students at risk for emotional and behavioral disorders. *Journal of School Psychology, 86*, 78-99. https://doi.org/10.1016/ j.jsp.2021.03.004.

[55] Freedman, S. (2018). Forgiveness as an educational goal with at-risk adolescents. *Journal of Moral Education, 47*(4), 415-431. https://doi.org/10.1080/03057240.2017.1399869.

[56] Ramirez, T., Brush, K., Raisch, N., Bailey, R., & Jones, S. M. (2021). Equity in social emotional learning programs: a content analysis of equitable practices in PreK-5 SEL programs. *Frontiers in Education, 6*, 679467. https://doi.org/10.3389/feduc.2021.679467.

[57] CASEL. (n.d.). *Transformative SEL*. Retrieved from https://casel.org/fundamentals-of-sel/how-does-sel-support-educational-equity-and-excellence/transformative-sel/.

[58] Steiner, R. J., Sheremenko, G., Lesesne, C., Dittus, P. J., Sieving, R. E., & Ethier, K. A. (2019). Adolescent connectedness and adult health outcomes. *Pediatrics, 144*(1). https://doi.org/10.1542/peds.2018-3766.

[59] CDC. (2022). *Adolescent and school health: School connectedness helps students thrive*. Retrieved from https://www.cdc.gov/healthyyouth/protective/school_connectedness.htm.

[60] Eisenhower, A., Taylor, H., & Baker, B. L. (2016). Starting strong: A school-based indicated prevention program during the transition to kindergarten. *School Psychology Review, 45(2*), 141-170. https://doi.org/10.17105/spr45-2.141-170.

[61] Ohye, B. Y., Jakubovic, R. J., Zakarian, R., & Bui, E. (2020). Staying strong with schools: Testing an Elementary school-based intervention for military-connected children. *Journal of Clinical Child and Adolescent Psychology, 49*(5), 595-602. https://doi.org/10.1080/15374416.2018.1547971.

[62] Wilkins, N. J., Krause, K. H., Verlenden, J. V., Szucs, L. E., Ussery, E. N., Allen, C. T., . . . Ethier, K. A. (2023). School connectedness and risk behaviors and experiences among high school students—Youth Risk Behavior Survey, United States, 2021. *MMWR Supplements, 72*(1), 13-21. https://doi.org/10.15585/ mmwr.su7201a2.

[63] Mpofu, J. J., Cooper, A. C., Ashley, C., Geda, S., Harding, R. L., Johns, M. M., . . . Underwood, J. M. (2022). Perceived racism and demographic, mental health, and behavioral characteristics among high school students during the COVID-19 pandemic—Adolescent Behaviors and Experiences Survey, United States, January–June 2021. *MMWR Supplements, 71*(3), 22-27. https://doi.org/10.15585/mmwr.su7103a4.

[64] Schaeffer, K. (2021, December 10). *America's public school teachers are far less racially and ethnically diverse than their students*. Retrieved from https://www.pewresearch.org/short-reads/2021/12/10/americas-public-school-teachers-are-far-less-racially-and-ethnically-diverse-than-their-students/.

[65] Atkins, D. N., Fertig, A. R., & Wilkins, V. M. (2014). Connectedness and expectations: How minority teachers can improve educational outcomes for minority students. *Public Management Review, 16*(4), 503-526. https://doi.org/10.1080/14719037.2013.841981.

[66] Terry, J. D., Weist, M. D., Strait, G. G., & Miller, M. (2021). Motivational interviewing to promote the effectiveness of selective prevention: An integrated school-based approach. *Prevention Science, 22*(6), 799-810. https://doi.org/10.1007/s11121-020-01124-4.

[67] Smith, S. W., Daunic, A. P., Barber, B. R., Aydin, B., Van Loan, C. L., & Taylor, G. G. (2014). Preventing risk for significant behavior problems through a cognitive-behavioral intervention: Effects of the tools for getting along curriculum at one-year follow-up. *Journal of Primary Prevention, 35*(5), 371-387. https://doi.org/10.1007/s10935-014-0357-0.

[68] Sumi, W. C., Woodbridge, M. W., Wei, X., Thornton, S. P., & Roundfield, K. D. (2021). Measuring the impact of trauma-focused, cognitive behavioral group therapy with middle school students. *School Mental Health, 13*(4), 680-694. https://doi.org/10.1007/s12310-021-09452-8.

[69] Masia Warner, C., Colognori, D., Brice, C., Herzig, K., Mufson, L., Lynch, C., . . . Klein, R. G. (2016). Can school counselors deliver cognitive-behavioral treatment for social anxiety effectively? A randomized controlled trial. *Journal of Child Psychology and Psychiatry, 57*(11), 1229-1238. https://doi.org/10.1111/jcpp.12550.

[70] Galla, B. M., Wood, J. J., Chiu, A. W., Langer, D. A., Jacobs, J., Ifekwunigwe, M., & Larkins, C. (2012). One year follow-up to modular cognitive behavioral therapy for the treatment of pediatric anxiety disorders in an elementary school setting. *Child Psychiatry and Human Development, 43*(2), 219-226. https://doi.org/10.1007/s10578-011-0258-x.

[71] Blickenstaff, H. R., Bastin, T. J., & Byram, J. N. (2022). Exploring Resilience Factors in Medical Students with Adverse Childhood Experiences: a Pilot Study. *Academic Psychiatry, 46*(2), 218-222. https://doi.org/10.1007/ s40596-021-01560-6.

[72] Langley, A. K., Gonzalez, A., Sugar, C. A., Solis, D., & Jaycox, L. (2015). Bounce back: Effectiveness of an elementary school-based intervention for multicultural children exposed to traumatic events. *Journal of Consulting and Clinical Psychology, 83*(5), 853-865. https://doi.org/10.1037/ccp0000051.

[73] Pössel, P., Martin, N. C., Garber, J., & Hautzinger, M. (2013). A randomized controlled trial of a cognitive-behavioral program for the prevention of depression in adolescents compared with

nonspecific and no-intervention control conditions. *Journal of Counseling Psychology, 60*(3), 432-438. https://doi.org/10.1037/ a0032308.

[74] Ros, A. M., Brewer, S. K., Raviv, T., & Santiago, C. D. (2019). How do parent psychopathology and family income impact treatment gains in a school-based intervention for trauma? *School Mental Health, 11*(4), 777-789. https://doi.org/10.1007/s12310-019-09324-2.

[75] Santiago, C. D., Lennon, J. M., Fuller, A. K., Brewer, S. K., & Kataoka, S. H. (2014). Examining the impact of a family treatment component for CBITS: When and for whom is it helpful? *Journal of Family Psychology, 28*(4), 560-570. https://doi.org/10.1037/a0037329.

[76] Ginsburg, G. S., Pella, J. E., Pikulski, P. J., Tein, J.-Y., & Drake, K. L. (2020). School-based treatment for anxiety research study (STARS): A randomized controlled effectiveness trial. *Journal of Abnormal Child Psychology, 48*(3), 407-417. https://doi.org/10.1007/s10802-019-00596-5.

[77] Bruns, E. J., Pullmann, M. D., Nicodimos, S., Lyon, A. R., Ludwig, K., Namkung, N., & McCauley, E. (2019). Pilot test of an engagement, triage, and brief intervention strategy for school mental health. *School Mental Health, 11*(1), 148-162. https://doi.org/10.1007/s12310-018-9277-0.

[78] Cooley-Strickland, M. R., Griffin, R. S., Darney, D., Otte, K., & Ko, J. (2011). Urban African American youth exposed to community violence: a school-based anxiety preventive intervention efficacy study. *Journal of Prevention & Intervention in the Community, 39*(2), 149-166. https://doi.org/10.1080/ 10852352.2011.556573.

[79] Powell, T., & Thompson, S. J. (2016). Enhancing coping and supporting protective factors after a disaster: Findings from a quasi-experimental study. *Research on Social Work Practice, 26*(5), 539-549. https://doi.org/10.1177/1049731514559422.

[80] Theodore-Oklota, C., Orsillo, S. M., Lee, J. K., & Vernig, P. M. (2014). A pilot of an acceptance-based risk reduction program for relational aggression for adolescents. *Journal of Contextual Behavioral Science, 3*(2), 109-116. https://doi.org/10.1016/j.jcbs.2014.03.001.

[81] Ricard, R. J., Lerma, E., & Heard, C. C. C. (2013). Piloting a dialectical behavioral therapy (DBT) infused skills group in a disciplinary alternative education program (DAEP). *Journal for Specialists in Group Work, 38*(4), 285-306. https://doi.org/10.1080/01933922.2013.834402.

[82] Steiner, E. D., Doan, S., Woo, A., Gittens, A. D., Lawrence, R. A., Berdie, L., . . . Schwartz, H. L. (2022). *Restoring teacher and principal well-being is an essential step for rebuilding schools: Findings from the State of the American Teacher and State of the American Principal Surveys*. Santa Monica, CA: RAND Corporation. https://www.rand.org/pubs/research_reports/RRA1108-4.html.

[83] Madigan, D. J., & Kim, L. E. (2021). Does teacher burnout affect students? A systematic review of its association with academic achievement and student-reported outcomes. *International Journal of Educational Research, 105*, 101714. https://doi.org/10.1016/j.ijer.2020.101714.

[84] Kaspereen, D. (2012). Relaxation intervention for stress reduction among teachers and staff. *International Journal of Stress Management, 19*(3), 238-250. https://doi.org/10.1037/a0029195.

[85] Kemeny, M. E., Foltz, C., Cavanagh, J. F., Cullen, M., Giese-Davis, J., Jennings, P., . . . Ekman, P. (2012). Contemplative/emotion training reduces negative emotional behavior and promotes prosocial responses. *Emotion, 12*(2), 338-350. https://doi.org/10.1037/a0026118.

[86] Benn, R., Akiva, T., Arel, S., & Roeser, R. W. (2012). Mindfulness training effects for parents and educators of children with special needs. *Developmental Psychology, 48*(5), 1476-1487. https://doi.org/10.1037/a0027537.

[87] Hirshberg, M. J., Frye, C., Dahl, C. J., Riordan, K. M., Vack, N. J., Sachs, J., . . . Goldberg, S. B. A randomized controlled trial of a Smartphone-based well-being training in public school system employees during the COVID-19 pandemic. *Journal of Educational Psychology*, 18. https://doi.org/10.1037/edu0000739.

[88] Jennings, P. A., Brown, J. L., Frank, J. L., Doyle, S., Oh, Y., Davis, R., . . . Greenberg, M. T. (2017). Impacts of the CARE for Teachers Program on teachers' social and emotional competence and classroom interactions. *Journal of Educational Psychology, 109*(7), 1010-1028. https://doi.org/10.1037/ edu0000187.

[89] Jeffcoat, T., & Hayes, S. C. (2012). A randomized trial of ACT bibliotherapy on the mental health of K-12 teachers and staff. *Behaviour Research and Therapy, 50*(9), 571-579. https://doi.org/10.1016/ j.brat.2012.05.008.

[90] Hirshberg, M. J., Frye, C., Dahl, C. J., Riordan, K. M., Vack, N. J., Sachs, J., . . . Goldberg, S. B. (2022). A randomized controlled trial of a Smartphone-based well-being training in public school system employees during the COVID-19 pandemic. *Journal of Educational Psychology, 114*(8), 1895-1911. https://doi.org/ 10.1037/edu0000739.

[91] Lewis, S. (2009). *Improving school climate: Findings from schools implementing restorative practices. Bethlehem, PA: International Institute of Restorative Practices*. Retrieved from https://www.iirp.edu/pdf/IIRP-Improving-School-Climate.pdf.

[92] Skiba, R. J., Arredondo, M. I., & Rausch, M. K. (2014). *New and developing research on disparities in discipline*. Bloomington, In: The Equity Project at Indiana University. https://www.njjn.org/uploads/digital-library/OSF_Discipline-Disparities_Disparity_NewResearch_3.18.14.pdf.

[93] Curran, F. C. (2020). A matter of measurement: How different ways of measuring racial gaps in school discipline can yield drastically different conclusions about racial disparities in discipline. *Educational Researcher, 49*(5), 382-387. https://doi.org/10.3102/0013189X20923348.

[94] Skiba, R. J., Arredondo, M. I., Gray, C., & Rausch, M. K. (2018). Discipline disparities: New and emerging research in the *United States The Palgrave international handbook of school discipline, surveillance, and social control* (pp. 235-252): Palgrave Macmillan, Cham.

[95] Lodi, E., Perrella, L., Lepri, G. L., Scarpa, M. L., & Patrizi, P. (2022). Use of restorative justice and restorative practices at school: A systematic literature review. *International Journal of Environmental Research and Public Health, 19*(1), 96. https://doi.org/10.3390/ijerph19010096.

[96] Augustine, C. H., Engberg, J., Grimm, G. E., Lee, E., Wang, E. L., Christianson, K., & Joseph, A. A. (2018). *Can restorative practices improve school climate and curb suspensions: An evaluation of the impact of restorative practices in a mid-sized urban school district*. RAND Corporation, RR-2840-DOJ. Retrieved from https://www.rand.org/pubs/research_reports/RR2840.html.

[97] Acosta, J., Chinman, M., Ebener, P., Malone, P. S., Phillips, A., & Wilks, A. (2019). Evaluation of a whole-school change intervention: Findings from a two-year cluster-randomized trial of the restorative practices intervention. *Journal of Youth and Adolescence, 48*, 876-890. https://doi.org/10.1007/s10964-019-01013-2.

[98] Harper, C. R., Johns, M. M., Orenstein, D., Pampati, S., Jones, T. M., Leonard, S., . . . Robin, L. (2022). Association between LGBTQ student nondiscrimination laws in selected states and school district support for gay-straight alliances. *Journal of Adolescent Health, 70*(4), 584-587. https://doi.org/10.1016/j.jadohealth.2021.11.032.

[99] Wright, M. F., Wachs, S., & Gámez-Guadix, M. (2022). The role of perceived gay-straight alliance social support in the longitudinal association between homophobic cyberbullying and LGBTQIA adolescents' depressive and anxiety symptoms. *Journal of Youth and Adolescence, 51*(7), 1388-1396. https://doi.org/10.1007/s10964-022-01585-6.

## Chapter 3

# Caring for Our Kids: Supporting Mental Health in the Transition from High School to College*

## Committee on Health, Education, Labor, and Pensions

Wednesday, November 30, 2022
U.S. Senate, Subcommittee on Children and Families,
Committee on Health, Education, Labor, and Pensions,
Washington, DC.

The Subcommittee met, pursuant to notice, at 10:01 a.m., in room 430, Dirksen Senate Office Building, Hon Robert Casey, Chairman of the Subcommittee, presiding.

Present: Senators Casey [presiding], Murphy, Kaine, Hassan, Smith, Cassidy, Marshall, and Tuberville.

### Opening Statement of Senator Casey

The CHAIRMAN. This hearing will come to order. I want to thank everyone for being here, especially our witnesses, for their testimony today and the expertise they bring to bear, as well as traveling to be with us.

I want to thank Ranking Member Cassidy for his leadership on these issues, as well as working with us and our two staffs to arrange this Subcommittee hearing. I don't think it comes as news to many Americans that our Nation faces a crisis in adolescent mental health.

At any given time, 1 in 5—1 in 5 adolescents are experiencing a mental, developmental, or behavioral disorder. The COVID–19 pandemic placed a heavy burden on young people struggling with their mental health.

One survey of high school students found that 44 percent persistently felt sad or hopeless. In addition to that survey, we know of other surveys that find similar results. We know, for

---

* This is an edited, reformatted and augmented version of Hearing before the Subcommittee on Children and Families, of the Committee on Health, Education, Labor, and Pensions, United States Senate, One Hundred Seventeenth Congress, Second Session, on Examining Caring for Our Kids, Focusing on Supporting Mental Health in the Transition from High School to College, Publication No. S. HRG. 117–557, dated November 30, 2022.

In: Understanding Youth Mental Health
Editor: Michael A. Post
ISBN: 979-8-89530-700-7

example, that about half of all people who experience a mental health condition begin presenting symptoms by the age of 14, making high school a critical intervention point.

The Biden administration and the 117th Congress has recognized the importance of mental health support in our schools and have made critical investments in our communities to this end. It is critical that students, particularly those with disabilities, feel both academically and emotionally supported in their schools.

Most schools have some mental health supports in place, like peer support, one on one counseling, and outside care referrals. But many students are falling through the cracks. To reach every student, we need all hands on deck.

That means far more mental health professionals and making every student, every caregiver, teacher, and school staff member a part of the solution to teen mental health crisis. In 2021, the average ratio of students to school counselors was 415 to 1, despite a recommended ratio of 250 to 1.

We cannot expect progress in addressing this crisis without lifting up professionals in such high impact settings. We must do more to identify and help secondary students in need of mental health support, especially as they prepare for college. The transition to college is, of course, both exciting but also very stressful and a very stressful time for our teens.

Living away from home and an emotional support system for the first time, it is easy for students to be caught up in their new life and not get the mental health care that they need. When students arrive on campus, they may confront new challenges to adjusting to hectic schedules, making new friends, and keeping up with academic expectations, which can compound feelings of stress and despair.

The social isolation of the pandemic left students unprepared for the social transition to college and less likely to establish connections with peers and mentors at school. These forces are compounded for students entering college with a mental health condition.

Without supports in place, these students care can and often does lapse just when they need it the most. The task of navigating a switch to telehealth or finding a new provider in college largely falls on the students, and if available, their parents.

Students are left to maneuver the complexities of the health care system, including insurance coverage. With a shortage of providers in most areas and many not covered by insurance, finding an affordable and timely care can be very onerous.

Data shows that when college students don't get the mental health care that they need, it can lead to major disruptions in their education, as unaddressed mental health needs are associated with poorer academic performance and lower rates of degree completion.

In a survey conducted in 2021, over 70 percent of bachelor's and associate degree students who had considered taking a break from school in the past 6 months said emotional stress was an important reason.

In order to set students up for success in college, early identification of mental health needs and ready access to treatment are, of course, critical. When students move away from home and transition to college and adult life, continuity of care and reasonable accommodations help them manage new stressors and lead—new stressors and lead meaningful, productive lives.

That kind of support shouldn't be a luxury for students experiencing mental health conditions, but today, unfortunately, it is. Families are getting priced out of timely mental health care and the evaluations needed for mental health accommodations can cost thousands of dollars out-of-pocket.

Because of gaps in our pediatric mental health care system, many needs are not being addressed until far too late, if at all. Accessing timely mental health care that is covered by insurance shouldn't feel like winning the lottery. It should be the same as getting care for any other health condition.

That is why Ranking Member Cassidy and I introduced the Health Care Capacity for Pediatric Mental Health Act, which would establish grant programs to expand mental health integration, workforce training, and care capacity among providers to treat young people.

Senator Cassidy and I also introduced the RISE Act, which would provide information to students with mental health disabilities and their families to help them select the right college and streamline disability documentation requirements so that the cost of repetitive testing is not a barrier to reasonable accommodations.

In addition, Senator Portman and I introduced the Investing in Kids Mental Health Now Act, which would provide guidance to states on expanding pediatric mental health care capacity, and a Medicaid payment increase for pediatric behavioral health services to strengthen the continuum of care for many children.

While we have made strides this Congress to address the mental health crisis among our youngest Americans, it is clear that more work needs to be done. When pediatric emergency departments across the country are overwhelmed with children in need of mental health care, it is a cry for help.

Young people experiencing mental health challenges need somewhere to go and get the care they really need in a supportive environment where they can thrive. So I look forward to hearing from today's witnesses about how we can expand mental health support in preparation for and in the transition to college.

I will now turn to Ranking Member Cassidy for his opening statement.

## Opening Statement of Senator Cassidy

Senator CASSIDY. Somewhere there is a teenager who will one day be sitting in that chair, in this chair, and be speaking of ranking members and chairs and be sitting on the dais, and she or he is our future leader.

Our obligation to that person is how do we best equip she or he in order to be the person sitting there are sitting here? And of course, I hope they are all Republicans, but maybe you can only hope for so much. And so we have to take that within the context of what we are currently addressing.

The context which we are currently addressing is that 3 years of COVID have just had their toll upon the mental health of adolescents and college students. The isolation that formerly was kind of never there because you were always with others, under COVID it became so pronounced that those who had issues could not convey them to others, but rather kept them within themselves, and we see, if you will, despair.

Now, the studies—the statistics bear out the intuition. Suicide, third leading cause of death among those 15 to 24 in 2021. Mental health emergency room visits increased 25 percent in children, 30 percent in teens in 2020. And I go back, this is more than a statistic, it is our future. So the question is, how do we care for those teens who are our future?

Now, several people on the dais here, we have worked together. We need to reauthorize the Mental Health Reform Reauthorization Act of 2022, which Senator Murphy and I worked back on in 2016, and we need to reauthorize it. It expired in September.

There is an urgency here that we need to accomplish. I will point out, since this law passed, all 50 states now have wraparound, coordinated specialty care for teens with early psychosis.

Previewing my question for Dr. Weiss will be, why has the reach been so limited? When we put this in, we wished to have those wraparound services so that when the young person has his first psychotic episode at 16, it is his last psychotic episode because everything he needs to return him to wholeness is wrapped around and it becomes a distant memory, but not a life defining event.

We need to ensure that would occur. We also, as my co-sponsor of the legislation, Senator Casey spoke out, need to help with that transition to college from high school. And again, the Mental Health Reform Reauthorization Act of 2022 can help achieve this.

Now, we have had success on, aside from the bill I just talked about, recent success addressing mental health issues. In response to the Uvalde shooting, there are resources that are put in that response bill, which are for troubled youth at risk of suicide, at risk of addiction, of harming others, and other mental health issues that would be in high schools.

We have increased access to mental health and crisis intervention services, telemental health and in-school mental health services. I would just echo what Senator Casey just said, two bills that we put forward, Health Care Capacity for Pediatric Mental Health Act, to increase mental health access outside of hospitals so children can stay at home and don't miss school.

The RISE Act. A child will get an IEP in a high school, say, for example, for dyslexia. Then they got to get them redone when they go to college. The underlying problem leading to the IEP has not changed.

Why are we putting this obstacle as they transition from high school to college? Oh, you got to go through it again. If the condition is not permanent, that can be indicated. But usually, for example, with dyslexia, the condition is permanent.

Why do we put obstacles for people to receive the interventions they need as they are on their pathway to be filling these halls to be our future leaders. Now, it is so wonderful you see young people stepping forward.

Ms. Williams, thank you for your example that we will hear of how you have used grief in your life in order to lead people your age to mental health wholeness. An example from my own state, Emma Benoit, who attempted suicide, but after coming out of that, has used her experience and the kind of the process of events that led her to that terrible state to help others, to help her peers avoid it.

That is the way our democracy works, in which it is not just the folks on this dais helping those younger people who are our future leaders, but those younger people providing leadership in and of themselves, so they help prepare themselves to be our future leader.

With that, I yield.

The CHAIRMAN. Thank you, Ranking Member Cassidy. Now we will turn to our witness introductions. I will provide several and Ranking Member Cassidy will provide some as well. Our first witness is Dr. Sharon Hoover.

Dr. Hoover is a licensed clinical psychologist and professor at the University of Maryland School of Medicine, Division of Child and Adult Psychiatry. Dr. Hoover is also the co-director of the National Center for School Mental Health and the Director of the National Child Traumatic Stress Network's Center for Safe, Supportive Schools.

We want to thank Dr. Hoover for being here. Maybe hadn't had to travel as long as some of the others. We are grateful she could be with us to bring her expertise. For our second and third witnesses, I will turn to Ranking Member Cassidy.

Senator CASSIDY. I get to introduce two people today, two folks from Louisiana. I will begin with Dr. Curtis Wright. Dr. Wright is a Vice President for Student Affairs at Xavier University in New Orleans. He oversees numerous programs dedicated to improving student life, including education, wellness, campus safety, and athletics.

Before joining Xavier, Dr. Wright served as the Dean of Campus Life at Wagner College in New York City, and oversaw multicultural affairs at New York University, and in residence education at the University of Arkansas at Little Rock.

Dr. Wright earned his B.A. in Sociology, a Master's of Education in Adult Education from the University of Arkansas, and a Doctorate in Higher Education Management from the University of Pennsylvania. Dr. Wright's experience will allow him to speak with a wealth of knowledge and experience to us. Thank you.

Dr. Ashley Weiss. Dr. Weiss is an Associate Professor of Psychiatry and the Director of Medical Student Education and Psychiatry at Tulane University School of Medicine. She received her Bachelor of Science at Loyola University in New Orleans, and a Master of Public Health at Tulane.

Attended medical school at Lake Erie College of Osteopathic Medicine in Florida, returned to New Orleans to do a Residency in Psychiatry and Subspecialty Fellowship in Child and Adolescent Psychiatry at Tulane.

After developing expertise and caring for the young person's mental health during her medical training, Dr. Weiss built the first comprehensive first episode psychosis care program in New Orleans called Epic NOLA.

She also launched Calm, which is a community education campaign to increase people in Louisiana's awareness about emerging psychosis symptoms and available treatment. In my medical practice, I worked in the same setting as Dr. Weiss, taking care of the uninsured and the chronically mentally ill.

They would have, I tell you, benefited from your expertise, Dr. Weiss, so I am grateful that you are here, and we look forward to hearing how your experience and your education can improve the support for our youth. Mr. Casey.

The CHAIRMAN. Thank you, Ranking Member Cassidy. Our final witnesses, Ms. Brooklyn Williams. Brooklyn is a high school senior at Baldwin High School in Pittsburgh, Pennsylvania, where she has founded the Chill Club, an offshoot of the Allegheny Health Network's Chill Project.

The Chill Club is an open door mindfulness club aimed at supporting students coping with the stresses and anxieties of high school. Brooklyn, we are very pleased to welcome you here today.

We will turn to our witnesses for their opening statements. We will begin with Dr. Hoover.

## Statement of Sharon Hoover, Ph.D., Professor of Psychiatry and Co-Director of the National Center for School Mental Health, University of Maryland School of Medicine, Baltimore, MD

Dr. HOOVER. Good morning, thank you. I want to express my thanks to you, Chairman Casey, Ranking Member Cassidy, and to all the Members of the Subcommittee for inviting me here to speak with you about these important issues, and for your commitment to the mental health and well-being of our young people.

Again, my name is Sharon Hoover, and I will be speaking to you today from my perspective as a Professor of Child and Adolescent Psychiatry and also the co-Director of the National Center for School Mental Health and the National Center for Safe, Supportive Schools, both funded by the U.S. Department of Health and Human Services.

I also speak to you through my lens as a parent of three young people, a 9th grader, an 11th grader, and a freshman in college, so these issues are near and dear to my own heart. We are all concerned about the growing mental health needs of our young people.

The good news is that there are many strategies and effective programs to support and promote youth mental health and to also support their effective transition from high school to college. And I hope we can get into some of those programs today. I am going to share three important ideas with you this morning.

No. 1, invest early in nurturing environments for families and schools. We have incontrovertible evidence that the vast majority of challenges impacting our adolescents and young adults could be prevented by diminishing, or diminished rather by creating nurturing environment, starting early, and continuing into middle school and high school and beyond.

In Dr. Anthony Bacon's book, The Nurture Effect, he details decades of scientific research into actionable steps to reduce youth problems and to produce caring—to reduce youth problems rather, and to produce caring and productive young people.

Just as we were able to reduce the prevalence of smoking decades ago with a national public health movement, at this point in time, we need a relentless public health movement to increase the prevalence of nurturing environments that minimize toxic conditions and promote pro-social behavior in our young people.

In the earliest years of children's development, effective family interventions include things like the incredible years, nurse family partnerships, the triple-p parenting program, which exist in many of the states across our Nation but are not really at full scale as they should be. In elementary years and beyond, interventions like Family Checkup are helpful to support parents as they handle some of the common problems of their children, as they use reinforcement to promote pro-social behavior, as they monitor their children's behavior and help set limits, and as they improve family communication and problem solving.

Students who receive the family checkup program in sixth grade are much less likely to be depressed, to use substances, and to actually graduate from high school, and to not be arrested by the time they are 18.

Schoolwide systems to minimize punitive interactions and to teach and promote and ritually reinforce pro-social behaviors, and these include programs like the good behavior game, like positive behavior interventions and supports, where we have decades of research, have demonstrated long term positive impacts on adolescent risk behavior and engagement in college and career.

First, to optimize the success of our high school and college students, we must invest in nurturing environments at every level of their development. No. 2, establish comprehensive school mental health systems in all schools.

This includes supporting the mental health of all students in their classrooms through teaching social and emotional skills and mental health literacy schoolwide, and providing mental health interventions where they are, in partnership with families in schools.

Comprehensive school mental health systems not only improve mental health outcomes for our young people, but they also have, again, demonstrated success in improving really important academic indicators like attendance and grades.

In my written testimony, I provide specific examples of policies to advance mental health in schools, such as establishing mental health as a state required component of K through 12 education, like those we see in New York and Virginia, and requiring health plans to reimburse for mental health screenings that are conducted on campus.

The Hopeful Futures campaign this year released school mental health report cards across all 50 states and an accompanying legislative guide, and this is a great starting point for policymakers who wish to strengthen school mental health in their own communities, and it is detailed in my written testimony.

No. 3, we must equip high school to college transition skills for all of our students, like self-determination, time management, emotion regulation, help seeking and navigating adversity. And again, we have evidence based strategies to do all of these.

This should begin by middle school and extend into college and include efforts like self-guided modules to support emotional health, free well-being screenings at high school and college campuses, peer to peer mental health education and support, and texting warm lines where students can report concerns about themselves or others.

For youth with mental health challenges, we need to provide tailored transition supports for in-person centered planning. And two such exemplary programs include the Renew Program which was developed and studied out of the University of New Hampshire, and a program called Got Transitioned, developed by the National Alliance to Advance Adolescent Health.

I want to thank you again for the time to speak. I look forward to hearing from my fellow panelists and to our further discussion.

[The prepared statement of Dr. Hoover follows:]

## Prepared Statement of Sharon Hoover

I want to express my thanks to you, Chairman Casey, and Ranking Member Cassidy, and to all Members of the Subcommittee, for the invitation to speak with you today and for your commitment to supporting the mental health and well-being of our Nation's youth. It is a privilege to be here with you today to discuss these important issues.

My name is Sharon Hoover, and I am speaking to you from my perspective as a Professor of Child and Adolescent Psychiatry at the University of Maryland School of Medicine. I am the Co-Director of the National Center for School Mental Health and Director of the National Center for Safe Supportive Schools, both funded by the US Department of Health and Human Services. I also speak to you through my lens as a parent to three teenagers, 9th and 11th graders in high school, and a freshman in college. So, my remarks are informed by my 25 years of working with children, adolescents, and their families and schools, and are also personally meaningful to me as someone who is navigating the high school and college years of our own children.

## Youth Mental Health Needs Are Urgent and Rising

We are all concerned about the growing mental health challenges among our children and adolescents.

This year, U.S. Surgeon General Vivek Murthy as well as some of our most valued child-serving national institutions including the American Academy of Pediatrics, the American Academy of Child and Adolescent Psychiatry, and the Children's Hospital Association have highlighted the urgency of youth mental health needs.[1,2]

Youth mental health has worsened over the past decade, and this has only been exacerbated during the pandemic,[3] with increased rates of anxiety and depression symptoms and positive suicide risk screens among youth.[4,5]

*Many youth lack the fundamental skills and supports necessary to transition from high school to college and career.*

*The good news is that there are many best practices and strategies to promote student mental health and successful transition.*

As you consider opportunities to promote the well-being of our youth and set them on a path to successful college and career, I will share *three important ideas* for you to consider:

### *1. Invest Early in Nurturing Environments in Families and Schools*

Especially in the wake of the pandemic, young people have not had adequate exposure to well-being promotion. Ask kindergarten and first grade teachers right now and they will tell you that their students are not adequately learning and demonstrating the critical social, emotional, and behavioral skills that will help them to succeed at home and in school and eventually in career and college. These need to be taught both at home and in school.

I recognize that we are here today talking about high school and college students. However, I would argue that the environment of our youngest learners is what will foster or hinder their ultimate success at this critical transition. The data would back me up.

---

[1] Office of the Surgeon General. (2021). Protecting Youth Mental Health: The U.S. Surgeon General's Advisory. U.S. Department of Health and Human Services. Washington, DC.

[2] American Academy of Pediatrics. (2021, October 19). AAP-AACAP-CHA Declaration of a National Emergency in Child and Adolescent Mental Health. *https://www.aap.org/en/advocacy/child-and-adolescent-healthy-mental-development/aap-aacap-cha-declaration-of-a-national-emergency-in-child-and-adolescent-mental-health/.*

[3] Centers for Disease Control and Prevention. (2020). Youth Risk Behavior Surveillance Data Summary & Trends Report: 2009–2019. *https://www.cdc.gov/nchhstp/dear-colleague/2020/dcl-102320-YRBS2009-2019-report.html.*

[4] Mayne, S. L., Hannan, C., Davis, M., Young, J. F., Kelly, M. K., Powell, M., Dalembert, G., McPeak, K.E., Jenssen, B.P., & Fiks, A.G., (2021). COVID–19 and adolescent depression and suicide risk screening outcomes. Pediatrics, 148(3), e2021051507. *https://publications.aap.org/ pediatrics/article/148/3/e2021051507/ 179708/COVID-19-andAdolescent-Depression-and-Suicide.*

[5] Lantos, J. D., Yeh, H-W., Raza, F., Connelly, M., Goggin, K., & Sullivant, S. A. (2022). Suicide risk in adolescents during the COVID–19 pandemic. Pediatrics, 149(2), e2021053486. *https://publications.aap.org/pediatrics/ article/149/2/e2021053486/184349/Suicide-RiskinAdolescents-During-the-COVID-19.*

We have incontrovertible evidence at our fingertips that the vast majority of challenges impacting our adolescents and young adults, those transitioning from high school to college, could be prevented or diminished by creating nurturing environments starting early and continuing into middle and high school and beyond.

If I can urge you to add one book to your bookshelf today, it would be "The Nurture Effect: How the Science of Human Behavior Can Improve Our Lives and Our World" by Dr. Anthony Biglan.[6] Dr. Biglan is a Senior Scientist at the Oregon Research Institute and has been conducting research on the development and prevention of child and adolescent problem behavior for the past 30 years.

This book distills down decades of scientific research from our fields of psychology and prevention science into tangible, actionable steps that policymakers, families, and institutions like schools can take to reduce youth problems and to produce caring and productive young people.

In a nutshell, the research from years of rigorous randomized trials tells us that all successful interventions make environments more nurturing in at least three of four ways:

- Promoting and reinforcing prosocial behavior
- Minimizing socially and biologically toxic conditions, like poor nutrition and housing insecurity
- Monitoring and setting limits on influences and opportunities to engage in problem behavior
- Promoting the mindful, flexible, and pragmatic pursuit of prosocial values

These interventions can and should be implemented with both families and schools.

In the earliest years of children's development, effective interventions include things like *Incredible Years, Nurse-Family Partnerships, and the Triple P Parenting Program.* In elementary years and beyond, interventions like *Family Check Up* are helpful to support parents in handling common problems, using reinforcement to promote positive behavior, monitoring their child's behavior and setting limits, and improving family communication and problem solving. In a randomized trial of this program in middle schools in Oregon, the program significantly increased parents' monitoring and reduced family conflict. Even more striking is that although this program was implemented in 6th grade, those young people who received the program were less likely to use alcohol, tobacco, or marijuana and less likely to be arrested when they were 18 years old.

Schoolwide systems to minimize coercive and punitive interactions and to teach, promote, and richly reinforce prosocial behaviors have demonstrated long-term positive impacts on adolescent risk behavior and engagement in college and career. When implemented with fidelity, the promise of programs like *Good Behavior Game, Positive Action*, and *Positive Behavioral Interventions and Supports* to promote prosocial outcomes in our adolescents and young adults is tremendous.

*An ounce of prevention is worth a pound of cure*. Every time you move to invest in downstream interventions, first consider the root causes and reallocate investment upstream.

---

[6] Biglan, A. (2015). *The nurture effect: How the science of human behavior can improve our lives and our world.* New Harbinger Publications.

***(2) Establish Comprehensive School Mental Health Systems in All Schools***

Increasingly, schools have *comprehensive school mental health systems*, reflecting partnerships between the education and behavioral health sectors to support a full continuum of mental health supports and services, from promotion to treatment.[7] These school-based mental health supports improve vital academic indicators, including attendance, grades, and test scores.[8] Every child deserves to have this type of mental health support in their school.

Below, I provide specific examples of policies to promote universal mental health promotion for all students and to expand early identification and intervention services in schools.

**Policies to Support Universal Mental Health Promotion and Prevention Policies**

- *Require the selection of indicators of student mental health and well-being* as a core metric of school performance under federal education funding, with provisions to assist schools as they strive to perform well on these indicators. Indicators may include school climate, student-reported subjective well-being and distress, and reports of school connectedness.
- *Incentivize teaching education programs to include mental health literacy* to improve the capacity of the educator workforce to: promote mental health of all students in the classroom, including teaching of social-emotional learning competencies; identify mental health concerns and link students to needed supports and services; reduce stigma related to mental illness; and promote student and family help-seeking.
- *Establish mental health as a state-required component of K-12 curricula,* with efforts in New York and Virginia as examples. The federal government could support this state-level effort by passing a resolution encouraging states to follow existing state efforts to integrate mental health into curricula and by providing direct funding for educator training and ongoing professional development.
- *Leverage Federal Title I and Title IV funding to provide universal mental health programming for students,* including social-emotional learning programming. Joint guidance by the U.S. Department of Education and the U.S. Department of Health and Human Services could support states as they navigate these funding mechanisms to support universal mental health in schools.
- *Expand federal grants to state and local education and behavioral health authorities to increase mental health awareness and promotion in schools.* This could include the expansion of grant programming initiated in recent years by SAMHSA (e.g., Project AWARE) and the U.S. Department of Education (School Climate Transformation) that require funded states to partner with three local jurisdictions to promote student well-being and mental health training and awareness for school staff, and then to scale successful efforts statewide.

---

[7] Hoover, S. A., Lever, N. A., Sachdev, N., Bravo, N., Schlitt, J. J., Price, O. A., . . . & Cashman, J. (2019). *Advancing Comprehensive School Mental Health Systems: Guidance from the Field.* National Center for School Mental Health, University of Maryland School of Medicine.

[8] Kase C, Hoover S, Boyd G, et al: Educational outcomes associated with school behavioral health interventions: a review of the literature. J Sch Health 2017; 87:554–562.

**Policies to Support Early Identification, Intervention, and Treatment in Schools**

- *Expand existing federal workforce development programs* (e.g., Behavioral Health Workforce Education and Training Program, National Health Service Corps, Minority Fellowship Program) to increase the school mental health workforce. This strategy can also be applied to federal loan repayment programs by increasing incentives for providers who choose schools as a service setting.
- *Expand federal, state, and local funding to ensure adequate staffing and professional development for student instructional support personnel,* including school psychologists, school social workers, school counselors and school nurses. Funding expansion could include increased investments in Title I of the Every Student Succeeds Act (ESSA) to provide additional mental health staffing for students living in poverty and in Title I, Title II, and Title IV of ESSA and IDEA to increase opportunities for professional development. State and local investments could include competitive salary and benefits packages to recruit and retain school mental health providers and supplementing federal funding for staffing and professional development.
- *Strengthen and support funding for mental health services by investing in school Medicaid programs.* Ensure states and school districts are fully participating in school Medicaid by modernizing existing guidance for schools to provide clarity and best practices in school Medicaid, including those that address mental health prevention and early intervention.
- *Require health plans to reimburse for mental health screenings conducted in schools.* Follow guidance from the American Academy of Pediatrics and the American Academy of Child and Adolescent Psychiatry to cover universal mental health screening as a mechanism for improving mental health and reducing mental illness. Coverage should include screening conducted during well-child exams in pediatric primary care, and also extended screening conducted in schools.
- *Maximize Medicaid, Children's Health Insurance Program (CHIP) and private reimbursement for school mental health services,* including early identification, intervention, and treatment. This may include better understanding and leveraging existing state Medicaid allowances for school mental health or the initiation of state plan amendments to improve school mental health coverage. As outlined in the 2019 Joint Informational Bulletin from The Centers for Medicaid and Medicare Services (CMS) and SAMHSA, several states already access Medicaid and other payers, including private insurers, to cover school and community professionals' delivery of mental health services in schools. The Centers for Medicaid and Medicare Services (CMS), the U.S. Department of Education and the U.S. Department of Health and Human Services could offer technical assistance to states seeking to improve Medicaid and other payer coverage of school mental health.
- *Expand reimbursement and technical assistance for telemental health services in schools.* Given the current national shortage of mental health specialists, particularly in rural settings, schools will benefit from access to telemental health consultation and direct service, facilitated by public and private insurance coverage and federaland state-supported technical assistance.
- *Implement accountability mechanisms that require the implementation of high-quality, evidence-based practices that align with national performance standards for school*

*mental health.* Federal, state, and local investments should shift their metrics away from counting frequency and duration of services to measuring the implementation of national best practices for school mental health care and impacts of school mental health services provision on psychosocial and academic outcomes (see *www.theSHAPEsystem.com*).

The *Hopeful Futures Campaign*, a coalition of national organizations committed to ensuring that every student has access to effective and supportive school mental health care, released this year the first ever "America's School Mental Health Report Card and Action Center," with *individual report cards* for all 50 states and the District of Columbia. These school mental health report cards highlight accomplishments and provide important action steps to help address the children's mental health crisis in every state. They serve as a great starting point for policymakers who want to strengthen school mental health supports and policies in their communities. I also urge you to review The Hopeful Futures Campaign *School Mental Health Legislative Guide* released just a few weeks ago.[9] This guide offers exemplar legislation across eight key dimensions of school mental health (detailed below) and can serve as a roadmap for states and Federal policymakers to advance school mental health.

**School Mental Health Legislative Guide Recommendations and Examples**

1. *School Mental Health Professionals*—We urge states to meet nationally recommended ratios for school psychologists, counselors, and social workers, and to ensure that these providers reflect the diversity of the students they serve. We also urge you to consider how to broaden your workforce beyond these specialists to include peer supports, community health workers, and bachelors level professionals that can receive a certificate in youth mental health.
   Delaware and Arizona both passed bills to implement a process of reaching national ratios for school counselors and psychologists or licensed mental health professionals. Alabama requires each local board of education to establish a school mental health service coordinator.
2. *Teacher and Staff Training*—Regular training in mental health, substance use, and suicide prevention can help educators and staff feel better equipped to identify warning signs of mental health or substance use problems, to respond appropriately, and to have knowledge of available resources and effective interventions. While many states have training in one or more of these topics, few states specifically require all three topics.
   North Dakota is notable for requiring a minimum of eight hours of youth behavioral health training every two years for teachers and staff, and specifying a range of topics, including trauma, resiliency, suicide prevention, bullying, understanding of the prevalence and impact of youth behavioral health wellness, behavioral health symptoms and risks, referral sources and evidenced-based interventions, strategies to reduce risk factors, and evidence-based behavior prevention or mitigation techniques.
3. *Funding Supports*—Sustainable funding for school mental health services is critical and Medicaid can play an important role, bringing federal matching funds that help

---

9 Hopeful Futures Campaign. State legislative guide for school mental health. August 2022. *https://hopefulfutures.us/wp-content/uploads/2022/09/State-Legislative-Guide-for-School-Mental-Health-1.pdf.*

state dollars go further. Multiple state Medicaid programs cover school mental health services, including via telehealth, for all Medicaid-enrolled students, but many others limit coverage to students on an Individualized Education Programs (IEP). Some states have taken the additional step of ensuring that all school mental health professionals are eligible to bill under their state's Medicaid program.

Michigan has taken a further step by also including certified school psychologists and licensed school social workers as Medicaid-billable providers.

4. *Well-Being Checks*—Regular checks of mental wellness can help identify students and staff who may need support. With high rates of trauma, anxiety, depression, and other mental health and substance use challenges, it's important to be able to intervene early and provide the services and supports.

   New Jersey stands out for taking a step in the right direction on well-being checks. In 2021, New Jersey created a $1 million Mental Health Screening in Schools Grant Program that provides funds for schools to administer annual depression screenings for students in grades 7–12.

   Illinois followed suit by recently Establishing the Wellness Checks in Schools Collaborative for school districts that wish to implement wellness checks to identify students in grades 7 through 12 who are at risk of mental health conditions.

5. *Healthy School Climate*—This involves policies that foster safe, supportive schools help create a positive learning environment and foster mental wellness for all students, but especially for LGBTQ students, students of color, and other highly impacted populations.

   As of last year, Arkansas Requires every school district to conduct a school safety audit every three years, including an audit of the school climate and culture.

   In 2019, Utah passed legislation that Requires creating a model school climate survey that may be used by a local education agency to assess stakeholder perception of a school environment.

6. *Skills for Life Success*—Life skills competencies, such as developing healthy relationships, responsible decision-making, and self-management, can help students at every age succeed in school and life. Washington State has gone the extra mile to support students in gaining age-appropriate K–12 life skills through multiple statutes. Many states have taken promising steps by adopting life skills competencies in K–12 but have yet to establish them in statute. One example is Arkansas, which offers the G.U.I.D.E. for Life program, which is designed to help K–12 students develop skills in growth (manage yourself), understanding (know yourself), interaction (build relationships), decisions (make responsible choices), and empathy (be aware of others).

7. *Mental Health Education*—Mental health education, when well-implemented and fully integrated into K–12 health education, can increase awareness and understanding and promote help-seeking behavior. While many states mention mental health concepts in their health education, states are increasingly passing legislation to ensure comprehensive, age-appropriate mental health education in every grade.

   New York deserves continued praise for its widely lauded mental health education law, which requires that all schools' health education programs include mental health.

Utah just passed legislation that Requires the Huntsman Mental Health Institute and the State Board of Education to coordinate to develop a youth mental health curriculum in schools.

I love that Utah was intentional about not only sharing this curriculum with schools, but also with parents and families and other youth-serving organizations so that we can all be in this together.

8. *School-Family-Community Partnerships*—Partnering with and effectively engaging families, youth, and community stakeholders, including community-based mental health providers, is vital to successfully implementing and sustaining a comprehensive school mental health system.

   Youth Behavioral Health Initiative with multiple requirements, including competitive grants to support school-linked behavioral health services for children and youth 25 years of age and younger. The bill also requires health insurance plans to cover mental health and substance use disorder treatment delivered at schools.

   Support Partnerships to fund community partnerships to meet students' behavioral health needs, to ensure partnerships provide services in a holistic and non-stigmatized manner and coordinate with youth-serving government agencies, and to develop a model for expanding school behavioral health services and maximize Medicaid and private insurance participation.

### *3. Equip Students with High School-to-College Transition Skills Using Evidence-Based Strategies*

In addition to providing early nurturing environments at home and in school and installing comprehensive school mental health systems in every school in the Nation, we can invest in evidence-based programming to equip our students with transition skills like self-determination, time management, emotion regulation, and coping with adversity.

This programming can begin in high school and extend into college, and can be fostered at home and in school, including through self-guided modules.

## Examples of Programs to Support High Schooler Mental Health as They Prepare for College and Career

- *Postsecondary Resilience Education Program (PREP)* is designed to help ease the transition to college. In this course, students master the skills needed to reach their academic goals. The structure of PREP lets students access the content in any order and to any depth, so they can focus on the skills that they would most benefit from mastering.
- *Student Curriculum on Resilience Education (SCoRE)*—Self-Paced helps students cope with the personal, social, and academic challenges of college life and prepare for future success. This online course can be purchased by individual students or offered by colleges and universities as part of a counseling program, first-year experience curriculum, wellness program, or student retention initiative.
- The JED Foundation (nonprofit that protects emotional health and prevents suicide for our nation's teens and young adults):
  - *"Set to Go"*—information and resources specific to the transition from high school to college

   - *The Transition of Care Guide,* provides a detailed steps for students and families to take during each year in high school and in college in order to transition their care. Major steps outlined: learn the details of your condition and treatment; discuss, discover, and define your personal needs to find the best college for you; manage the transition of care.
- *NAMI Mental Health College Guide* (developed in collaboration with the JED Foundation). Provides guidance about transition from high school to college focused on relationships and self-care; self-advocacy, HIPAA & FERPA; mental health, identity, race; taking care of your mental health; staying safe.
- *Guidance from American Academy of Child and Adolescent Psychiatry* Provides guidance for students with mental health challenges and their families on considerations for colleges (e.g., mental health supports on the campus, developing expectations about academic workload etc.)

**Examples of Programs to Support College Student Well-Being and Mental Health**

- *Free mental health screenings.* Drexel University's Recreation Center has a mental health screening kiosk. Students can complete a private, short mental health screening. At the end of the screening, students receive information for mental health resources and supports, if needed. The work is a product of collaboration between Drexel, the *Thomas Scattergood Foundation*, a local grant-making organization; *Screening for Mental Health, Inc.*, a nonprofit geared toward large-scale mental health screenings; and the *Philadelphia Department of Behavioral Health and Intellectual disAbility Services*.
- *Developing and fostering resilience.* Florida State University launched an online trauma resilience training tool developed through the Institute of Family Violence Studies and their College of Social Work. The Student Resilience Project developers recognized that many students coming to their university have experienced "significant family and community stress" and that stress can affect their learning. Florida State University now requires all incoming freshmen and transfer students to participate in the training, which features videos, animations, and TED-talk-style informational sessions to foster student strengths and coping strategies. Student Resilience Project: *https://strong.fsu.edu/*.
- *Encouraging talking about mental health (personal challenges and talking with peers).*
   - Kognito Program. At least 350 colleges use Kognito's "HigherEd Mental Health Suite" that "prepares learners to lead real-life conversations around mental health and suicide prevention that build resilience, a strong campus culture and strengthens relationships." Kognito Mental Health Suite: *https://kognito.com/mental-health-suite/*
- *Texting programs.* University of Sioux Falls—one of the first universities to offer free texting hotline for students called Text4Hope. Aims to guide students who are concerned about a peer or about themselves. *https://mentalhealthfoundation.ca/text4hope/*
- *Peer-to-peer approaches.*
   - Active Minds is a national organization supporting mental health awareness and education for young adults. Hundreds of college campus chapters across the

country. Active Minds changes the conversation about mental health among adolescents and young adults, reduces stigma associated with mental health conditions, and establishes a culture of caring on college and university campuses. Programs and resources are built for students, faculty, staff, administrators, and the broad campus community to ensure long-term change at the individual, campus community, and policy levels. Active Minds prioritizes the student voice to ensure a student-driven and student-focused approach in mental health promotion. We inspire mental health advocates to have conversations that have the potential to save lives. Link to information for specific higher ed programming here: *https://www.activeminds.org/programs/colleges-universities/*

- UVA Project RISE is a peer counseling service that was established in 2006 by a small group of Black students. It is a university-sponsored program that provides free, one-on-one, confidential services to enrolled University of Virginia students. Program directly connected through both the Office of African American Affairs and to the department of Counseling and Psychological Services in Elson Student Health More information here: *https://oaaa.virginia.edu/project-rise*

- *Training/resources for university faculty and staff.*
  - University of North Carolina recently trained 900 faculty and staff in *Mental Health First Aid*—aimed to provide basic skills to support students with mental health and substance use challenges
  - Penn State "*Red Folder Campaign*"—guides faculty, staff, student leaders, and others who are interacting with students to recognize, respond effectively to, and refer Penn State Students in various states of distress (high, moderate, low)
- *Rapid access to support.*
  - *Let's Talk Programs.* Many universities across the country use "Let's Talk" programs to facilitate rapid access to support. Let's Talk encourages informal one-on-one sessions with a university counselor. Many universities offer tele options.
- *College orientation.* More colleges beginning to share mental health information with students during orientation sessions. Approaches to these sessions include traditional presentations and panel discussions, role plays, short videos, and student testimonials. Goal of these sessions is for students to understand how to recognize signs of mental health challenges, know where to access resources and supports, and learn how to talk with friends who might be struggling with their mental health. Example from Northwestern University: Originally, mental health orientation sessions included information provided by expert speakers. Based on feedback from students, orientation organizers shifted to student testimonials that included narratives of alumni sharing their mental health challenges and how they received help.

In addition to programming for all students to navigate the high school-to-college transition, it is important to invest in tailored supports for students at risk for or with mental health needs. There is good evidence that providing person-centered planning and transition support for students with specific health care needs, including mental health, can significantly improve the probability of a successful transition to college and career.

As one example, colleagues at the University of New Hampshire demonstrated the success of the *RENEW program* to promote college and career readiness for students with significant emotional and behavioral disorders.

Similarly, the National Alliance to Advance Adolescent Health developed the *Got Transition* program to facilitate the health care transition of youth with special health care needs from pediatric to adult health care.

Colleagues at the University of Washington have demonstrated the success of weaving mental health education and support into a *comprehensive college preparation program* that supports vulnerable youth from middle school through successful college graduation.

I want to express my gratitude to you all for opening up this important discussion and I look forward to hearing from my fellow panelists and engaging in discussion with you all.

* * *

The CHAIRMAN. Thank you, Dr. Hoover.

Now we will turn to Dr. Wright.

## Statement of Curtis Wright, Ed.D., Vice President of Student Affairs, Xavier University of Louisiana, New Orleans, LA

Dr. WRIGHT. Subcommittee Chair Casey, Subcommittee Ranking Member Cassidy, and the Members of the Committee on Health, Education, Labor, and Pensions Subcommittee on Children and Families, thank you for the opportunity to testify today.

It is an honor and privilege to sit before you this morning as the Vice President for Student Affairs and Interim Vice President for Enrollment Management at Xavier University of Louisiana, the Nation's only Black and Catholic institution of higher education.

I was asked to testify this morning to address the importance of strengthening the continuum of mental health support for all adolescents, particularly in the years leading up to and during the transition to college. I will do that, and of course, I will also offer a particular lens which allows me to address the issues confronted by those students who choose to matriculate at HBCUs.

Chairman Casey, most students who entered Xavier University in August have never known a world without Facebook or war. While I learned how to exit the building in a single file line in preparation for a potential fire, my students have learned how to run, hide, or fight their ways out of an active shooter situation.

They are all too familiar with social, political, and racial unrest in this country, and they have probably participated in more marches or rallies than most of us in this room. They have lived through global economic recessions that resulted in family members losing their jobs, homes, and overall financial instability.

They are also still in the midst of a global pandemic that caused the entire world to stand still and reimagine what normal looks like. Some of these young people lost multiple family members due to COVID related illness, in part because they lacked access to affordable health care, and also had family members whose primary source of income meant their status as a front line worker was non-negotiable.

Our students were well acquainted with loss long before the pandemic as they routinely attended candlelight vigils, memorials, and funerals for friends who died due to gun violence, drug addiction, and suicide. What our student at Xavier experience mirrors what their peers across the country are experiencing.

The prevalence of anxiety and depression is rising across the Nation, particularly among young people. College students of all ages are more distressed than ever before, and increasing shares are enrolling with mental health histories in terms of diagnosis, treatment, and medication.

Institutions like Xavier are challenged to recreate systems of care and support to meet the growing needs of a very different student body. While students and their lived experiences they bring to campus have changed, the funds who take care of them have not.

The number of students seeking help at campus counseling centers have increased almost 40 percent between 2009 and 2015 and continued to rise until the pandemic began. This is according to data from Penn State University's Center for Collegiate Mental Health.

We, like so many of our peers, know that we can't do it alone and are developing strategic relationships with our K through 12 partners and our parent community. Access to health care, specifically mental health care, is not always readily available to students who come from rural areas, inner cities, or economically depressed communities.

Most colleges and universities were the direct beneficiary of the CARES Act, the HERF II of the Consolidated Appropriations Act of 2021, and HERF III authorized by the American Rescue Plan. These critical legislative lifelines allow us to maintain university life for our students throughout the pandemic.

The HBCU bond thrust of 2022 have altered the higher educational landscape for every single student studying at historically Black college to better their lives. For this specific set of institutions, not only to be singled out and threatened repeatedly, have caused our students untold mental anguish and stress.

Although the prosecution of those who maliciously caused the situation is a law enforcement issue, the impact on our students is not. Specific mental health focus should be directed to us as the sole recipients of these threats.

Senator Casey, over 20 years ago, a mentor asked me if I knew the difference between a high school senior and a college freshman. After often what I considered to be these profound responses, she replied without emotion, 3 months.

For incoming students, 3 months is the only thing for separate high school from college. Yet we believe that these students should arrive on campus fully prepared to not only make adult decisions, but more importantly, to live within those adult consequences. It is our responsibility to help them navigate the contested intersections of university life.

While the landscape as it relates to mental health with young people can appear bleak, I like my fellow Arkansan President William Jefferson Clinton still believe in a place called hope. I am hopeful because of the resilience of our students and the generation from which they have come.

However, for them to achieve success, we must dismantle our outdated systems that were not designed for their success. So, Mr. Chairman, I want to leave you with some recommendations.

First, similar to the guidance offered by the Office of Civil Rights related to Title IX, the Department of Education should consider offering guidance on mental health first aid to support educators and administrators for all K through 16 institutions which receive Federal funding.

No. 2, the Department of Education should extend the funding period for HERF I, II, and III, as well as the HBCU, TCU, and MSI set aside funding until August 31st, 2026. HELP must push the Senate to red line House Resolution 6893, IGNITE HBCU and MSI Act to improve HBCU facilities in response to the HBCU bomb threats and increase the sense of security on our campuses.

No. 4, financial stress is one of the most prevalent causes of anxiety for students entering college across the country. Congress should continue to advance common sense legislation to reduce the costs of higher education and support President Biden's plan to address college debt through limited student loan forgiveness.

Last, Congress should follow the lead of Senator Casey and the distinguished gentleman from the great State of Louisiana to Senator Cassidy and pass the Health Care Capacity Act for Pediatric Mental Health and the RISE Act. It has been an honor to present this testimony, and I thank the Committee for addressing this important issue.

As a leader in higher education, I know the benefits of early screening, the impact of developing coping strategies, and the importance of empowering families to train their children to become problem solvers.

We must address this mental health concern of our youth as the stakes have never been higher and our collective work should be a priority for every American. I am grateful to the Committee for leaning into this very difficult conversation, and Xavier University of Louisiana stands ready to serve as a resource and Committee partner.

For more information and details regarding my remarks, I ask that you read my written testimony for support for your review.

[The prepared statement of Dr. Wright follows:]

## Prepared Statement of Curtis Wright

### Introduction

Subcommittee Chairman Casey, Subcommittee Ranking Member Cassidy, Committee Chair Murray, Ranking Member Burr, and Members of the U.S. Senate Committee on Health, Education, Labor, and Pension's Subcommittee on Children and Families, thank you for the opportunity to testify today.

It is an honor and privilege to sit before you this morning as the Vice President for Student Affairs and Interim Vice President for Enrollment Management at Xavier University of Louisiana. Xavier was founded by Saint Katharine Drexel of the sisters of the Blessed Sacrament and is the only institution of higher education in the country that is both Catholic and a historically Black college or university (HBCU).

Xavier's mission since 1925, in part, has been to contribute to the promotion of a more just and humane society by preparing our students to assume roles of leadership and service in a global society. We do this by cultivating a diverse learning and teaching environment that incorporates all relevant educational means—including research and community service. Our students can engage in a world class practical liberal arts curriculum while living out the mission of our university.

Before the Committee today, I will address the importance of strengthening the continuum of mental health support for all adolescents, particularly in the years leading up to and during the transition from high school to college. I will also address unique challenges of students who are first generation college students, students who come from lower socio-economic backgrounds, and those who are attending HBCUs.

Chairman Casey, most students who entered Xavier University of Louisiana in August, have never known a world without Facebook or war. While I learned how to exit the building in a single file line in preparation for a potential fire, my students have learned how to "run, hide or fight" their way out of an active shooter situation. They are all too familiar with social, political and racial unrest in this country, and they have probably participated in more marches or rallies than most of us in this room. They have lived through global economic recessions that resulted in some family members losing their jobs, homes and overall financial instability. They are also emerging from a global pandemic that caused the entire world to stand still and reimagine what normal looks like. These young people have lost multiple family members due to COVID related illnesses, in part, because they lacked access to affordable healthcare. Additionally, for the student population we serve, the vast majority of their parents were front line workers, and because of that the members of their households have been more exposed to the coronavirus pandemic. Whether they are from Staten Island, Chicago or New Orleans, these students were well acquainted with loss, long before the pandemic as they routinely attended candlelight vigils, memorials, and funerals for friends who died due to gun violence, drug addiction, or suicide.

We, like so many of our peers, know that we cannot confront our students mental health challenges alone, and we are developing strategic relationships with our K– 12 partners and our parent community. We have learned that the habits of self-care that our students bring with them are informed, in part, by their environment. Access to healthcare, specifically mental healthcare, is not always readily available to students who come from rural areas, inner cities or economically depressed communities. Most colleges and universities are the direct beneficiaries of the Coronavirus Aid, Recovery, and Economic Security (CARES) Act, Public Law 116–136; the Consolidated Appropriations Act of 2021 and its Higher Education Emergency Relief Fund II (HEERF II), Public Law 116–260; and the HEERF III which was authorized by the American Rescue Plan (ARP), Public Law 117–2. These critical legislative lifelines allowed colleges and universities, like ours, to maintain university life for our students throughout the pandemic. In fact, at Xavier, we were able to expand the reach of our Counseling and Wellness office by adding additional therapists, offering enhanced services and training our community on mental health first aid. In addition to the HEERF funding received by almost every college and university, the specific funding allotted only to HBCUs, Tribal Colleges and Universities (TCUs), and Minority Serving Institutions (MSIs) has been instrumental in the accomplishments above. We are acutely aware that the provisions of three pieces of legislation have an expiration date and are working alongside community partners to identify other resources that may fill the gaps that will be left as the funding sunsets. However, we would like the Senate HELP Committee to consider passing an extension of the funding through August 31, 2026.

## Mental Health on College Campuses

What our students at Xavier experience mirrors, what their peers are experiencing across the country, even though there are some real, unique, and necessary to mention experiences recently at HBCUs. In a 2022 *Chronicle of Higher Education* article entitled, "Overwhelmed: The real campus mental-health crisis and new models for well-being," Researchers suggests the following:

> The prevalence of anxiety and depression is rising across the country, particularly among young people. College students of all ages are more distressed than ever before, and increasing shares are enrolling with mental-health histories, in terms of diagnoses, treatment, and medication." Institutions like Xavier University are challenged to recreate systems of care and support to meet the growing needs of a very different student body.

According to data cited in a 2022 article in the *Journal of Affective Disorders*, "By nearly every metric, student mental health is worsening." During the 2020–2021 school year, more than 60 percent of college students met the criteria for at least one mental health problem, according to the Healthy Minds Study, which collects data from 373 campuses nationwide (Lipson, S. K., et al., Journal of Affective Disorders, Vol. 306, 2022). In another national survey, almost three quarters of students reported moderate or severe psychological distress (National College Health Assessment, American College Health Association, 2021). While students and the lived experiences they bring to campus have evolved and changed, the funding to take good care of those students has not although the demands for that funding have increased dramatically.

Penn State's Center for Collegiate Mental Health shared, "That rising demand (for mental health care) hasn't been matched by a corresponding rise in funding, which has led to higher caseloads." nationwide, the average annual caseload for a typical full-time college counselor is about 120 students, with some centers averaging more than 300 students per counselor (CCMH Annual Report, 2021). The number of students seeking help at campus counseling centers increased almost 40 percent between 2009 and 2015 and continued to rise until the pandemic began, this is according to data from Penn State University's Center for Collegiate Mental Health (CCMH), a research-practice network of more than 700 college and university counseling centers (CCMH Annual Report, 2015).

## The Xavier University Community Response

At Xavier University of Louisiana, and institutions like us, we are working across the campus to address the growing mental health challenges of our students. At Xavier specifically, we have expanded the reach of our Counseling and Wellness office by using HEERF funding to add additional therapists and mental health counselors. Relatedly we expanded offerings around campus to empower students with the tools to address commonly known stressors, which include:

- Mindfulness and Meditation
- Time Management/Study Skills/Financial Literacy Workshops

- Creating Virtual Parent Communities
- Enhanced Fitness and Wellness Options

Recognizing the need to deepen the pool of individuals prepared to respond in emergency situations, we engage in Mental Health First Aid training. These workshops provide student leaders, faculty, and staff with basic skills in identifying mental health concerns and connected them with resources to support students before a crisis arises.

One of the major projects introduced at Xavier University is the "Take A Minute RU Ok" campaign. Guided by the notions of connection, commitment and community, students, faculty and staff are encouraged to engage in intentional self-care. Through workshops, social media and random acts of kindness, the community is routinely exposed to information about how to connect to something outside of themselves, challenged to follow-through on commitments, and invited to be involved in a community that cares.

Our unfinished work requires us to build alliances with faith communities, K–12 partners, and community groups, to share resources. We know that our students come to us from communities that have not always placed value on asking for help. Central to our efforts will be exposing our students and families to resources in their communities along with the need to reduce the stigma attached to accessing mental healthcare. We are heartened by the work that lies ahead.

## HBCU Bomb Threats

The HBCU bomb threats of 2022 have altered the higher education landscape for every student studying at an historically Black college to better their life. For this specific set of institutions, only, to be singled out and threatened repeatedly has caused our students—Black students already who have likely overcome significant societal pressures to find themselves on the verge of a life changing degree—untold mental anguish and stress. Although the prosecution of those who maliciously caused this situation is a law enforcement issue, the impact on our students is not. Specific mental health focus should be directed to us as the sole recipients of these threats. The Commerce, Justice, and Science (CJS) Appropriations bill for fiscal year 2023 should have language that guides the funding for National Joint Terrorism Task Force's ability to harden campuses specifically to HBCUs instead of generally extending the funds to states who do not report back to Congress which institutions receive it and likely award the funding to their "flagship institutions." Additionally, the Senate HELP Committee must pass the IGNITE HBCU and MSI Excellence Act (H.R. 6893) to improve HBCU facilities, harden the campuses to reduce the likelihood of these kinds of threats, and allow the cyber-related infrastructure to be strengthened enough to track these threats when they occur.

## Commonsense Solutions

As it relates to mental health and our young people, the national landscape can appear bleak. However, I have much in common with my fellow Arkansan, President William Jefferson Clinton: *I still believe in a place called Hope*. I'm hopeful because of the resilience of our students and their generation. For them to achieve success, we must dismantle outdated systems that were not designed for their success. So, Chairman Casey and Ranking Member Cassidy, I want to leave you with some recommendations:

- Similar to guidance offered by the Office of Civil Rights related to Title IX, the Department of Education should consider offering guidance on mental health first aid to support educators and administrators for all K– 16 institutions which receive Federal funding.
- The Department of Education should consider extending the funding period for the HEERF I, II, and III as well as the HBCU, TCU, and MSI set aside funding until August 31, 2026, which will allow colleges and universities to continue to provide uninterrupted coordinated care to our students as they transition to campus.
- HELP must push the Senate to "redline" H.R. 6893, the IGNITE HBCU and MSI Act to improve HBCU facilities in response the HBCU bomb threats and increase a sense of security on the campuses. The fiscal year 2023 CJS Appropriations bill must also include guiding language to direct funding to HBCUs to harden their campuses in response to the HBCU bomb threats.
- Financial stress is one the of most prevalent causes of anxiety for students entering college across the country. Congress should continue to advance common-sense legislation to reduce the costs of higher education and support President Biden's plan to address college debt through limited student loan forgiveness.
- As previously mentioned, students arrive on campus with few coping skills as well as co-morbidities that impact their academic success. Earlier intervention would provide those students with the strategies and resources that they could equip them with tools for success. With that being said, Congress should follow the lead of Senators Casey and Cassidy and pass S. 4472 the Health Care Capacity for Pediatric Mental Health Act and S. 2550, the RISE Act.

**Conclusion**

It has been an honor to present this testimony. I thank the Committee for addressing this important issue. As a leader in higher education, I know the benefits of early screening, the impact of developing coping strategies, and the importance of empowering families to train their children to become problem solvers. We must address the mental health concerns of our youth as the stakes have never been higher and our collective work should be a priority of every American. I'm grateful to the Committee for leaning into this very difficult conversation and Xavier University of Louisiana stands ready to serve as a resource and community partner.

## [Summary Statement of Curtis Wright]

Subcommittee Chairman Casey, Subcommittee Ranking Member Cassidy, Chair Murray, Ranking Member Burr, and Members of the U.S. Senate Committee on Health, Education,

Labor, and Pension's (HELP) Subcommittee on Children and Families, thank you for the opportunity to testify today.

It is an honor and privilege to sit before you this morning as the Vice President for Student Affairs and Interim Vice President for Enrollment Management at Xavier University of Louisiana. Xavier was founded by Saint Katharine Drexel of the sisters of the Blessed Sacrament and is the only institution of higher education in the country that is both Catholic and a historically Black college or university (HBCU).

Xavier's mission since 1925, in part, has been to contribute to the promotion of a more just and humane society by preparing our students to assume roles of leadership and service in a global society. We do this by cultivating a diverse learning and teaching environment that incorporates all relevant educational means—including research and community service. Our students can engage in a world class practical liberal arts curriculum while living out the mission of our university.

I was asked to testify before the Committee today to address the importance of strengthening the continuum of mental health support for all adolescents, particularly in the years leading up to and during the transition from high school to college. I will do that, and of course I will also offer a particular lens which allows me to address the issues confronted by African Americans and those choosing to matriculate at HBCUs.

Chairman Casey, most students who entered Xavier University of Louisiana in August, have never known a world without Facebook or war. While I learned how to exit the building in a single file line in preparation for a potential fire, my students have learned how to "run, hide or fight" their way out of an active shooter situation. They are all too familiar with social, political and racial unrest in this country, and they have probably participated in more marches or rallies than most of us in this room. They have lived through global economic recessions that resulted in some family members losing their jobs, homes and overall financial instability. They are also still in the midst of a global pandemic that caused the entire world to stand still and reimagine what normal looks like. Some of these young people lost multiple family members due to COVID related illnesses, in part, because they lacked access to affordable healthcare and, also, had family members whose primary source of income meant their status as front line workers was non-negotiable. Whether they are from Staten Island, Chicago or New Orleans, they were well acquainted with loss, long before the pandemic as they routinely attended candlelight vigils, memorials and funerals for friends who died due to gun violence, drug addiction, or suicide.

What our students at Xavier experience mirrors what their peers are experiencing across the country. In a 2022 *Chronicle of Higher Education* article entitled, "Overwhelmed: The real campus mental-health crisis and new models for well-being," researchers suggest:

> The prevalence of anxiety and depression is rising across the country, particularly among young people. College students of all ages are more distressed than ever before, and increasing shares are enrolling with mental-health histories, in terms of diagnoses, treatment, and medication." Institutions like Xavier University are challenged to recreate systems of care and support to meet the growing needs of a very different student body.

According to data cited in a 2022 article in the *Journal of Affective Disorders*, "By nearly every metric, student mental health is worsening." During the 2020—2021 academic year, more than 60 percent of college students met the criteria for at least one mental health problem, according to the Healthy Minds Study, which collects data from 373 campuses nationwide (Lipson, S. K., et al., Journal of Affective Disorders, Vol. 306, 2022). In another national survey, almost three quarters of students reported moderate or severe psychological distress (National College Health Assessment, American College Health Association, 2021). While students and the lived experiences they bring to campus have evolved and changed, the funding to take good care of those students has not although the demands for that funding have increased dramatically.

Penn State's Center for Collegiate Mental Health shared, "That rising demand (for mental health care) hasn't been matched by a corresponding rise in funding, which has led to higher caseloads." nationwide, the average annual caseload for a typical full-time college counselor is about 120 students, with some centers averaging more than 300 students per counselor (CCMH Annual Report, 2021). The number of students seeking help at campus counseling centers increased almost 40 percent between 2009 and 2015 and continued to rise until the pandemic began, this is according to data from Penn State University's Center for Collegiate Mental Health (CCMH), a research-practice network of more than 700 college and university counseling centers (CCMH Annual Report, 2015).

We, like so many of our peers, know that we can't do it alone and are developing strategic relationships with our K–12 partners and our parent community. We've learned that the habits of self-care that our students bring with them are informed, in part, by their environment. Access to healthcare, specifically mental healthcare, is not always readily available to students who come from rural areas, inner cities or economically depressed communities. Most colleges and universities are the direct beneficiaries of the Coronavirus Aid, Recovery, and Economic Security (CARES) Act, Public Law 116–136; the Higher Education Emergency Relief Fund (HERF II) of the Consolidated Appropriations Act of 2021, Public Law 116–260; and the HEERF III authorized by the American Rescue Plan (ARP), Public Law 117–2. These critical legislative lifelines allowed colleges and universities to maintain university life for our students throughout the pandemic. In fact, at Xavier, we were able to expand the reach of our Counseling and Wellness office by adding additional therapists, offering enhanced services and training our community on mental health first aid. The traditional HEERF funding along with the funding allotted specifically to HBCUS, Tribal Colleges and Universities, and Minority Serving Institutions (MSI) were used to increase these services. We are acutely aware that these funding sources have an expiration date, and while we are working alongside community partners to identify other resources that may fill the gaps that will be left as the funding sunsets, one of our asks today is that sunset deadline be extended through at least August 31, 2026.

The HBCU bomb threats of 2022 have altered the higher education landscape for every student studying at an historically Black college to better their life. For this specific set of institutions, only, to be singled out and threatened repeatedly has caused our students—Black students already who have likely overcome significant societal pressures to find themselves on the verge of a life changing degree—untold mental anguish and stress. Although the prosecution of those who maliciously caused this situation is a law enforcement issue, the impact on our students is not. Specific mental health focus should be directed to us as the sole recipients of these threats. The Commerce, Justice, and Science (CJS) Appropriations bill for fiscal year 2023 should have language that guides the funding for National Joint Terrorism Task Force's ability to harden campuses specifically to HBCUs instead of generally extending the funds to states who do not report back to Congress which institutions receive it and likely award the funding to their "flagship institutions." Additionally, the Senate HELP Committee must pass the IGNITE HBCU and MSI Excellence Act (H.R. 6893) to improve HBCU facilities, harden the campuses to reduce the likelihood of these kinds of threats, and allow the cyber-related infrastructure to be strengthened enough to track these threats when they occur.

While the national landscape as it relates to mental health with young people can appear bleak, I like my fellow Arkansan, President William Jefferson Clinton, *still believe in a place called Hope*. I'm hopeful because of the resilience of our students and the generation from which they come. However, for them to achieve success, we must dismantle outdated systems that were not designed for their success. So, Madam Chair, I want to leave you with some recommendations:

- Similar to guidance offered by the Office of Civil Rights related to Title IX, the Department of Education should consider offering guidance on mental health first aid to support educators and administrators for all K– 16 institutions which receive Federal funding.
- The Department of Education should consider extending the funding period for the HEERF I, II, and III as well as the HBCU, TCU, and MSI set aside funding until August 31, 2026, which will allow colleges and universities to continue to provide uninterrupted coordinated care to our students as they transition to campus.
- HELP must push the Senate to "redline" H.R. 6893, the IGNITE HBCU and MSI Act to improve HBCU facilities in response the HBCU bomb threats and increase a sense of security on the campuses. The fiscal year 2023 CJS Appropriations bill must also include guiding language to direct funding to HBCUs to harden their campuses in response to the HBCU bomb threats.
- Financial stress is one the of most prevalent causes of anxiety for students entering college across the country. Congress should continue to advance common-sense legislation to reduce the costs of higher education and support President Biden's plan to address college debt through limited student loan forgiveness.
- As previously mentioned, students arrive on campus with few coping skills as well as co-morbidities that impact their academic success. Earlier intervention would provide those students with the strategies and resources that they could equip them with tools for success. With that being said, Congress should follow the lead of Senators Casey and Cassidy and pass S. 4472 the Health Care Capacity for Pediatric Mental Health Act and S. 2550, the RISE Act.

For more information and details regarding my remarks, I ask that you read my written testimony submitted for your review.

The CHAIRMAN. Dr. Wright, thanks very much for your testimony.

Dr. Weiss.

## Statement of Ashley Weiss, DO, Mph, Director of Medical Student Education in Psychiatry, Tulane University School of Medicine, New Orleans, LA

Dr. WEISS. Thank you for having me here, Chairman Casey, and Ranking Member, Dr. Cassidy, and the rest of the Committee.

Again, my name is Ashley Weiss. I am a Child and Adolescent Psychiatrist at Tulane School of Medicine in New Orleans, Louisiana. I specialize in first episode psychosis. Psychosis is a symptom typically associated with the onset of schizophrenia and bipolar disorder.

These illnesses can have devastating consequences, from the increased risk of cardiovascular disease and premature death, to the ramifications of being chronically marginalized by society. Why am I bringing up illnesses like schizophrenia in a hearing about mental health and high school and college students? It is because this is where they start, in our young people and not by any fault of their own.

Adolescence is a time of incredible brain maturation, and for some, this maturing process goes awry, leading to the emergence of severe psychiatric disorders. These illnesses don't discriminate. They were present pre-COVID, and they are still present now with a little bit of a different context.

Globally, these illnesses lead to the greatest costs, both directly and indirectly. So what is psychosis? Psychosis can be described as a loss of touch with reality. Examples of psychosis symptoms are hallucinations, confusion, and delusions.

These experiences start small, like mishearing sounds as voices or beginning to feel as if people are watching you. This paranoid feeling could turn into a belief, a delusion, where one is convinced the world is literally out to get them. And it is difficult but very necessary to imagine what this might feel like for a young person.

Some facts about psychosis. 3 out of 100 people will experience psychosis in their lifetimes, mostly occurring for the first time between ages 16 and 25. For every one person experiencing psychosis, six other friends or family are directly impacted.

In the U.S., the average time one experiences psychosis prior to treatment is 72 weeks, not days, weeks. 1 in 10 will attempt or complete suicide with the highest risk being after the first episode.

To give these statistics a local context, George Washington University enrollment is about 26,000 students, which means almost 800 will experience psychosis annually and will not receive appropriate care for over a year.

Over 4,500 friends and family are impacted. Nearly 80 will attempt or complete suicide. So there is a sense of urgency because time is not on our side. The impact of the brain can be deteriorating.

The last three decades of research show that specialized intervention as early as possible after psychosis onset improves outcomes across the board. There is no time to wait. The same philosophy is already accepted in stroke intervention and should be accepted in psychosis intervention as well.

In 2015, I started the Early Psychosis Intervention Clinic in New Orleans. We have treated nearly 100—nearly 1,000 people since we opened our doors. Our multidisciplinary team provides coordinated specialty care, including medication management from psychiatrists, individual family, and group therapy, and wellness coaching.

All treatment is deeply individualized, with the goal of getting young people back on track, and that often means back to school or graduating or to their first job. But what we do in the clinic is not enough. Because of the need for early treatment in psychosis, we are forced to think about early detection.

We have a robust early detection campaign called Calm, which was mentioned, and this aims to educate the community about psychosis, debunk myths, reduce stigma so hopefully people will feel comfortable and safe coming forward for treatment.

Our goal is that an individual comes forth on their own and they don't have to wait for someone else to bring them in, and they certainly don't have to wait for the police to pick them up having an acute psychosis and take them to the emergency room.

There are significant challenges and barriers that must be considered. For most people, recovery can take many, many months, but time continues to pass for everyone else in their lives. Their friends have often moved on, graduated, moved away to college, or started their first job. They often feel misunderstood, ashamed, quickly leading to the loss of confidence and increased isolation.

There is a conspicuous gap in school based recognition of these needs for these individuals and keeping them engaged or even welcoming them back after their recovery. I have multiple college students in my program.

Students in every college in Louisiana, actually, which makes me very proud, who didn't even know that they were eligible for retroactive medical leave that would erase incompletes from their transcripts, who have crushing student loan debt from the semesters that they became ill. We are often the first place to provide guidance in how to approach these issues. There are financial threats to programs like ours.

Although our program is committed to long term care, most programs like ours don't go beyond two to 3 years. We are now realizing that people lose their gains when they lose specialized care. But how do we pay for continued care?

We have subsidized our growth through the Congressional legislation mandating a portion of the SAMHSA block grant be set aside for early, severe mental illness. We appreciate this opportunity because it covers the necessary care that is not covered by insurances.

In our State of Louisiana, Medicaid and commercial insurers do not reimburse any of the coordination of care that is required to provide this model. No case management, no record review, no coordination with community partners like schools or hospitals, no treatment team meetings.

Without the coordination, the risk of relapse increases exponentially. And commercially insured patients might have two co-pays a week, that will quickly add up after a month, and that becomes unattainable.

People in this age group fall off their parents' insurances and they might not even qualify for Medicaid. And then barriers exist beyond our clinic. There is a pervasive lack of education coupled with ample misinformation about psychosis and what it even is.

This gap in education exists in the general public but extends even to mental health professionals. Psychosis is not a topic in health education curriculums for high school or college students, even though their age group is most at risk.

Psychosis education is not a prominent part of the curriculum for those interfacing with high risk groups. Psychosis intervention is far from being considered an essential part——

The CHAIRMAN. Doctor, we have to wrap up.

Dr. WEISS. Okay. Can I have a 10 second wrap up?

The CHAIRMAN. Sure.

Dr. WEISS. Okay. I am here today to say out loud for the record that our youth and young adults are the vulnerable ones to these illnesses, and we cannot ignore this fact as a society any longer.

These illnesses are not curable, but they should not be associated with an inevitable lack of productivity and institutionalization. They are not preventable, but there are strategies to mitigate risks, such as early detection. They are manageable, and management does not mean doing the bare minimum.

That approach has not served us well historically, and we need to do better for our people. It is a necessity for them. We must be ambitious in our commitment to these youth and young adults so that their recovery is supported while they explore their opportunities that they deserve and expand their futures.

[The prepared statement of Dr. Weiss follows:]

## Prepared Statement of Ashley Weiss

My name is Ashley Weiss. I am a child and adolescent psychiatrist at Tulane School of Medicine in New Orleans, Louisiana. I specialize in first-episode psychosis. Psychosis is a symptom typically associated with onset of schizophrenia or bipolar disorder. These illnesses can have devastating consequences, from the increased risk of cardiovascular disease and premature death, to the ramifications of being marginalized by society. Why am I bringing up illnesses like schizophrenia in a hearing about mental health in high school and college students? Because this is where they start, in our young people, and not by any fault of their own. Adolescence is time of incredible brain maturation, and for some, this maturing process goes awry, leading to the emergence of severe psychiatric disorders.

What is psychosis? Psychosis can be described as the loss of touch with reality. Examples of psychosis symptoms are hallucinations, confusion, and delusions. These experiences start small, like mis-hearing sounds as voices, or beginning to feel as if people are watching you. This paranoid feeling could then turn into a belief, a delusion, where one is *convinced* the world is literally out to hurt them. It is difficult, but necessary, to imagine what this may feel like.

Some facts about psychosis:

- 3 out of 100 people will experience psychosis in their lifetimes
  - Mostly occurring for the *first time* between 16 and 25 years old.
- For every 1 person experiencing psychosis, 6 more friends and family are directly impacted.
- In the US, the average time one experiences psychosis prior to treatment is 72 weeks
- 1 in 10 will attempt or complete suicide with the highest risk after the first episode

To give these statistics a local context:

- George Washington University enrollment is about 26,000 students
- Which means, almost 800 will experience psychosis annually and will not receive appropriate care for over a year

- Over 4500 friends and family are impacted
- Nearly 80 will attempt or complete suicide.

There is a sense of urgency because time is not on our side when it comes to psychosis and its impact on the brain. But the last 3 decades of research shows that *specialized* intervention as early as possible after psychosis onset improves outcomes across the board. There is no time to wait. The same philosophy is already accepted in stroke intervention and should be in psychosis intervention as well.

In 2015, I started the Early Psychosis Intervention Clinic in New Orleans. We have treated nearly 1000 people since we opened our doors. Our multi-disciplinary team provides coordinated specialty care, including medication management from psychiatrists, individual and family therapy, groups, and wellness coaching. All treatment is deeply individualized, with the goal of getting young people back on track, and often this means back in school.

But what we do in the clinic is not enough. Because of need for early *treatment* of psychosis, we are forced to think about early *detection*. We have a robust early detection campaign called CALM-Clear Answers to Louisiana Mental Health that aims to educate the community about psychosis, debunk myths and reduce stigma, so hopefully people will seek help for themselves or their loved ones sooner than later.

There are significant challenges and barriers that must be considered. For most people, recovery can take many months, but time continues to pass for everyone else in their lives. Their friends have often moved on, graduated, moved away to college, or started their first job. They often feel very misunderstood and ashamed, quickly leading to loss of confidence and increased isolation. And there is a conspicuous gap in school-based recognition of the needs of these individuals, in keeping them engaged, or welcoming them back during recovery. I have multiple college students in my program who didn't know they were eligible for retroactive medical leave that may erase incompletes from transcripts, who have crushing student loan debt from the semesters they became ill. We are often the first place to provide guidance in approaching these issues.

There are financial threats to programs like ours. Although our program has committed to long-term care, most programs like ours do not go beyond 2 or 3 years, and we are realizing now that people lose their gains when they lose specialized care. But how do we pay for continued care? We have subsidized our growth through the congressional legislation mandating a portion of a SAMSHA block grant be 'set-aside' for early severe mental illness. We are appreciative of this opportunity because it covers the necessary care that is NOT covered by insurances. In our state, Medicaid and commercial insurers do not reimburse ANY of the *coordination of care* services-no case management, no record review, no coordination with community partners like hospitals and schools, no treatment team meetings-and without the coordination, the risk of relapse increases exponentially. If commercially insured, patients may have 2 co-pays a week for treatment which quickly adds up and becomes a burden. People in this age group also fall off their parents' insurance but may not qualify for Medicaid.

Barriers exist beyond the clinic. There is a pervasive lack of education (coupled with ample misinformation) about what psychosis even is. This gap in education exists in the general public but extends even to mental health professionals. Psychosis is not a topic in health education curriculums for high school or college students, even though their age-group is the *most* at-risk. Psychosis education is not a prominent part of the curriculum for those *interfacing* with the high-risk groups, for instance teachers and school-based mental health professionals. Psychosis *intervention* is far from being considered an essential part of school-based healthcare. At this point, we should not be surprised when a college freshman experiences psychosis, we should be *anticipating* this, working to disseminate knowledge about early warning signs, and strategically planning with community partners to ensure students get back on track once well.

I'm here today, to say out loud and for the record, that our youth and young adults that are the topic of this hearing are the vulnerable ones, where the *severe* mental illnesses strike. We cannot ignore this fact as a society any longer. These illnesses are *not curable* but they should not be associated with inevitable lack of productivity and institutionalization. They are *not preventable* but there are strategies to mitigate risks associated with earlier onset such as substance use. They *are manageable* but management doesn't mean doing the bare minimum. That approach has not served us well historically. A specialized approach may require a weekly meeting with their team for years, however, if that means individuals have more opportunities, more graduations, more jobs, more meaningful relationships, improved quality of life, then we are in a better place. If our communities have fewer suicides, fewer inpatient psychiatric hospitalizations, fewer ER visits, fewer people living in poverty, then we are in a better place. We collectively benefit from a progressive and more accurate narrative about psychosis, but for our young people, it is necessity. We must be *ambitious* in our commitment to these youth and young adults, so that their recovery is supported while they explore opportunities and expand their futures.

The CHAIRMAN. Doctor, thanks very much.
We will conclude now with Brooklyn Williams.

## Statement of Brooklyn Williams, High School Senior and Founder of the Chill Club, Pittsburgh, PA

Ms. WILLIAMS. Senator Casey, Senator Cassidy, thank you for listening to my story. And everyone else here, thank you for listening to my testimony. Looking at me, you might not suspect that I am dealing with a lot of internal struggles.

I am speaking in public so you might not suspect that I have severe social anxiety. I cover my eye bags, and no one tells that I struggle with insomnia. I ate my entire breakfast this morning, but I still have bulimia.

I got out of bed and did my hair, so to not look depressed. Just because I did not fit the description of someone with mental health problems that does not mean that I am fine, and I feel like we as a society overlook people with these health issues because they do not fit into the concrete mold in the textbooks of mental health symptoms.

There is a fluidity in the way each of us experience mental health, and I feel like schools and communities only intervene when it becomes intensely severe, or in unfortunate cases too late. In my experience, mental health highs and lows happen in waves, always sporadic, and most recently due to being a high school senior, in my last year of childhood.

As a child, I do not remember feeling there was any disordered thinking in my life. Yet looking back on it, I feel that mental health was not ever a topic of conversation at school or home until I was 18.

When I was 13, my mom passed away from stage four metastatic breast cancer after a 10 yearlong battle with the disease. Losing her devastated my family and I, and I felt like a portion of myself died with her. As much as I love my dad and my siblings, my mom was my lifeline and my best friend.

Although we tried to prepare as much as possible for her passing, it was the worst feeling that I have ever experienced. The following year was a blur of numbness and therapy sessions, but the pandemic caused everything to shut down and I felt alone.

To combat those feelings of grief, depression, and isolation, I started to paint and do crafts to cope. It helped me express and lose myself in an activity rather than sulk in my emotions. Once school started up again, I thought, if this is making me feel better, then maybe it will make others feel better too.

I started the Chill Club where we do activities like meditation, yoga, crafts and painting every month as a group to come together and talk about our shared emotions and not worry about the problems in our lives.

From starting my club 2 years ago, I have been graced with many opportunities that helped me to share my story and cope with the loss of my mom and the struggles resulting from that, but I feel there is a long way to go. Incorporating mental health topics from an early age would be the first steppingstone I would take to support people's needs.

Talking about these issues with teens before they are reaching for help. Providing more accessible outreach professionals in schools, having all students speak to these professionals and not only the ones that come for help.

Allowing for mental health absent days to be excused, just like having physical illnesses, because mental health and physical health are equally as important. Allowing for anonymous assistance would also be effective because it is evident that most teens do not want to ask for help publicly.

Last, professionals working with teenagers should be more open and equipped to talk about mental health struggles by being provided with the correct necessities to help teens work through their problems. As a high school senior, I have grown to see that the process of moving from adolescence to adulthood is tricky enough with college essays, picking a major, and knowing that I will leave my childhood behind.

Providing teens with assessable professionals to speak with will only benefit our communities. Everyone needs to be aware of their mental health because it is not selective or to be stigmatized or to be put aside because it is too hard to understand.

Working through these issues will not only give opportunities for teens to grow and flourish into adults, but also to allow our communities to be stronger as we improve the way of life one kid at a time. Thank you.

[The prepared statement of Ms. Williams follows:]

## Prepared Statement of Brooklyn Williams

Thank you to all who listen to my story. Looking at me you might not suspect I am dealing with a ton of internal struggles. I am speaking in public so you would not suspect that I have severe social anxiety. I cover my eye bags so no one can tell I struggle with insomnia. I ate my entire breakfast this morning but I still have bulimia. And I got out of bed and did my hair, but I do not "look depressed." Just because I do not fit the description of someone with mental health problems does not mean that I am fine and I feel we as a society overlook people with these health issues because not all of us fit into the concrete mold in the textbooks of mental health symptoms. There is a fluidity in the way each of us experience mental health, and I feel schools and communities only intervene when it becomes intensely severe or in unfortunate cases, too late.

In my experience, my mental health highs and lows happen in waves. Always sporadic and most recently due to me being a high school senior in my last year of childhood. As a child I do not remember feeling like there was any disordered thinking in my life, yet looking back on it, I feel that mental health was never a topic of conversation at school or home until I was a teen. When I was 13, my mother passed away from stage 4 metastatic breast cancer after a 10-year long battle with the disease. Losing her devastated my family and I felt like a portion of myself died with her. As much as I love my dad and my siblings, my mother was my lifeline and best friend and although we tried to prepare as much as possible for her passing it was still the worst feeling I have ever experienced. The following year was a blur of numbness and therapy sessions, but the pandemic caused everything to shut down and I felt alone.

To combat those feelings of grief, depression, and isolation, I started to paint and do crafts to cope. It helped me to express myself and lose myself in an activity rather than sulk in my emotions. Once school started again I thought "if this is making me feel better maybe others will feel better too." So I started the Chill Club where we do activities like meditation, yoga, crafts, and painting every month as a group to come together to talk about our shared emotions and not worry about the other problems in our lives.

From starting my club 2 years ago to now I have been graced with many opportunities that have helped me to share my story and cope with the loss of my mom and the struggles resulting from that, but I feel there is still a long way to go.

Incorporating mental health topics from an early age would be the first stepping stone I would take to support people's needs. Talking about these issues with teens before they are calling out for help. Providing more accessible outreach professionals in schools and having all students speak to these people, not just the ones that come for help. Allowing for mental health absent days to be excused just like having a physical illness because mental health and physical health are equally as important. Allowing for anonymous assistance would also be effective because it is evident that most teens do not want to ask for help publicly. Last, professionals working with teenagers should be more open and equipped to talk about mental health struggles by being provided the correct necessities to help teens work through their problems.

I have grown to see that the process of moving from adolescence to adulthood is tricky enough with college essays, picking a major, knowing I will have to leave my childhood behind. So providing teens with accessible professionals to speak with will only benefit our communities. Everyone needs to be aware of their mental health because it is not selective or to be stigmatized or put to the side because it is "too hard" to understand. Working through these issues will not only give opportunities for teens to grow and flourish into adults, but to also allow our communities to become stronger as we improve the way of life one child at a time.

* * *

The CHAIRMAN. Well, Ms. Williams, thanks very much for your testimony. And I want to thank the testimony of all our witnesses, and especially to you for demonstrating uncommon courage at any age, but we have rarely heard testimony like the testimony you presented today, so we are thankful that you are here with us.

I will start a round of questions. I will just do one question to expedite our schedule a little bit. I will start with Dr. Wright. In your testimony, you described how a large number of students at your university are struggling with mental health.

Given that around half of mental health conditions begin by age 14, it is likely that many of the challenges that you are seeing, of course, started long before college. In addition to school staff, parents can be a child's strongest advocate to help with getting the needed support that they require. But these families, these parents need to know what to watch out for in their children.

How should we begin engaging families so that they are aware of the signs that their child may have a mental health, developmental, or learning disability?

Dr. WRIGHT. Thank you, Senator. That is an amazingly profound question. And when you think about the intersections of our students and their families, where they are coming from.

Many of our students come with these undiagnosed challenges. So when they first have their first moment, we don't know what to do, and neither do they.

I really believe that the work that you all are advancing in your bill, the Pediatric Access Act, will help with that because providing more touch points, training folks from the very beginning, having mental health first aid in our high schools and our elementary schools, but also in our community centers and in our churches.

Faith communities. I think so many of our families have been told that mental health is a secret, and they won't allow their students or kids to get help. So we have got to create some level of understanding that mental health is tantamount to having diabetes.

If someone has a heart attack, we don't keep them hidden away but we rush them to the hospital. And when someone is having these symptoms, we need to do it. So removing the stigma of mental health is one of the first things, but then educating their parents on how to connect them with folks in the community.

In rural spaces that might be harder. So working with them in their schools, with their counselors, working with them in their— in some spaces in their housing authority places or their therapist or their counselors there, but I do think being able to expand the reach of qualified mental health professionals in these spaces will allow those parents to see those warning signs, because many of our students' parents may not have been trained to know what to look for.

But providing schools, community organizations, resources to help them, I think will be essential in that.

The CHAIRMAN. Great. Doctor, thank you very much. I will turn to Ranking Member Cassidy. I will reclaim some of my time later.

Senator CASSIDY. I will defer to Senator Tuberville and allow a colleague to go.

Senator TUBERVILLE. Thank you very much. Thank you for being here today. This is important. I don't think people really know how important it is. I coached for 40 years. I coached in eight states.

I went to high schools all over this country, and in the 80's and 90's we had a mental health problem. But after 2000, after the internet and this thing right here came out, it has devastated our kids, and I saw it every day. So this is a huge problem. It is going to get worse before it gets better.

Dr. Wright, I am like you, faith based family—I mean, that is how we are going to overcome a lot of this. It is going to have to come through that, but we have got to be prepared. We have got to be able to recognize a problem.

Dr. Hoover, for years I saw kids come play for me and a lot of them came in, and early in my career, with very little problems. Last 20 years, they came in and they had ADHD. They said they did, and we were giving them drugs right and the left. We weren't—the doctor were prescribing them.

Do we have a medication problem in this country when it comes to mental health?

Dr. HOOVER. It is a good question. And first of all, Senator Tuberville, I want to thank you for your coaching years, because we know that all of the adults, as was said earlier, by Chairman Casey, all of the adults have a responsibility to take care of the mental health of our young people, including our coaches.

I was on a plane yesterday next to a school bus driver, and I was telling her that she has one of the most important jobs when it comes to actually supporting the everyday experience of our young people and their mental health.

In terms of medication and the diagnoses that seem to be increasing, part of it, I would argue, is really that we are just becoming more aware of the mental health needs of our young people. I would say that our medications are far from perfect.

In fact, many would argue that they are imperfect solutions to the mental health challenges of our young people.

But there is also strong evidence that some of the medications for our children and adolescents, including for ADHD, as you mentioned, and other mental health challenges, have been effective, but they are most effective when combined with other interventions, and that includes mental health interventions provided by licensed counselors, social workers and psychologists, but also the everyday supports, whether it is from the faith community, from families, or from schools.

It is not a one size fits all approach and it is not a one intervention approach. In fact, most of the data would agree that medication, combined with other interventions, is probably the most effective for some of our most debilitating disorders.

Senator TUBERVILLE. Thank you. Dr. Weiss, we locked these kids down for several years. Fortunately, in Alabama, we didn't do as much. And we had a study come out not too long ago.

We went from 49 to 39 in some areas of our scores improving. We went from 40th in the country to first in the country in graduation rate because we stayed in school. My question is, we have already spent so much money on a lot of these problems.

In your opinion, how do we best direct these funds in the future to help with mental health?

Dr. WEISS. I have to—full disclosure, I am from Alabama and grew up with Auburn football, so——

[Laughter.]

Senator TUBERVILLE. Well you did good. I should have asked you in the first place——

[Laughter.]

Dr. WEISS. The work that I do is addressing severe mental illnesses that have long been underfunded. This—we don't have a good track record historically of taking care of those with the most severe mental illnesses and they really weren't given opportunities to complete school, to go to higher education.

Now we have them actually getting well after their first episode with a severe illness, just like you could get well with diabetes diagnosis early, just like you could get well with other major medical problems.

The cost needs to be reflective and encompass what it takes to scaffold them into these opportunities that they really haven't had before. And that might be more costly than to support a kid with ADHD from high school to college.

However, we are just really learning now in the last 10 years what that is going to look like for this country. So because early intervention and severe mental illnesses is such a new concept, and literally we are talking about the last 10 years of clinics, the last 20 years of research.

Senator TUBERVILLE. Dr. Hoover, I know we are talking about going to high school to college. Half the kids in this country don't go to college. They get a job. They get in the military. How do we help them? How do we evaluate them? Because most kids that go to college get some kind of valuation through the process of higher education. How do we help those kids don't go to college?

Dr. HOOVER. It is a great question. And when I saw the subject of today's hearing, I was hoping that it was—it would go beyond just college, because we know so many young people don't go on to college.

I would wish that we had better supports in place for them. I mean, I do think it really speaks to the first issue that was brought up that we need to start earlier. The supports that we are talking about from high school to college are critical.

But what is more critical is that we put systems in place from pre-K to K–12 to actually identify and provide scaffolding and structured support for their mental health. And that doesn't just mean—I think our young panelist, as usual, said it best, which was we can't wait until there is a crisis.

We can't wait until things get really bad to provide services. We need to be doing mental health literacy in the classroom. We need to be putting systems of identification into their hands, whether it is in schools, on college campuses, or in their communities. I think the efforts to support integration into primary care are critical.

For those who do go on to career, maybe not college, they can get some of those same supports in their primary care setting. Or in other natural settings, whether that is their faith community, whether that is their family.

There are many interventions that can support families to better equip them to support their young people, including as they transition to adulthood. So we need to not just put these services in schools or primary care, but we need to put them in the hands of families.

Senator TUBERVILLE. Dr. Wright, you got to comment on any of that, about kids that don't go to college? You see probably a lot of those.

Dr. WRIGHT. We do in just—in communities in general. And I think as she was describing, being able to put those—have them access those resources in other spaces. There is dignity and honor in our work but sometimes we privilege, this transition. The way that—my profession.

But being able to make sure that they have access to an affordable health care so that they can afford to take advantage of that, whether it is through state sponsored Medicaid or private insurance. But I do think that being able to recognize that we all live within the context of our lives and learn within the context of our lives, that there is support in their spaces of work and worship.

Then they have the ability to talk with their family because, again, secrets are the things that kill us. And so but, yes, I absolutely agree with what she said.

Senator TUBERVILLE. Thank you.

Thank you, Mr. Chairman.

The CHAIRMAN. Thank you, Senator Tuberville.

We turn next to Senator Smith.

Senator SMITH. Well, thank you, Senator Casey and to Senator Cassidy, who I believe had to leave, for pulling together. I really appreciate. It is a great panel.

I think the people here in this room today believe that mental health care is health care and that every young person deserves access to the mental health care that they need. And yet, I think we also know that we failed in that mission, but we are working hard on it.

Everybody in this room, I think, in one way or another on this side has been working to expand access to mental health care in schools. I certainly have with legislation that I have introduced.

Let me ask you, Ms. Williams, if I could, so I first realized that I was suffering from depression when I was in college. I am quite sure now that I was having that experience when I was in high school, but I didn't quite understand what was going on. I didn't really see how it was incapacitating me.

I am quite sure now that my experience wasn't unique. It seems like with physical health care we do a lot of thinking around preventative care and early intervention, but yet what happens with mental health care is you get to a crisis point where you are really incapacitated and then you are sort of starting from behind.

I am wondering if you could just say from your perspective, like what that might look like in a high school setting where you are getting at it, getting at people's challenges earlier rather than later?

Ms. WILLIAMS. Yes, so I feel like in my experience, I really—I was behind like how you said. I started becoming really low in my depressive state before I thought to seek help. But I feel like now, nowadays there is a lot more—it is a lot more noticeable because of social media or being online and talking.

Like people just say anything nowadays and they talk about all the things in their lives. So like really just getting out there and saying that they are not feeling like the way they should or something. It really brings out the topic more. But I feel like starting at a young age, I feel like that would be a lot more beneficial for kids to learn about what is going on and start seeing the signs.

If they don't feel like they want to go outside or go to school or not feel the way they should feel, or they feel like they might be a little bit different, they should always have someone to talk to. And I feel like the first step to do that is to get everyone, get everyone like the care they need beforehand so nothing will escalate and get too great that no one can control it.

Unfortunately, there is so many cases of suicides and people going to psychiatric wards and stuff like that because they haven't got the help that they needed. And I have definitely seen that in my personal life. There is a lot of kids in my surrounding schools and even in my school that have lost their battle to depression or anxiety and stuff.

I feel like that should be a lot more preventable if we take the steps to reach out to their therapists and get them into schools more. Because I definitely see that also we have a school therapist on my school, but there is not that many people that are aware that there is a school therapist or have access or know the way to get to the therapy that they need or talk to the counselors, because there are thousands of kids inside one school at one time and there are four or five counselors for those thousands of kids.

Senator SMITH. Right, right. The part of it is not having enough—not having enough providers of therapy in schools. And part of it is making sure that people see the pathway from the way that they are feeling to the help that is there that they might not even realize is there, right?

Ms. WILLIAMS. Yes.

Senator SMITH. Let me just ask really any of the other panelists, I am very interested in how we can integrate physical health care and mental health care in a doctor's office setting too. And at the pediatric level, what kind of integration can we do there?

I am just wondering if you have any insight for us as we think about that, because it seems to me that a lot of folks, assuming they have access to health care, and God knows not everybody in this Country does have access to health care, physical health care. Kind of what we have seen.

Maybe, Dr. Hoover, you would like to address that.

Dr. HOOVER. I would be happy to. Thank you for the question, and I appreciate your asking, again, our youngest member of the panel first, because I think when we speak to our youth about kind of their ideas of how we can get services and supports to them, they usually have the best answers.

With respect to better integration into primary care, first of all, it can happen out in our pediatric, mental health clinics, and our young adult clinics. We often have this bifurcation. It is a really artificial bifurcation between pediatric medical care and adult medical care.

I would argue that we shouldn't just drop young people off at the age of 18 and say that they have to switch to an adult provider, that is No. 1. But in terms of integration into primary care, it can happen both in those health care settings, but also in health care settings in schools.

School based health centers, I appreciate the investment in school based health care. More young people are able to access primary care when it is offered in the context of school based health.

Whether it is out in the community, in primary care, or in the context of a school based health center, we have wonderful examples of mental health, behavioral health providers situated in those settings, but we also have many examples, especially in a more rural or smaller campuses, where they don't have the provider network to be situated physically in the building.

We actually have wonderful examples of effectively using telemental health to integrate right there into the mental health—or excuse me, into the primary care setting. And the last thing I will note is just the increased investment in the child psychiatry access programs are now called the primary care, the mental health and primary care access, where you have primary care providers that can pick up a phone or get on tele and actually reach out to a specialty mental health provider, have been instrumental.

I really appreciate the expanded coverage of that. We have seen it not only in primary care can be critical, but also in the context of schools.

Senator SMITH. Thank you. Chairman Casey, I know I am out of time. I am going to submit for the record a question that I have also around the sort of—the plethora proliferation of mental health care apps. And I am trying to understand the efficacy of those and what kinds of consumer protections we need to think about for those. Thank you very much.

The CHAIRMAN. Thank you, Senator Smith.

I will turn next to Ranking Member Cassidy.

Senator CASSIDY. I will defer to Dr. Marshall.

Senator MARSHALL. Thank you, Senator Casey. Thank you, Senator Cassidy. Again, thanks to all of our panel for being here. And especially Ms. Williams, thank you for coming. You are absolutely the most courageous person I will meet today, to come and share your story. You may be the most courageous person I will meet all week and all month, and I got a question for you in a second.

My first question is going to be for Dr. Weiss and Dr. Hoover. Prior authorization, access to care has been a bigger issue—is the No. 1 physician administrative concern in America. As an obstetrician, I saw the issue delay care for infertility patients, for high risk patients.

My friends in orthopedic surgery tell me that it is getting harder and harder to get the joint replaced and maybe that the process delays it three or 4 months' time. And meanwhile, we get the patient addicted to two narcotics.

I am just curious, in your clinical experience, when it comes to mental health issues, are you seeing any challenges in the prior authorization realm? Dr. Weiss, why don't you go first.

Dr. WEISS. It is mind numbing.

Senator MARSHALL. Mind numbing.

Dr. WEISS. Yes our clinic bills for services and we also have some money that subsidizes what is not covered.

But even the services that are covered, and I deal with a lot of antipsychotic medication and long acting antipsychotic injectables that are not preferred on formulary, but that are the best medications of certain classes of medications that are more appropriate for young patients versus the older ones for many, many more reasons, like less side effects.

It will take weeks sometimes. Getting prior authorization for community based mental health services can sometimes take weeks, and then every 3 months they want you to repeat the authorization.

In Louisiana, Medicaid has been privatized, so there are five companies that provide Medicaid services, each requiring a different type of pre-authorization or prior authorization for services. So this is a job of two or three people.

We have a census of about 170, so it is hard to finance that because I am, aware that businesses need to be financed in a fiscally responsible manner. But the amount of administrative support you need to get these things done is astronomical.

Senator MARSHALL. Yes. Dr. Hoover, do you have anything to add?

Dr. HOOVER. The only thing I would add is I certainly agree with everything you said. And yet, of course, we need some authorization in place, especially for our most vulnerable youth, who may, for example, experience polypharmacy.

Young people in the foster care system, for example, we know may be on multiple medications. There needs to be some authorization and process for understanding the medications that they have been prescribed so that it is done responsibly.

But the wait times for getting into mental health care, as you said, it is mind numbing, astronomical, and for families can be really impossible to navigate.

Senator MARSHALL. In my experiences, what was most frustrating is after my nurses had spent days and days in the back and forth with faxes, not emails or on online, but faxes, eventually I get to talk to a person and maybe it was a neurologist trying to explain to me why we shouldn't be using progesterone for pre-term—have you ever had that same frustration? I wouldn't begin to want to tell you the drugs you should be using.

Dr. HOOVER. Yes. I left inpatient work specifically because of this. I would be told that someone did not qualify for inpatient psychiatric hospitalization because they weren't actively trying to kill themselves or someone else.

I would say, so what about like hearing the demon and coming to get you, and you can't even get out of your bed or go to your house or eat food—you don't qualify for inpatient services. And I just——

Senator MARSHALL. I just want to reassure you that we do have legislation that we could get across the finish line that would impact Medicare, this prior authorization issue. And then we will go after CHIP and Medicaid and some of those others.

I am running out of time. I want to go to Dr. Wright and Ms. Williams for a second as well. One of the tragedies in this country is fentanyl poisoning. And this is an editorial written by a mom from Kansas who lost her son, Cooper Davis, a little bit over a year ago.

A 16 year old who ordered a half of a Percocet tablet via Snapchat, unknowingly laced with fentanyl and the child died. Dr. Wright are you seeing any problems with—the high risk group we are talking about, I am afraid oftentimes they are trying to find Xanax or Adderall or uppers, downers, and they are being laced with fentanyl.

Are you seeing any of this in your world, Dr. Wright?

Dr. WRIGHT. Specifically at my institution, no. We don't see— that is not the drug of choice for our student population. However, prior to Xavier, I lived in Staten Island, and I worked in a private liberal arts college on Staten Island where we saw a huge problem with the drugs that were laced with fentanyl.

Students who were—whose prescriptions had lapsed, and so now they are going out and finding other ways. And so, yes, that is a huge problem that our young people are dealing with.

It is partly because as Senator Tuberville said, they came medicated, and now they don't have access to those medicines now, and they are trying to find it any way they can. But it is a growing problem, particularly for students who are trying to take care of themselves.

Senator MARSHALL. Sure. Thank you. Ms. Williams, and I certainly don't want to get too personal. I always tell my patients, you can pass on any of my questions, but are do you see any problems, any—are students able to find those types of things online? Do you see it in your school or any concerns about it?

Ms. WILLIAMS. You mean drugs?

Senator MARSHALL. The specifically fake pills laced with fentanyl. Like people are trying to find Xanax or Adderall and my goodness, it has been laced with fentanyl.

Ms. WILLIAMS. Never in my experience have I heard of anyone doing that, no.

Senator MARSHALL. All right. All right. Well, thank you so much. Dr. Weiss, you want—do you have anything to add?

Dr. WEISS. I just—I think one thing that you bring up is important, that every community is different in terms of what very emergent substance use problem is going on. In New Orleans, we have a major problem with synthetics and people smoking mojo and becoming psychotic——

Senator MARSHALL. I don't know what that is.

Dr. WEISS. The point that you can't get them—well, it is just a fake marijuana. I can buy it in a grocery store. I mean, just and it can ruin your kidneys. So you have to be attentive to what is happening in different areas for sure.

The CHAIRMAN. Senator Marshall, thank you. We will next turn to Senator Kaine.

Senator KAINE. Well, thanks to Senator Casey and Cassidy for pulling this together. And what a great panel. I want to talk a little bit about before college and then want to talk about the transition of college.

I spent Thanksgiving with family and friends, and one of the friends I spent time with is an administrator in the St. John County Florida school system, which includes Saint Augustine, and her responsibility includes all the guidance counselors.

She was telling me, we don't have enough, and they are doing college guidance and helping people with financial aid forms and trying to be counselors. And there are some Florida laws now that are making it even harder because they can't talk about everything with the student without letting parents know.

But setting that aside, the point she was making is there is just not enough people here. So, Ms. Williams, let me just ask you. You go to Baldwin High School in Pittsburgh. How big is Baldwin High School? How many kids?

Ms. WILLIAMS. It is like 1,400, but it is also with the middle school and high school.

Senator KAINE. It is all—that is all together.

Ms. WILLIAMS. Yes.

Senator KAINE. When you decided, hey, I need to seek help from somebody because of the many issues I am dealing with. And as you described, death of your mom and COVID and there are so many, was it—where did you go? And was it easy to get help or was it hard to get help?

Ms. WILLIAMS. I think I did it the wrong way. But I went to my principal first because I was having trouble with like just trying to get to school and get to do things I wanted to do with my friends and everything. So I went to the principal first because I was closer to him because I didn't have the same guidance counselor of years in my high school.

Senator KAINE. You were getting assigned a different one?

Ms. WILLIAMS. Yes. There was—I think I have had five in the past 4 years, so it was just a little——

Senator KAINE. Is that because you get assigned a different one each year, but also just there is some turnover and people coming in and out.

Ms. WILLIAMS. Yes. It is because—we were supposed to have the same one all 4 years, but because of, COVID and everything, and some people taking maternity leave and different things like that, it was just not consistent, so we just didn't have the same——

Senator KAINE. Well, let me ask Dr. Hoover a question. I am going to come back to you in a minute about college, Ms. Williams. Dr. Hoover, do you think families utilize the IEP process sufficiently to help children deal with emotional and mental health issues?

I have been a Mayor and worked with my school system and am really familiar with IEPs. One of my three kids had an IEP. But commonly for something like a speech therapy or a very narrowly defined learning disability, families can use the IEP process for getting accommodations for students to deal with emotional mental health issues.

Do you think we use that enough in the K–12 space?

Dr. HOOVER. Thank you, Senator Kaine, for the question and for your support of mental health in schools. So the simple answer is, yes, families can use IEP process, and no, they don't use it probably as often or as well as they should have, in part because they are not often aware of how to do it. They don't have the family peer support to help them navigate the process. Of course the stigma——

Senator KAINE. To the extent that there is still any stigma about mental health issues too, that would probably be an additional variable——

Dr. HOOVER. Hugely detrimental. But the other point I want to make, so we need to increase awareness, decrease stigma about using special education accommodations to support mental, emotional, behavioral issues.

But we also need to provide supports that go outside of or beyond the special education system. There are a lot of young people who could get mental health supports in schools that would not require an IEP, but they can still get mental health support in schools.

Senator KAINE. I want to go over to the college side. So Ms. Williams, you are a senior. So when—are you thinking about going to college next year?

Ms. WILLIAMS. Yes.

Senator KAINE. When you go to college, with the experience you have had and you have now found some support systems that have helped you, and you have created support systems that have helped others, but you are going to show up on a campus where like you will be one of maybe hundreds or thousands and you will be kind of a free agent day one.

What are you going to do when you go to college to try to make sure you have the services that you need? And I ask you this because there might be a lot of people just like you listening to this hearing that would want to hear the way you are going to do it, since you have been appropriately sort of assertive in trying to find the help that you need.

Ms. WILLIAMS. I am thinking about joining different clubs and different social settings that will help me with mental health and other people that deal with the same things that I deal with, and different groups that deal with kids with a parent that passes or a person that deals with depression or anxiety or something like that.

I wanted to join different groups. But I also talked with my therapist a little bit about how to transition from her being my child therapist to becoming—having an adult therapist.

What they were planning on doing is like overlapping sort of the time between her leaving my life and having a new therapist so we can—so she can talk me through the way I should interact with the new therapist and try to overlap them and try to, I don't know, get a way through the——

Senator KAINE. I get you—the transition, yes——

Ms. WILLIAMS [continuing]. Process easier—the transition easier.

Senator KAINE. That is good advice for others. And Mr. Chairman, could I ask one more question of Dr. Wight. We have had two really tough situations in Virginia in recent years. One, when I was Governor, a tragic shooting at Virginia Tech, and then recently a tragic shooting on the University of Virginia campus.

In both instances, there is some differences, and I don't want to make them sound exactly similar when they are not. But in both instances, the individuals who carried out these grievous crimes had tough high school years but had found supports in high school where they were able to be successful, successful students, successful athletes.

But then when they went to college, it was like none of that information that helped them succeed in the high school setting, it is like none of it went to the university setting.

In each instance, and we are still learning more about the University of Virginia situation, it seems like there was sort of a downward spiral, and maybe partly because they didn't have the support services surrounding them that knew their situation and knew how to help them succeed when they were in high school.

The RISE Act, which you all have introduced, would take, if somebody has an IEP, it would take that information from high school and not just make it easier for them to continue it in a university setting, but it would also transfer the knowledge about how to help this young person succeed to the college setting.

But how do you deal with that in your institution? This coming into a place where you are brand new and it is all you were expecting after 3 months to be an independent adult, make good choices, and maybe you have a past history that doesn't really—it is not— it is not made known to anybody on campus.

How do you help students in that transition at Xavier?

Dr. WRIGHT. Sure. So there is peer to peer training that we conduct so that the freshmen are paired with what we call peer deans, who are upper class students who help connect them to not only the social side of university life, but also those resources that will help them navigate the university.

We also think about those spaces where students are going and try to marry. So we know that students are going to see our campus ministry office, right. So training those folks to be able to help identify when they hear things, get them the counseling.

Similarly doing that same work in the classroom because sometimes faculty will interact with students, and they will see something in a report that they have written.

Or they will come to them, and they will say, I missed class today because of x. Or they will also let us know when they start to see things that are different. But I do think that the other—one of the most important things that we have been doing is really engaging our students' parents.

We want to respect them as full adults, but we also recognize that we can't do it without a full support system for them. And so working with those parents will oftentimes get us information that we didn't know that will then help us connect with their previous therapist.

Senator KAINE. Thank you. Thank you for that. I appreciate your letting me go over.

The CHAIRMAN. Thank you, Senator Kaine. Senator Cassidy.

Senator CASSIDY. Dr. Wright, just to follow-up the kind of same thread as did Senator Kaine, and I think this is more for the audience watching so I just want you to kind of document by your testimony, if somebody does have an IEP as in a high school and they are trying to transfer to Xavier or another university, are you able to access that information at all? Can you access it even though there is difficulty in terms of utilizing or using that information. Can you comment on that, please?

Dr. WRIGHT. We can't access it unless they give it to us. So they have to bring it to us. And then when they bring it to us, even if it is outdated, what we will do is provisionally provide those accommodations and set them up with a coordinated care plan to get them the evaluations that they need.

But unless they bring it to us, we don't have access to that, because in our admissions process, we are not allowed to ask them information about their mental health. Doctor——

Dr. WEISS. I was just going to add, and what you I think demonstrated so beautifully, is that when there is a mental health team involved with a high school student that is going to be transitioning to college or to a job, whatever they want we are very aware of what is going on in the senior year of high school.

We are sort of anticipating and preparing ahead of time of where they are planning on going, the application process. I have had to read a lot of personal statements for college applications.

We have already identified the key players in their new community. Whether it is a—they need a first episode program in their community. We have already reached out to them. We don't have——

Senator CASSIDY. Sorry, excuse me. What you are telling me is a best practice is that the high school counselor would then be seeking a HIPPA form release that she or he could send the information to the college, and the college could just again continue that sort of enveloping we are going to support you?

Dr. WEISS. Yes.

Dr. WRIGHT. Correct.

Senator CASSIDY. Do you have a sense of——

Dr. WEISS. You can be clear about what——

Senator CASSIDY. Do you have a sense of how often this best practice is actually implemented?

Dr. WRIGHT. Very little.

Dr. WEISS. Very little. I mean, it is——

Senator CASSIDY. Is it not implemented well or implemented so little, is that the problem with the university or is that the problem of the high school? Or what is going on here?

Dr. WRIGHT. I think that there is many, many things going on depending on what the situation is that you are dealing with. Via if it is an academic disability, then it would be——

Senator CASSIDY. But we are speaking specifically of mental health.

Dr. WEISS. Mental health.

Senator CASSIDY. Now, by the way, our RISE Act, if you have dyslexia, that doesn't change with lifetime. Forever you are dyslexic.

Dr. WEISS. Right.

Senator CASSIDY. That is easily taken over.

Dr. WEISS. Right.

Senator CASSIDY. Mental health is obviously a different issue.

Dr. WEISS. Right.

Senator CASSIDY. Again, if you had to tell us what is the problem between the person who is helping someone like Ms. Williams, sending that information to the college which she chooses to attend, and then that seamlessly moving into the counseling that she needs. Because if not, it ends up with the tragic consequences that Senator Kaine just referred to. What is the problem there? What can we do?

Dr. WEISS. Coordinating care from both sides.

Senator CASSIDY. Yes, ma'am, I get that. But what is the——

Dr. WEISS. People are answering the phones——

Senator CASSIDY [continuing]. Mechanism where we forced that marriage, if you will. It sounds like it is just not happening, and it sounds like it is just not happening because, it is a too strong to say, a lack of effort? Dr. Hoover.

Dr. HOOVER. Well, I would just say that we have to have some protections in place for health care privacy and——

Senator CASSIDY. But signing a HIPPA form would be——

Dr. HOOVER. That is exactly right. So we need to educate our young people as they transition to adulthood about their privacy rights and how to sign a HIPPA form.

Senator CASSIDY [continuing]. Because that really should be. I am a health care doctor——

Dr. HOOVER. Yes.

Senator CASSIDY. If somebody comes to me and I know they are moving to another state, I say, listen, I need to send your records to Mississippi and I need you to sign this form. I don't think it is incumbent upon the patient to understand that there is a form which she needs to sign.

Dr. HOOVER. But it is incumbent upon them to understand whether they would wish to. A lot of college students, one of the biggest hindrances of college students to actually having the—to actually getting services is because they don't necessarily know or want those services when they get to college.

Senator CASSIDY. But we are talking about something different. What we are talking about, because you and Dr. Wright, I think, spoke of, and Dr. Weiss spoke of proactively reaching out.

But that suggests that they have been informed that there is an issue. Now, I will say that the nice thing about somebody being 17 or 18, mama is still there.

Dr. WRIGHT. Correct.

Senator CASSIDY. I find that mamas are—like we couldn't live without them.

[Laughter.]

Senator CASSIDY. But she can come in and make sure, dear, I know that you need to sign this form, and I am going to sign it with you if you are a minor, and we are going to send those records. I am not sure I will accept the excuse that the student is unaware. Yes, that is true——

Dr. HOOVER. Not an excuse. I just think they need to be educated and I wholeheartedly agree.

Senator CASSIDY. But the initial sending of that record should be incumbent upon the guidance counselor or the social worker or whomever.

Dr. HOOVER. With the permission of the family, absolutely.

Senator CASSIDY. Exactly. I think what is not—what I am pushing, but what I am not quite sure I am receiving a yes that is true from, is there a problem, is there a lack of follow through on the behalf of the typical high school guidance counselor or social worker to trigger that?

Dr. HOOVER. Yes.

Dr. WEISS. Yes.

Senator CASSIDY. Okay. Now, is there likewise a sufficient—insufficient pull through, the university gets it and what do we do with it? Oh, that is great, put it in the file.

Dr. HOOVER. Yes.

Dr. WEISS. Yes.

Senator CASSIDY. As opposed to we are going to jump on this and make sure it doesn't happen?

Dr. WEISS. Yes.

Dr. HOOVER. There is often a requirement for reassessment, which as you alluded to earlier, is often completely unnecessary.

Dr. WEISS. Right.

Senator CASSIDY. Right. Our RISE Act addresses some of this.

Dr. HOOVER. Correct.

Senator CASSIDY. By this, I hope all my colleagues now will claim co-sponsors. But there is also, beyond Federal law, there is the lack of awareness in the high school and the university as to their respective roles.

Dr. WRIGHT. Correct. Senator, it is skill versus will, can we or will we. And I—can we? Absolutely, we can. But I do think that we sometimes hide behind policies, that will limit what we will do.

Senator CASSIDY. No, I totally get you, Dr. Wright. Oh, my gosh, people retreat because they are just so scared of their shadow, and they use that as an excuse.

Dr. WRIGHT. Right.

Senator CASSIDY. It is an incredible frustration of mine.

Dr. WRIGHT. Right. But I do think the RISE Act would help provide some Federal guidance on what we should be doing. And so——

Senator CASSIDY. But it is more than that, and I don't quite know what it is—it is probably——

Dr. WRIGHT. I think clinically if you are a clinically astute therapist with a high schooler, then you should be talking about these things. And it shouldn't be the day before you go, oh, let's send your mental health information.

It should be this whole transition and what is going to happen to make them feel safe and comfortable with like continuing their mental health care in the next phase of their life.

Senator CASSIDY. I will say, on the Federal level, there are some times that we can do best practices and we judge different organizations by best practices. And can you do an audit of your charts and see how many X, Y and Z?

I just say that for my colleagues, for us to start thinking about. I am out of time. I actually had other questions for you all, but I will submit those for the records, particularly for you, Dr. Weiss, as regards to how you are using the wraparound services and the need to augment Medicaid, which seems—just seems crazy. But we will get back to you. We will send you the letter for the record. Thank you.

The CHAIRMAN. Thank you, Senator Cassidy. And I will, I know we have to wrap up soon, but I will exercise a Chairman's prerogative by just adding maybe one more question for Brooklyn Williams.

But to our three doctors, if you can each, if you want to, provide anything else for the record that you hope you would—we have on the record, in 30 to 1—30 seconds to 1 minute each, if you can do that. This is kind of a quick lightning round before I will wrap up with Brooklyn, and then we will do our closings.

Dr. HOOVER. Glad to. So the one thing that I want to emphasize is that while we do need to invest in child mental health specialists and increase the numbers of counselors in schools, psychologists, etcetera, we really do need to make it that every adult and peer has education and training to support mental health.

That can be through things like mental health first aid and youth mental health first aid. There is also a free, federally funded mental health training for all educators called Classroom Well-Being Information and Strategies for educators or classroom wise.

We have many tools at our fingertips to train everybody in the system, and that would include in mental health literacy in the K through 12 curriculum. It can't rely—we can't rely solely on mental health specialists to cure our way out of this mental health crisis.

The CHAIRMAN. Thanks, Dr. Hoover. Dr. Wright.

Dr. WRIGHT. I also want to echo Dr. Hoover in the need for mental health first aid. As someone who has sat and attended far too many funerals of students over the course of my career who had bright, brilliant futures but they weren't able to see that, this is an important conversation, and I am so grateful to the Committee for engaging in it.

But we also need to recognize that teacher preparation should involve a certain level of understanding how to navigate these spaces because they are the front line. So, thank you.

The CHAIRMAN. Thank you. Thank you, Dr. Wright.

Dr. Weiss.

Dr. WEISS. I echo as well and think that this mental health first stage should also include specific and more severe illnesses and not just be a generic approach, because dealing with some of these more misunderstood mental health conditions can be very challenging for someone that doesn't have the background.

I just want to stress that while we talk about early intervention, we have to think about early detection and beyond schools, like to the communities.

The CHAIRMAN. Doctor, thanks very much. I am told Senator Kaine, you had something you wanted to say.

Senator KAINE. If I could just quick, and this is back to Senator Cassidy, this point on best practices. A university probably wouldn't want to try to get a student's medical record before the student was admitted because the student and family might wonder, well, maybe they will turn me down if they see something in my metal record they don't like.

But once a university admits a student the first letter that goes out is, hey, you have been admitted and here is the deposit you have to put down, and it has a whole lot of other information in it.

That letter from a college could say, we can help provide services on day one that will help your students succeed if we know as much as we can about what services help the students succeed in high school, if you will fill out this HIPPA form and send it back to us, we can get the schools full record, not just the transcript, but the full record so we can do that.

There are—the RISE Act is a really good one. But I also think there is best practices at that moment. Everybody is going to eagerly devour that letter, you are in and here is the deposit, but here is information, and that is a good moment to have that discussion.

I just kind of wanted to put that on the record for anybody from colleges that might be listening to this hearing.

The CHAIRMAN. Good point. Well, Brooklyn, you are going to be the last answer of the hearing. But I want to particularly thank you for not only being here. That is difficult enough. I could never do what you are doing when I was your age. Not even close.

But also, as much as it is inspiring to have you here and to hear your testimony, and to listen to the answers to questions, your story, what you have had to overcome personally is not just inspiring to people here but will inspire countless young people across the country. So we want to commend you for that.

I guess sometimes we don't often—often we don't listen enough here in Washington. We don't take enough time to hear the perspectives of young people. So I guess just by way of conclusion, what was your hope that we would hear? What point do you want to make before we conclude?

Ms. WILLIAMS. I would say just like try to take advantage of the young people that want to come and work with you guys, and just try to get them to reach out to the people around their age more because talking to people that are around your age is a lot I would say easier than trying to talk to people that have not like grown up the same way you have.

There is a lot of different experiences from when I would say when everyone here is like younger than whenever, like me now, like being a 17 year old in 2022. I would say just having more like ears and having the constant communication is very beneficial.

Without that, I feel like there is a lot—there would be a lot less good in what we are trying to accomplish. And I just wanted to say thank you for letting me talk among these doctors and all of you very insightful, like professional people.

It is just a really nice experience, and I am eternally grateful.

The CHAIRMAN. Brooklyn, thanks so much. We are honored by your presence as we are by all of our witnesses. I will have a closing statement and then I will turn to Ranking Member Cassidy for his. We know that in today's hearing we heard very, very powerful testimony about how to address the crisis in adolescent mental health and set our Nation's young people up for success in college and in life.

We also discussed creating systems of comprehensive mental health support in schools and communities to identify and respond to unprecedented mental health needs among our young people.

We also talked about gaps in the continuum of mental health care that must be filled through care integration in health care, and health workforce development, and a greater variety of timely care options. Long before the pandemic, there was a significant rise in mental health conditions among our Nation's young people.

Their mental health challenges have only been exacerbated by isolation and stress in recent years. Too many of our young people are not even able to show up as their full selves to fully enjoy the many experiences that make high school and college special.

Too often they don't have that opportunity to perform at their best and to achieve meaningful goals. Young people across our Country have unbounded potential and their whole lives ahead of them, and yet suicide is the second leading cause of death among people ages 10 to 14, and the third leading cause of death among young people ages 15 to 24.

We can't accept this. We must do more. We must do more here in Washington and across the country to help get young people the support they need. Congress must continue to support successful programs and legislation like those we have talked about today.

I look forward to working with my colleagues to achieve that, and to make sure that young people have the future that they deserve. So I will turn to Ranking Member Cassidy for his closing remarks.

Senator CASSIDY. Very briefly. Thank you all. What a great conference. In one sense, oh my gosh, there is so much to do. But there are tangible things that can be done that came out of this.

This room, as your example, of youth groups, peer to peer, if you will, helping others. The whole conversation regarding pre-authorization and how that can be better. And the whole idea that maybe we get to have Medicaid provide those sorts of services, those kind of coordination services, that therefore the SAMHSA grant would not be used for a lower calling, if you will, but could be a higher level of service.

Dr. Wright, thank you so much for Xavier doing best practices. Dr. Weiss too as regards how to take a child who is leaving high school in those 3 months later enrolling. Dr. Hoover, you have kind of seen the whole spectrum.

Thank you all. I think what we learned from this is a set of— a set of measures that, if taken, can make the situation better. And there is nothing more we could have asked for from this hearing. Thank you once more.

The CHAIRMAN. Thank you, Ranking Member Cassidy, and thanks for your work in helping us arrange this hearing.

# Additional Material: Excerpt from the 2020 National Survey on Drug Use and Health

**Table 11.1A.** Settings where mental health services were received in past year: among people aged 12 to 17; Numbers in thousands, 2002-2020

| Setting Where Mental Health Service Was Received | 2002 | 2003 | 2004 | 2005 | 2006 | 2007 | 2008 | 2009 | 2010 | 2011 | 2012 | 2013 | 2014 | 2015 | 2016 | 2017 | 2018 | 2019 | 2020 |
|---|---|---|---|---|---|---|---|---|---|---|---|---|---|---|---|---|---|---|---|
| SPECIALTY MENTAL HEALTH SERVICE[1] | 2,898 | 3,065 | 3,348 | 3,362 | 3,255 | 3,104 | 3,129 | 2,925 | 2,920 | 3,101 | 3,118 | 3,341 | 3,369 | 3,253 | 3,598 | 3,646 | 3,901 | 4,088 | *4,246* |
| Outpatient | 2,662 | 2,795 | 3,015 | 3,048 | 2,931 | 2,787 | 2,837 | 2,650 | 2,635 | 2,842 | 2,846 | 3,064 | 3,110 | 2,958 | 3,239 | 3,328 | 3,547 | 3,747 | *4,088* |
| Private Therapist, Psychologist, Psychiatrist, Social Worker, or Counselor | 2,254 | 2,347 | 2,523 | 2,573 | 2,416 | 2,365 | 2,408 | 2,296 | 2,265 | 2,409 | 2,427 | 2,572 | 2,698 | 2,532 | 2,819 | 2,908 | 3,080 | 3,213 | *3,491* |
| Mental Health Clinic or Center | 611 | 635 | 716 | 657 | 587 | 583 | 567 | 537 | 547 | 547 | 610 | 731 | 760 | 792 | 929 | 995 | 977 | 1,169 | *1,187* |
| Partial Day Hospital or Day Treatment Program | 440 | 425 | 439 | 449 | 471 | 416 | 374 | 340 | 362 | 393 | 431 | 477 | 467 | 455 | 489 | 505 | 484 | 517 | *354* |
| In-Home Therapist, Counselor, or Family Preservation Worker | 693 | 656 | 762 | 731 | 719 | 707 | 716 | 657 | 674 | 767 | 776 | 787 | 836 | 830 | 845 | 840 | 951 | 1,091 | *939* |
| Inpatient or Residential[1] | 509 | 542 | 629 | 619 | 596 | 581 | 539 | 524 | 531 | 526 | 547 | 574 | 606 | 642 | 737 | 708 | 683 | 701 | *510* |
| Hospital | 422 | 467 | 515 | 529 | 516 | 511 | 469 | 440 | 447 | 438 | 463 | 504 | 547 | 588 | 666 | 622 | 608 | 618 | *429* |
| Residential Treatment Center | 224 | 233 | 299 | 229 | 225 | 199 | 198 | 213 | 217 | 240 | 238 | 206 | 252 | 271 | 311 | 318 | 300 | 293 | *277* |
| NONSPECIALTY MENTAL HEALTH SERVICE[2] | nc | nc | nc | nc | nc | nc | nc | 3,430 | 3,465 | 3,463 | 3,649 | 3,634 | 3,736 | 3,691 | 3,732 | 3,810 | 3,977 | 4,371 | *3,651* |
| Education[2,3] | nc | nc | nc | nc | nc | nc | nc | 2,931 | 2,957 | 2,920 | 3,157 | 3,147 | 3,229 | 3,206 | 3,193 | 3,231 | 3,444 | 3,727 | *3,136* |
| School Social Worker, School Psychologist, or School Counselor | nc | nc | nc | nc | nc | nc | nc | 2,286 | 2,214 | 2,188 | 2,389 | 2,284 | 2,379 | 2,239 | 2,278 | 2,249 | 2,395 | 2,698 | *2,354* |
| Special School or Program within a Regular School for Students with Emotional or Behavioral Problems | nc | nc | nc | nc | nc | nc | nc | 975 | 1,054 | 1,063 | 1,142 | 1,218 | 1,207 | 1,357 | 1,319 | 1,345 | 1,461 | 1,477 | *1,061* |
| General Medicine | | | | | | | | | | | | | | | | | | | |
| Pediatrician or Other Family Doctor | 657 | 732 | 840 | 810 | 694 | 692 | 710 | 605 | 601 | 619 | 629 | 686 | 700 | 668 | 708 | 805 | 767 | 902 | *762* |
| Juvenile Justice | | | | | | | | | | | | | | | | | | | |
| Juvenile Detention Center, Prison, or Jail | -- | -- | -- | -- | -- | -- | -- | 109 | 80 | 103 | 83 | 59 | 63 | 53 | 53 | 45 | 48 | 49 | *22* |
| Child Welfare | 157 | 179 | 158 | 143 | 129 | 114 | 118 | 92 | 108 | 140 | 96 | 99 | 92 | 79 | 108 | 92 | 94 | 97 | *66* |

**Table 11.1A.** (Continued)

| Setting Where Mental Health Service Was Received | 2002 | 2003 | 2004 | 2005 | 2006 | 2007 | 2008 | 2009 | 2010 | 2011 | 2012 | 2013 | 2014 | 2015 | 2016 | 2017 | 2018 | 2019 | 2020 |
|---|---|---|---|---|---|---|---|---|---|---|---|---|---|---|---|---|---|---|---|
| Foster Care or Therapeutic Foster Care | | | | | | | | | | | | | | | | | | | |
| SPECIALTY MENTAL HEALTH SERVICES AND EDUCATION, GENERAL MEDICINE OR CHILD WELFARE SERVICES[1,2,3] | nc | nc | nc | nc | nc | nc | nc | 1,226 | 1,283 | 1,328 | 1,397 | 1,490 | 1,457 | 1,408 | 1,513 | 1,615 | 1,706 | 1,910 | *1,678* |

* = low precision; -= not available; da = does not apply; nc = not comparable due to methodological changes; nr = not reported due to measurement issues.

NOTE: Estimates in the 2020 column are italicized to indicate caution should be used when comparing estimates between 2020 and prior years because of methodological changes for 2020. Due to these changes, significance testing between 2020 and prior years was not performed. See the *2020 National Survey on Drug Use and Health: Methodological Summary and Definitions* for details.

NOTE: Some 2006 to 2010 estimates may differ from previously published estimates due to updates (see Chapter 3 of the *2020 National Survey on Drug Use and Health: Methodological Summary and Definitions*).

NOTE: Mental health services for people aged 12 to 17 includes treatment/counseling for emotional or behavioral problems not caused by drug or alcohol use. Respondents with unknown mental health service information were excluded. Questions on virtual services were added in Quarter 4 of 2020. Estimates in this table do not include data from these questions. See the *2020 National Survey on Drug Use and Health: Methodological Summary and Definitions* for details.

NOTE: Respondents could indicate multiple service settings; thus, the response categories are not mutually exclusive.

[1]Because of revisions in 2013 to Specialty Mental Health Service estimates, these 2002 to 2012 estimates may differ from estimates published prior to the 2013 NSDUH.

[2]Because of revisions in 2009 to the questions on the Source of Youth Mental Health Education Services, these estimates are not comparable with the education services estimates published prior to the 2009 NSDUH.

[3]Respondents who did not report their school enrollment status, who reported not being enrolled in school in the past 12 months, or who reported being home-schooled were not asked about receipt of mental health services from this setting; however, respondents who reported not being enrolled in school in the past 12 months were classified as not having received mental health services from this setting.

Definitions: Measures and terms are defined in Appendix A.

Source: SAMHSA, Center for Behavioral Health Statistics and Quality, National Survey on Drug Use and Health, 2002-2019, and Quarters 1 and 4, 2020.

**Table 11.1B.** Settings where mental health services were received in past year: among people aged 12 to 17; percentages, 2002-2020

| Setting Where Mental Health Service Was Received | 2002 | 2003 | 2004 | 2005 | 2006 | 2007 | 2008 | 2009 | 2010 | 2011 | 2012 | 2013 | 2014 | 2015 | 2016 | 2017 | 2018 | 2019 | 2020 |
|---|---|---|---|---|---|---|---|---|---|---|---|---|---|---|---|---|---|---|---|
| SPECIALTY MENTAL HEALTH SERVICE1 | 11.8 | 12.4 | 13.4 | 13.4 | 13.0 | 12.4 | 12.7 | 12.0 | 12.1 | 12.6 | 12.7 | 13.6 | 13.7 | 13.3 | 14.7 | 14.8 | 16.0 | 16.7 | *17.3* |
| Outpatient | 10.8 | 11.3 | 12.1 | 12.1 | 11.7 | 11.2 | 11.5 | 10.9 | 10.9 | 11.5 | 11.5 | 12.5 | 12.7 | 12.0 | 13.2 | 13.6 | 14.5 | 15.3 | *16.6* |
| Private Therapist, Psychologist, Psychiatrist, Social Worker, or Counselor | 9.2 | 9.5 | 10.1 | 10.2 | 9.6 | 9.5 | 9.8 | 9.4 | 9.4 | 9.8 | 9.8 | 10.5 | 11.0 | 10.3 | 11.5 | 11.8 | 12.6 | 13.1 | *14.2* |
| Mental Health Clinic or Center | 2.5 | 2.6 | 2.9 | 2.6 | 2.3 | 2.3 | 2.3 | 2.2 | 2.3 | 2.2 | 2.5 | 3.0 | 3.1 | 3.2 | 3.8 | 4.0 | 4.0 | 4.8 | *4.8* |
| Partial Day Hospital or Day Treatment Program | 1.8 | 1.7 | 1.8 | 1.8 | 1.9 | 1.7 | 1.5 | 1.4 | 1.5 | 1.6 | 1.7 | 1.9 | 1.9 | 1.8 | 2.0 | 2.0 | 2.0 | 2.1 | *1.4* |
| In-Home Therapist, Counselor, or Family Preservation Worker | 2.8 | 2.6 | 3.0 | 2.9 | 2.9 | 2.8 | 2.9 | 2.7 | 2.8 | 3.1 | 3.1 | 3.2 | 3.4 | 3.4 | 3.4 | 3.4 | 3.9 | 4.5 | *3.8* |
| Inpatient or Residential[1] | 2.1 | 2.2 | 2.5 | 2.5 | 2.4 | 2.3 | 2.2 | 2.1 | 2.2 | 2.1 | 2.2 | 2.3 | 2.5 | 2.6 | 3.0 | 2.9 | 2.8 | 2.9 | *2.1* |
| Hospital | 1.7 | 1.9 | 2.1 | 2.1 | 2.0 | 2.0 | 1.9 | 1.8 | 1.8 | 1.8 | 1.9 | 2.0 | 2.2 | 2.4 | 2.7 | 2.5 | 2.5 | 2.5 | *1.7* |
| Residential Treatment Center | 0.9 | 0.9 | 1.2 | 0.9 | 0.9 | 0.8 | 0.8 | 0.9 | 0.9 | 1.0 | 1.0 | 0.8 | 1.0 | 1.1 | 1.3 | 1.3 | 1.2 | 1.2 | *1.1* |
| NONSPECIALTY MENTAL HEALTH SERVICE[2] | nc | nc | nc | nc | nc | nc | nc | 14.2 | 14.5 | 14.2 | 15.0 | 15.0 | 15.4 | 15.2 | 15.4 | 15.7 | 16.5 | 18.1 | *15.0* |
| Education[2,3] | nc | nc | nc | nc | nc | nc | nc | 12.1 | 12.4 | 11.9 | 12.9 | 13.0 | 13.2 | 13.2 | 13.1 | 13.3 | 14.2 | 15.4 | *12.8* |
| School Social Worker, School Psychologist, or School Counselor | nc | nc | nc | nc | nc | nc | nc | 9.4 | 9.2 | 8.9 | 9.7 | 9.4 | 9.7 | 9.2 | 9.3 | 9.2 | 9.9 | 11.1 | *9.6* |
| Special School or Program within a Regular School for Students with Emotional or Behavioral Problems | nc | nc | nc | nc | nc | nc | nc | 4.0 | 4.4 | 4.3 | 4.7 | 5.0 | 4.9 | 5.6 | 5.4 | 5.5 | 6.0 | 6.1 | *4.3* |
| General Medicine | | | | | | | | | | | | | | | | | | | |
| Pediatrician or Other Family Doctor | 2.7 | 2.9 | 3.4 | 3.2 | 2.8 | 2.8 | 2.9 | 2.5 | 2.5 | 2.5 | 2.5 | 2.8 | 2.9 | 2.7 | 2.9 | 3.3 | 3.1 | 3.7 | *3.1* |
| Juvenile Justice | -- | -- | -- | -- | -- | -- | -- | 0.4 | 0.3 | 0.4 | 0.3 | 0.2 | 0.3 | 0.2 | 0.2 | 0.2 | 0.2 | 0.2 | *0.1* |
| Juvenile Detention Center, Prison, or Jail | | | | | | | | | | | | | | | | | | | |
| Child Welfare | 0.6 | 0.7 | 0.6 | 0.6 | 0.5 | 0.5 | 0.5 | 0.4 | 0.4 | 0.6 | 0.4 | 0.4 | 0.4 | 0.3 | 0.4 | 0.4 | 0.4 | 0.4 | *0.3* |

**Table 11.1B.** (Continued)

| Setting Where Mental Health Service Was Received | 2002 | 2003 | 2004 | 2005 | 2006 | 2007 | 2008 | 2009 | 2010 | 2011 | 2012 | 2013 | 2014 | 2015 | 2016 | 2017 | 2018 | 2019 | 2020 |
|---|---|---|---|---|---|---|---|---|---|---|---|---|---|---|---|---|---|---|---|
| Foster Care or Therapeutic Foster Care | | | | | | | | | | | | | | | | | | | |
| SPECIALTY MENTAL HEALTH SERVICES AND EDUCATION, GENERAL MEDICINE OR CHILD WELFARE SERVICES[1,2,3] | nc | nc | nc | nc | nc | nc | nc | 5.0 | 5.3 | 5.4 | 5.7 | 6.1 | 5.9 | 5.7 | 6.2 | 6.6 | 7.0 | 7.8 | *6.8* |

* = low precision; -= not available; da = does not apply; nc = not comparable due to methodological changes; nr = not reported due to measurement issues.

NOTE: Estimates in the 2020 column are italicized to indicate caution should be used when comparing estimates between 2020 and prior years because of methodological changes for 2020. Due to these changes, significance testing between 2020 and prior years was not performed. See the *2020 National Survey on Drug Use and Health: Methodological Summary and Definitions* for details.

NOTE: Some 2006 to 2010 estimates may differ from previously published estimates due to updates (see Chapter 3 of the *2020 National Survey on Drug Use and Health: Methodological Summary and Definitions*).

NOTE: Mental health services for people aged 12 to 17 includes treatment/counseling for emotional or behavioral problems not caused by drug or alcohol use. Respondents with unknown mental health service information were excluded. Questions on virtual services were added in Quarter 4 of 2020. Estimates in this table do not include data from these questions. See the *2020 National Survey on Drug Use and Health: Methodological Summary and Definitions* for details.

NOTE: Respondents could indicate multiple service settings; thus, the response categories are not mutually exclusive.

[1] Because of revisions in 2013 to Specialty Mental Health Service estimates, these 2002 to 2012 estimates may differ from estimates published prior to the 2013 NSDUH.

[2] Because of revisions in 2009 to the questions on the Source of Youth Mental Health Education Services, these estimates are not comparable with the education services estimates published prior to the 2009 NSDUH.

[3] Respondents who did not report their school enrollment status, who reported not being enrolled in school in the past 12 months, or who reported being home-schooled were not asked about receipt of mental health services from this setting; however, respondents who reported not being enrolled in school in the past 12 months were classified as not having received mental health services from this setting.

Definitions: Measures and terms are defined in Appendix A.

Source: SAMHSA, Center for Behavioral Health Statistics and Quality, National Survey on Drug Use and Health, 2002-2019, and Quarters 1 and 4, 2020.

**Table 11.2A.** Major depressive episode in past year: among people aged 12 to 17; by demographic characteristics, numbers in thousands, 2004-2020

| Demographic Characteristic | 2004 | 2005 | 2006 | 2007 | 2008 | 2009 | 2010 | 2011 | 2012 | 2013 | 2014 | 2015 | 2016 | 2017 | 2018 | 2019 | 2020 |
|---|---|---|---|---|---|---|---|---|---|---|---|---|---|---|---|---|---|
| TOTAL | 2,225 | 2,191 | 1,970 | 2,016 | 2,027 | 1,954 | 1,911 | 2,011 | 2,213 | 2,587 | 2,751 | 3,031 | 3,089 | 3,214 | 3,482 | 3,783 | *4,131* |
| AGE GROUP | | | | | | | | | | | | | | | | | |
| 12-13 | 445 | 417 | 383 | 337 | 366 | 330 | 330 | 312 | 420 | 470 | 548 | 587 | 548 | 516 | 632 | 816 | *902* |
| 14-15 | 783 | 811 | 684 | 705 | 706 | 741 | 706 | 710 | 844 | 1,025 | 986 | 1,163 | 1,115 | 1,200 | 1,250 | 1,341 | *1,533* |
| 16-17 | 997 | 964 | 902 | 974 | 955 | 883 | 876 | 989 | 950 | 1,091 | 1,217 | 1,281 | 1,427 | 1,498 | 1,600 | 1,626 | *1,696* |
| GENDER | | | | | | | | | | | | | | | | | |
| Male | 637 | 571 | 539 | 586 | 540 | 577 | 536 | 566 | 581 | 657 | 710 | 725 | 786 | 845 | 946 | 1,076 | *1,135* |
| Female | 1,588 | 1,620 | 1,431 | 1,430 | 1,487 | 1,377 | 1,375 | 1,446 | 1,632 | 1,930 | 2,042 | 2,306 | 2,303 | 2,369 | 2,537 | 2,708 | *2,996* |
| HISPANIC ORIGIN AND RACE | | | | | | | | | | | | | | | | | |
| Not Hispanic or Latino | 1,848 | 1,802 | 1,614 | 1,691 | 1,681 | 1,594 | 1,537 | 1,586 | 1,648 | 1,970 | 2,123 | 2,323 | 2,366 | 2,419 | 2,601 | 2,755 | *3,176* |
| White | 1,413 | 1,390 | 1,220 | 1,284 | 1,266 | 1,180 | 1,186 | 1,167 | 1,231 | 1,449 | 1,578 | 1,742 | 1,781 | 1,785 | 1,905 | 1,975 | *2,330* |
| Black or African American | 287 | 288 | 245 | 292 | 261 | 285 | 236 | 238 | 269 | 289 | 306 | 302 | 301 | 313 | 334 | 367 | *392* |
| AIAN | 13 | 10 | 12 | 7 | 13 | 9 | 10 | 15 | 7 | 7 | 11 | * | 16 | 24 | 23 | 20 | * |
| NHOPI | * | * | * | * | * | * | 1 | * | * | * | * | * | * | * | * | * | * |
| Asian | 82 | 63 | 77 | 66 | 73 | 73 | 57 | 90 | 49 | 123 | 124 | 118 | 152 | 145 | 189 | 190 | *252* |
| Two or More Races | 51 | 41 | 52 | 41 | 59 | 41 | 48 | 75 | 81 | 95 | 93 | 121 | 109 | 138 | 137 | 189 | *179* |
| Hispanic or Latino | 377 | 389 | 356 | 325 | 347 | 360 | 374 | 425 | 566 | 617 | 628 | 708 | 724 | 795 | 882 | 1,028 | *956* |

* = low precision; -= not available; da = does not apply; nc = not comparable due to methodological changes; nr = not reported due to measurement issues.

NOTE: Estimates in the 2020 column are italicized to indicate caution should be used when comparing estimates between 2020 and prior years because of methodological changes for 2020. Due to these changes, significance testing between 2020 and prior years was not performed. See the *2020 National Survey on Drug Use and Health: Methodological Summary and Definitions* for details.

NOTE: Some 2006 to 2010 estimates may differ from previously published estimates due to updates (see Chapter 3 of the *2020 National Survey on Drug Use and Health: Methodological Summary and Definitions*).

NOTE: Respondents with unknown past year Major Depressive Episode (MDE) data were excluded.

Definitions: Measures and terms are defined in Appendix A.

Source: SAMHSA, Center for Behavioral Health Statistics and Quality, National Survey on Drug Use and Health, 2004-2019, and Quarters 1 and 4, 2020.

**Table 11.2B.** Major depressive episode in past year: among people aged 12 to 17; by demographic characteristics, percentages, 2004-2020

| Demographic Characteristic | 2004 | 2005 | 2006 | 2007 | 2008 | 2009 | 2010 | 2011 | 2012 | 2013 | 2014 | 2015 | 2016 | 2017 | 2018 | 2019 | 2020 |
|---|---|---|---|---|---|---|---|---|---|---|---|---|---|---|---|---|---|
| TOTAL | 9.0 | 8.8 | 7.9 | 8.2 | 8.3 | 8.1 | 8.0 | 8.2 | 9.1 | 10.7 | 11.4 | 12.5 | 12.8 | 13.3 | 14.4 | 15.7 | *17.0* |
| AGE GROUP | | | | | | | | | | | | | | | | | |
| 12-13 | 5.4 | 5.2 | 4.9 | 4.3 | 4.9 | 4.6 | 4.3 | 4.1 | 5.4 | 6.1 | 7.2 | 7.8 | 7.3 | 6.9 | 8.4 | 10.5 | *11.2* |
| 14-15 | 9.2 | 9.5 | 7.9 | 8.4 | 8.5 | 8.8 | 9.0 | 8.6 | 10.2 | 12.4 | 11.9 | 13.8 | 13.3 | 14.5 | 15.3 | 16.4 | *18.2* |
| 16-17 | 12.3 | 11.5 | 10.7 | 11.5 | 11.2 | 10.4 | 10.6 | 11.7 | 11.4 | 13.2 | 14.6 | 15.5 | 17.2 | 17.7 | 19.0 | 20.1 | *21.9* |
| GENDER | | | | | | | | | | | | | | | | | |
| Male | 5.0 | 4.5 | 4.2 | 4.6 | 4.3 | 4.7 | 4.4 | 4.5 | 4.7 | 5.3 | 5.7 | 5.8 | 6.4 | 6.8 | 7.7 | 8.8 | *9.2* |
| Female | 13.1 | 13.3 | 11.8 | 11.9 | 12.5 | 11.7 | 11.9 | 12.1 | 13.7 | 16.2 | 17.3 | 19.5 | 19.4 | 20.0 | 21.5 | 23.0 | *25.2* |
| HISPANIC ORIGIN AND RACE | | | | | | | | | | | | | | | | | |
| Not Hispanic or Latino | 8.9 | 8.7 | 7.9 | 8.4 | 8.5 | 8.2 | 8.1 | 8.3 | 8.7 | 10.4 | 11.3 | 12.5 | 12.8 | 13.1 | 14.2 | 15.2 | *17.5* |
| White | 9.2 | 9.1 | 8.2 | 8.7 | 8.8 | 8.4 | 8.6 | 8.6 | 9.1 | 10.9 | 12.0 | 13.4 | 13.8 | 14.0 | 15.1 | 15.9 | *18.7* |
| Black or African American | 7.7 | 7.6 | 6.4 | 7.8 | 7.1 | 7.9 | 6.8 | 7.0 | 7.9 | 8.6 | 9.1 | 9.0 | 9.1 | 9.5 | 10.3 | 11.4 | *12.9* |
| AIAN | 7.8 | 6.1 | 9.3 | 4.6 | 10.1 | 7.5 | 7.4 | 11.4 | 5.2 | 4.5 | 6.9 | * | 11.5 | 16.3 | 15.2 | 12.2 | * |
| NHOPI | * | * | * | * | * | * | 1.8 | * | * | * | * | * | * | * | * | * | * |
| Asian | 8.3 | 6.0 | 7.7 | 6.6 | 7.7 | 7.6 | 5.5 | 7.6 | 4.2 | 10.2 | 10.4 | 9.7 | 11.9 | 11.3 | 13.6 | 15.1 | *13.9* |
| Two or More Races | 11.7 | 10.5 | 13.0 | 9.9 | 12.0 | 8.0 | 9.4 | 10.6 | 11.3 | 13.0 | 12.5 | 15.6 | 13.8 | 16.9 | 17.7 | 20.9 | *29.9* |
| Hispanic or Latino | 9.1 | 9.1 | 8.0 | 7.1 | 7.5 | 7.7 | 7.8 | 8.1 | 10.5 | 11.4 | 11.5 | 12.6 | 12.7 | 13.8 | 15.1 | 17.3 | *15.7* |

* = low precision; -= not available; da = does not apply; nc = not comparable due to methodological changes; nr = not reported due to measurement issues.

NOTE: Estimates in the 2020 column are italicized to indicate caution should be used when comparing estimates between 2020 and prior years because of methodological changes for 2020. Due to these changes, significance testing between 2020 and prior years was not performed. See the *2020 National Survey on Drug Use and Health: Methodological Summary and Definitions* for details.

NOTE: Some 2006 to 2010 estimates may differ from previously published estimates due to updates (see Chapter 3 of the *2020 National Survey on Drug Use and Health: Methodological Summary and Definitions*). NOTE: Respondents with unknown past year Major Depressive Episode (MDE) data were excluded.

Definitions: Measures and terms are defined in Appendix A.

Source: SAMHSA, Center for Behavioral Health Statistics and Quality, National Survey on Drug Use and Health, 2004-2019, and Quarters 1 and 4, 2020.

**Table 11.3A.** Major depressive episode with severe impairment in past year: among people aged 12 to 17; by demographic characteristics, numbers in thousands, 2006-2020

| Demographic Characteristic | 2006 | 2007 | 2008 | 2009 | 2010 | 2011 | 2012 | 2013 | 2014 | 2015 | 2016 | 2017 | 2018 | 2019 | 2020 |
|---|---|---|---|---|---|---|---|---|---|---|---|---|---|---|---|
| TOTAL | 1,358 | 1,371 | 1,460 | 1,404 | 1,350 | 1,388 | 1,544 | 1,868 | 1,990 | 2,129 | 2,168 | 2,265 | 2,423 | 2,671 | *2,919* |
| AGE GROUP | | | | | | | | | | | | | | | |
| 12-13 | 211 | 200 | 239 | 235 | 232 | 218 | 285 | 314 | 375 | 388 | 354 | 332 | 382 | 530 | *641* |
| 14-15 | 518 | 500 | 505 | 521 | 479 | 487 | 590 | 752 | 707 | 826 | 789 | 861 | 891 | 970 | *1,094* |
| 16-17 | 629 | 671 | 716 | 648 | 639 | 683 | 669 | 801 | 909 | 915 | 1,025 | 1,072 | 1,150 | 1,171 | *1,184* |
| GENDER | | | | | | | | | | | | | | | |
| Male | 335 | 386 | 359 | 391 | 395 | 397 | 373 | 435 | 461 | 477 | 539 | 581 | 628 | 736 | *732* |
| Female | 1,023 | 986 | 1,101 | 1,013 | 954 | 991 | 1,172 | 1,432 | 1,529 | 1,652 | 1,629 | 1,684 | 1,795 | 1,935 | *2,187* |
| HISPANIC ORIGIN AND RACE | | | | | | | | | | | | | | | |
| Not Hispanic or Latino | 1,118 | 1,141 | 1,226 | 1,150 | 1,093 | 1,113 | 1,152 | 1,425 | 1,540 | 1,651 | 1,703 | 1,694 | 1,841 | 1,981 | *2,230* |
| White | 871 | 873 | 944 | 858 | 853 | 799 | 883 | 1,046 | 1,167 | 1,258 | 1,290 | 1,256 | 1,354 | 1,415 | *1,616* |
| Black or African American | 150 | 193 | 171 | 204 | 157 | 183 | 164 | 207 | 214 | 198 | 196 | 233 | 225 | 256 | *294* |
| AIAN | 9 | 4 | 8 | 5 | 7 | 13 | 4 | 6 | 8 | * | 8 | 6 | * | 19 | * |
| NHOPI | * | * | * | * | * | * | * | * | * | * | * | * | * | * | * |
| Asian | 54 | 39 | 44 | 48 | 44 | 60 | 30 | 98 | 80 | 67 | 118 | 101 | 127 | 142 | *186* |
| Two or More Races | 32 | 32 | 50 | 31 | 30 | 57 | 64 | 61 | 66 | 98 | 86 | 89 | 109 | 134 | *118* |
| Hispanic or Latino | 240 | 230 | 233 | 254 | 257 | 275 | 392 | 442 | 450 | 477 | 465 | 571 | 582 | 690 | *689* |

* = low precision; -= not available; da = does not apply; nc = not comparable due to methodological changes; nr = not reported due to measurement issues.

NOTE: Estimates in the 2020 column are italicized to indicate caution should be used when comparing estimates between 2020 and prior years because of methodological changes for 2020. Due to these changes, significance testing between 2020 and prior years was not performed. See the *2020 National Survey on Drug Use and Health: Methodological Summary and Definitions* for details.

NOTE: Some 2006 to 2010 estimates may differ from previously published estimates due to updates (see Chapter 3 of the *2020 National Survey on Drug Use and Health: Methodological Summary and Definitions*). NOTE: Respondents with unknown past year Major Depressive Episode (MDE) data were excluded.

NOTE: Respondents with unknown impairment data were excluded.

Definitions: Measures and terms are defined in Appendix A.

Source: SAMHSA, Center for Behavioral Health Statistics and Quality, National Survey on Drug Use and Health, 2006-2019, and Quarters 1 and 4, 2020.

**Table 11.3B.** Major depressive episode with severe impairment in past year: among people aged 12 to 17; by demographic characteristics, percentages, 2006-2020

| Demographic Characteristic | 2006 | 2007 | 2008 | 2009 | 2010 | 2011 | 2012 | 2013 | 2014 | 2015 | 2016 | 2017 | 2018 | 2019 | 2020 |
|---|---|---|---|---|---|---|---|---|---|---|---|---|---|---|---|
| TOTAL | 5.5 | 5.5 | 6.0 | 5.8 | 5.7 | 5.7 | 6.3 | 7.7 | 8.2 | 8.8 | 9.0 | 9.4 | 10.0 | 11.1 | *12.0* |
| AGE GROUP | | | | | | | | | | | | | | | |
| 12-13 | 2.7 | 2.5 | 3.2 | 3.2 | 3.0 | 2.8 | 3.7 | 4.1 | 4.9 | 5.1 | 4.7 | 4.4 | 5.1 | 6.8 | *7.9* |
| 14-15 | 6.0 | 6.0 | 6.1 | 6.2 | 6.1 | 5.9 | 7.1 | 9.1 | 8.5 | 9.8 | 9.4 | 10.4 | 10.9 | 11.9 | *13.0* |
| 16-17 | 7.5 | 7.9 | 8.4 | 7.7 | 7.7 | 8.1 | 8.0 | 9.7 | 10.9 | 11.1 | 12.4 | 12.7 | 13.7 | 14.5 | *15.3* |
| GENDER | | | | | | | | | | | | | | | |
| Male | 2.6 | 3.0 | 2.9 | 3.2 | 3.2 | 3.2 | 3.0 | 3.5 | 3.7 | 3.8 | 4.4 | 4.7 | 5.1 | 6.0 | *5.9* |
| Female | 8.4 | 8.2 | 9.3 | 8.6 | 8.2 | 8.3 | 9.8 | 12.0 | 13.0 | 14.0 | 13.7 | 14.2 | 15.2 | 16.5 | *18.4* |
| HISPANIC ORIGIN AND RACE | | | | | | | | | | | | | | | |
| Not Hispanic or Latino | 5.5 | 5.7 | 6.2 | 5.9 | 5.7 | 5.8 | 6.1 | 7.6 | 8.2 | 8.9 | 9.2 | 9.2 | 10.1 | 11.0 | *12.3* |
| White | 5.8 | 5.9 | 6.5 | 6.1 | 6.2 | 5.9 | 6.5 | 7.8 | 8.9 | 9.7 | 10.0 | 9.8 | 10.7 | 11.4 | *13.0* |
| Black or African American | 3.9 | 5.1 | 4.6 | 5.7 | 4.5 | 5.4 | 4.8 | 6.2 | 6.4 | 5.9 | 6.0 | 7.1 | 6.9 | 8.0 | *9.7* |
| AIAN | 6.6 | 2.6 | 6.5 | 4.3 | 5.4 | 9.8 | 2.6 | 3.8 | 4.9 | * | 5.7 | 3.9 | * | 11.5 | * |
| NHOPI | * | * | * | * | * | * | * | * | * | * | * | * | * | * | * |
| Asian | 5.3 | 3.9 | 4.7 | 5.0 | 4.3 | 5.0 | 2.6 | 8.1 | 6.6 | 5.5 | 9.3 | 7.9 | 9.2 | 11.3 | *10.3* |
| Two or More Races | 8.0 | 7.8 | 10.2 | 6.0 | 5.9 | 8.1 | 9.0 | 8.4 | 8.9 | 12.6 | 10.9 | 10.9 | 14.2 | 14.9 | *19.7* |
| Hispanic or Latino | 5.4 | 5.1 | 5.1 | 5.4 | 5.4 | 5.2 | 7.3 | 8.2 | 8.2 | 8.5 | 8.2 | 9.9 | 10.0 | 11.7 | *11.3* |

* = low precision; -= not available; da = does not apply; nc = not comparable due to methodological changes; nr = not reported due to measurement issues.

NOTE: Estimates in the 2020 column are italicized to indicate caution should be used when comparing estimates between 2020 and prior years because of methodological changes for 2020. Due to these changes, significance testing between 2020 and prior years was not performed. See the *2020 National Survey on Drug Use and Health: Methodological Summary and Definitions* for details.

NOTE: Some 2006 to 2010 estimates may differ from previously published estimates due to updates (see Chapter 3 of the *2020 National Survey on Drug Use and Health: Methodological Summary and Definitions*). NOTE: Respondents with unknown past year Major Depressive Episode (MDE) data were excluded.

NOTE: Respondents with unknown impairment data were excluded.

Definitions: Measures and terms are defined in Appendix A.

Source: SAMHSA, Center for Behavioral Health Statistics and Quality, National Survey on Drug Use and Health, 2006-2019, and Quarters 1 and 4, 2020.

**Table 11.4A.** Receipt of treatment for depression in past year: among people aged 12 to 17 with major depressive episode in past year; by demographic characteristics, numbers in thousands, 2004-2020

| Demographic Characteristic | 2004 | 2005 | 2006 | 2007 | 2008 | 2009 | 2010 | 2011 | 2012 | 2013 | 2014 | 2015 | 2016 | 2017 | 2018 | 2019 | 2020 |
|---|---|---|---|---|---|---|---|---|---|---|---|---|---|---|---|---|---|
| TOTAL | 895 | 822 | 760 | 782 | 764 | 673 | 721 | 769 | 813 | 977 | 1,122 | 1,186 | 1,249 | 1,330 | 1,432 | 1,627 | *1,710* |
| AGE GROUP | | | | | | | | | | | | | | | | | |
| 12-13 | 169 | 136 | 133 | 137 | 122 | 98 | 106 | 112 | 127 | 181 | 194 | 185 | 189 | 193 | 251 | 302 | * |
| 14-15 | 278 | 329 | 263 | 259 | 236 | 244 | 271 | 258 | 307 | 376 | 394 | 472 | 455 | 453 | 514 | 585 | *629* |
| 16-17 | 448 | 357 | 364 | 386 | 405 | 331 | 343 | 400 | 379 | 420 | 535 | 530 | 605 | 684 | 667 | 740 | *675* |
| GENDER | | | | | | | | | | | | | | | | | |
| Male | 239 | 193 | 189 | 214 | 183 | 168 | 171 | 199 | 163 | 193 | 265 | 262 | 260 | 274 | 351 | 391 | *448* |
| Female | 656 | 629 | 571 | 568 | 581 | 505 | 549 | 570 | 650 | 784 | 857 | 924 | 989 | 1,056 | 1,081 | 1,236 | *1,262* |
| HISPANIC ORIGIN AND RACE | | | | | | | | | | | | | | | | | |
| Not Hispanic or Latino | 756 | 700 | 634 | 691 | 658 | 555 | 577 | 645 | 642 | 753 | 918 | 936 | 1,008 | 1,072 | 1,100 | 1,251 | *1,357* |
| White | 633 | 544 | 502 | 545 | 545 | 444 | 487 | 482 | 500 | 598 | 723 | 702 | 799 | 847 | 870 | 985 | *1,133* |
| Black or African American | 82 | 113 | 70 | 116 | 85 | 67 | 54 | 97 | 90 | 83 | 123 | 127 | 102 | 110 | 115 | 130 | * |
| AIAN | * | * | * | * | * | * | * | * | * | * | * | * | * | * | * | * | * |
| NHOPI | * | * | * | * | * | * | * | * | * | * | * | * | * | * | * | * | * |
| Asian | * | * | * | * | * | * | * | * | * | * | * | * | * | * | * | * | * |
| Two or More Races | * | * | * | * | * | * | * | * | * | * | * | 55 | * | 62 | 48 | 83 | * |
| Hispanic or Latino | 139 | 122 | 126 | 91 | 105 | 118 | 144 | 125 | 171 | 224 | 204 | 251 | 241 | 258 | 332 | 376 | *354* |

* = low precision; -= not available; da = does not apply; nc = not comparable due to methodological changes; nr = not reported due to measurement issues.

NOTE: Estimates in the 2020 column are italicized to indicate caution should be used when comparing estimates between 2020 and prior years because of methodological changes for 2020. Due to these changes, significance testing between 2020 and prior years was not performed. See the *2020 National Survey on Drug Use and Health: Methodological Summary and Definitions* for details.

NOTE: Some 2006 to 2010 estimates may differ from previously published estimates due to updates (see Chapter 3 of the *2020 National Survey on Drug Use and Health: Methodological Summary and Definitions*). NOTE: Respondents with unknown past year treatment for depression data were excluded.

NOTE: Respondents with unknown past year Major Depressive Episode (MDE) data were excluded.

Definitions: Measures and terms are defined in Appendix A.

Source: SAMHSA, Center for Behavioral Health Statistics and Quality, National Survey on Drug Use and Health, 2004-2019, and Quarters 1 and 4, 2020.

**Table 11.4B.** Receipt of treatment for depression in past year: among people aged 12 to 17 with major depressive episode in past year; by demographic characteristics, percentages, 2004-2020

| Demographic Characteristic | 2004 | 2005 | 2006 | 2007 | 2008 | 2009 | 2010 | 2011 | 2012 | 2013 | 2014 | 2015 | 2016 | 2017 | 2018 | 2019 | 2020 |
|---|---|---|---|---|---|---|---|---|---|---|---|---|---|---|---|---|---|
| TOTAL | 40.3 | 37.8 | 38.8 | 39.0 | 37.7 | 34.6 | 37.8 | 38.4 | 37.0 | 38.1 | 41.2 | 39.3 | 40.9 | 41.5 | 41.4 | 43.3 | *41.6* |
| AGE GROUP | | | | | | | | | | | | | | | | | |
| 12-13 | 38.2 | 32.9 | 35.1 | 41.5 | 33.5 | 30.0 | 32.5 | 36.3 | 30.7 | 39.1 | 35.9 | 31.9 | 35.3 | 37.6 | 40.7 | 37.5 | * |
| 14-15 | 35.5 | 41.1 | 38.4 | 36.8 | 33.6 | 33.2 | 38.4 | 36.3 | 36.6 | 37.2 | 40.1 | 40.6 | 41.3 | 37.9 | 41.2 | 43.9 | *41.5* |
| 16-17 | 45.0 | 37.1 | 40.7 | 39.8 | 42.4 | 37.5 | 39.3 | 40.5 | 40.0 | 38.6 | 44.4 | 41.5 | 42.6 | 45.8 | 41.8 | 45.6 | *40.0* |
| GENDER | | | | | | | | | | | | | | | | | |
| Male | 37.7 | 34.1 | 35.3 | 36.7 | 34.0 | 29.2 | 32.0 | 35.3 | 28.3 | 29.7 | 37.7 | 36.3 | 33.5 | 32.5 | 37.5 | 36.8 | *39.7* |
| Female | 41.3 | 39.0 | 40.2 | 40.0 | 39.1 | 36.9 | 40.1 | 39.5 | 40.1 | 40.9 | 42.4 | 40.3 | 43.4 | 44.8 | 42.9 | 45.8 | *42.4* |
| HISPANIC ORIGIN AND RACE | | | | | | | | | | | | | | | | | |
| Not Hispanic or Latino | 41.0 | 39.0 | 39.5 | 41.1 | 39.3 | 35.0 | 37.6 | 40.7 | 39.0 | 38.5 | 43.5 | 40.5 | 42.9 | 44.4 | 42.6 | 45.7 | *43.1* |
| White | 44.9 | 39.3 | 41.3 | 42.7 | 43.1 | 37.7 | 41.1 | 41.4 | 40.7 | 41.6 | 46.1 | 40.6 | 45.1 | 47.5 | 46.1 | 50.3 | *49.1* |
| Black or African American | 28.9 | 39.3 | 29.1 | 39.7 | 32.4 | 23.9 | 23.0 | 41.0 | 33.5 | 28.6 | 40.6 | 42.0 | 34.5 | 35.1 | 34.6 | 35.6 | * |
| AIAN | * | * | * | * | * | * | * | * | * | * | * | * | * | * | * | * | * |
| NHOPI | * | * | * | * | * | * | * | * | * | * | * | * | * | * | * | * | * |
| Asian | * | * | * | * | * | * | * | * | * | * | * | * | * | * | * | * | * |
| Two or More Races | * | * | * | * | * | * | * | * | * | * | * | 46.7 | * | 44.8 | 34.8 | 44.4 | * |
| Hispanic or Latino | 36.8 | 31.8 | 35.9 | 28.2 | 30.4 | 33.0 | 38.4 | 29.4 | 30.8 | 36.9 | 33.1 | 35.5 | 34.1 | 32.7 | 37.9 | 36.8 | *37.0* |

* = low precision; -= not available; da = does not apply; nc = not comparable due to methodological changes; nr = not reported due to measurement issues.

NOTE: Estimates in the 2020 column are italicized to indicate caution should be used when comparing estimates between 2020 and prior years because of methodological changes for 2020. Due to these changes, significance testing between 2020 and prior years was not performed. See the *2020 National Survey on Drug Use and Health: Methodological Summary and Definitions* for details.

NOTE: Some 2006 to 2010 estimates may differ from previously published estimates due to updates (see Chapter 3 of the *2020 National Survey on Drug Use and Health: Methodological Summary and Definitions*). NOTE: Respondents with unknown past year treatment for depression data were excluded.

NOTE: Respondents with unknown past year Major Depressive Episode (MDE) data were excluded.

Definitions: Measures and terms are defined in Appendix A.

Source: SAMHSA, Center for Behavioral Health Statistics and Quality, National Survey on Drug Use and Health, 2004-2019, and Quarters 1 and 4, 2020.

**Table 11.5A.** Receipt of treatment for depression in past year: among people aged 12 to 17 with major depressive episode with severe impairment in past year; by demographic characteristics, numbers in thousands, 2006-2020

| Demographic Characteristic | 2006 | 2007 | 2008 | 2009 | 2010 | 2011 | 2012 | 2013 | 2014 | 2015 | 2016 | 2017 | 2018 | 2019 | 2020 |
|---|---|---|---|---|---|---|---|---|---|---|---|---|---|---|---|
| TOTAL | 627 | 601 | 622 | 542 | 554 | 602 | 633 | 832 | 882 | 945 | 1,001 | 1,074 | 1,133 | 1,321 | *1,361* |
| AGE GROUP | | | | | | | | | | | | | | | |
| 12-13 | 92 | 85 | 91 | 78 | 66 | 91 | 91 | 150 | 143 | 142 | 131 | 153 | 177 | 218 | * |
| 14-15 | 232 | 216 | 194 | 184 | 215 | 200 | 239 | 320 | 307 | 374 | 369 | 364 | 406 | 492 | *521* |
| 16-17 | 304 | 300 | 336 | 280 | 273 | 311 | 302 | 363 | 433 | 429 | 501 | 558 | 550 | 612 | *527* |
| GENDER | | | | | | | | | | | | | | | |
| Male | 134 | 154 | 132 | 132 | 132 | 147 | 127 | 157 | 189 | 206 | 208 | 208 | 274 | 300 | *341* |
| Female | 493 | 447 | 489 | 410 | 422 | 455 | 506 | 675 | 693 | 739 | 793 | 866 | 859 | 1,021 | *1,020* |
| HISPANIC ORIGIN AND RACE | | | | | | | | | | | | | | | |
| Not Hispanic or Latino | 535 | 534 | 550 | 443 | 448 | 502 | 506 | 645 | 725 | 755 | 827 | 868 | 882 | 1,018 | *1,088* |
| White | 432 | 439 | 461 | 352 | 380 | 379 | 403 | 504 | 572 | 563 | 668 | 679 | 695 | 800 | *917* |
| Black or African American | 53 | 72 | 65 | 58 | 42 | 82 | 56 | 72 | 99 | 97 | 71 | 97 | 90 | 108 | * |
| AIAN | * | * | * | * | * | * | * | * | * | * | * | * | * | * | * |
| NHOPI | * | * | * | * | * | * | * | * | * | * | * | * | * | * | * |
| Asian | * | * | * | * | * | * | * | * | * | * | * | * | * | * | * |
| Two or More Races | * | * | * | * | * | * | * | * | * | * | * | * | * | 63 | * |
| Hispanic or Latino | 92 | 67 | 72 | 99 | 106 | 100 | 127 | 187 | 158 | 190 | 174 | 206 | 251 | 304 | *273* |

* = low precision; -= not available; da = does not apply; nc = not comparable due to methodological changes; nr = not reported due to measurement issues.

NOTE: Estimates in the 2020 column are italicized to indicate caution should be used when comparing estimates between 2020 and prior years because of methodological changes for 2020. Due to these changes, significance testing between 2020 and prior years was not performed. See the *2020 National Survey on Drug Use and Health: Methodological Summary and Definitions* for details.

NOTE: Some 2006 to 2010 estimates may differ from previously published estimates due to updates (see Chapter 3 of the *2020 National Survey on Drug Use and Health: Methodological Summary and Definitions*). NOTE: Respondents with unknown past year treatment for depression data were excluded.

NOTE: Respondents with unknown past year Major Depressive Episode (MDE) data were excluded. NOTE: Respondents with unknown impairment data were excluded.

Definitions: Measures and terms are defined in Appendix A.

Source: SAMHSA, Center for Behavioral Health Statistics and Quality, National Survey on Drug Use and Health, 2006-2019, and Quarters 1 and 4, 2020.

**Table 11.5B.** Receipt of treatment for depression in past year: among people aged 12 to 17 with major depressive episode with severe impairment in past year; by demographic characteristics, percentages, 2006-2020

| Demographic Characteristic | 2006 | 2007 | 2008 | 2009 | 2010 | 2011 | 2012 | 2013 | 2014 | 2015 | 2016 | 2017 | 2018 | 2019 | 2020 |
|---|---|---|---|---|---|---|---|---|---|---|---|---|---|---|---|
| TOTAL | 46.5 | 43.9 | 42.6 | 38.8 | 41.1 | 43.5 | 41.0 | 45.0 | 44.7 | 44.6 | 46.7 | 47.5 | 46.9 | 49.7 | *46.9* |
| AGE GROUP | | | | | | | | | | | | | | | |
| 12-13 | 44.1 | 42.3 | 38.3 | 33.8 | 28.7 | 42.3 | 32.0 | 48.5 | 38.7 | 37.0 | 37.6 | 46.2 | 47.2 | 41.9 | * |
| 14-15 | 44.8 | 43.2 | 38.6 | 35.6 | 45.0 | 41.0 | 40.5 | 43.2 | 43.4 | 45.4 | 47.5 | 42.3 | 45.6 | 50.8 | *48.1* |
| 16-17 | 48.8 | 44.9 | 46.9 | 43.2 | 42.7 | 45.5 | 45.4 | 45.3 | 48.1 | 47.1 | 49.2 | 52.0 | 47.8 | 52.3 | *44.8* |
| GENDER | | | | | | | | | | | | | | | |
| Male | 40.1 | 40.2 | 36.9 | 34.0 | 33.4 | 37.3 | 34.4 | 36.4 | 41.2 | 43.1 | 39.0 | 35.8 | 43.7 | 41.2 | *46.6* |
| Female | 48.6 | 45.4 | 44.5 | 40.7 | 44.3 | 45.9 | 43.2 | 47.6 | 45.7 | 45.1 | 49.3 | 51.5 | 48.1 | 52.9 | *47.0* |
| HISPANIC ORIGIN AND RACE | | | | | | | | | | | | | | | |
| Not Hispanic or Latino | 48.0 | 46.8 | 44.9 | 38.7 | 41.1 | 45.2 | 43.9 | 45.6 | 47.3 | 46.0 | 48.9 | 51.3 | 48.1 | 51.7 | *49.2* |
| White | 49.8 | 50.4 | 48.9 | 41.1 | 44.5 | 47.4 | 45.7 | 48.6 | 49.2 | 45.0 | 52.1 | 54.1 | 51.6 | 57.0 | *57.3* |
| Black or African American | 35.5 | 37.4 | 38.0 | 28.9 | 26.9 | 44.6 | 34.4 | 34.9 | 46.9 | 48.8 | 37.1 | 41.6 | 40.1 | 42.3 | * |
| AIAN | * | * | * | * | * | * | * | * | * | * | * | * | * | * | * |
| NHOPI | * | * | * | * | * | * | * | * | * | * | * | * | * | * | * |
| Asian | * | * | * | * | * | * | * | * | * | * | * | * | * | * | * |
| Two or More Races | * | * | * | * | * | * | * | * | * | * | * | * | * | 47.3 | * |
| Hispanic or Latino | 39.4 | 29.4 | 30.8 | 39.3 | 41.3 | 36.4 | 32.6 | 43.1 | 35.6 | 40.0 | 38.4 | 36.1 | 43.2 | 44.0 | *39.6* |

* = low precision; -= not available; da = does not apply; nc = not comparable due to methodological changes; nr = not reported due to measurement issues.

NOTE: Estimates in the 2020 column are italicized to indicate caution should be used when comparing estimates between 2020 and prior years because of methodological changes for 2020. Due to these changes, significance testing between 2020 and prior years was not performed. See the *2020 National Survey on Drug Use and Health: Methodological Summary and Definitions* for details.

NOTE: Some 2006 to 2010 estimates may differ from previously published estimates due to updates (see Chapter 3 of the *2020 National Survey on Drug Use and Health: Methodological Summary and Definitions*). NOTE: Respondents with unknown past year treatment for depression data were excluded.

NOTE: Respondents with unknown past year Major Depressive Episode (MDE) data were excluded. NOTE: Respondents with unknown impairment data were excluded.

Definitions: Measures and terms are defined in Appendix A.

Source: SAMHSA, Center for Behavioral Health Statistics and Quality, National Survey on Drug Use and Health, 2006-2019, and Quarters 1 and 4, 2020.

**Table 11.6A.** Substance use in past year and past month: among people aged 12 to 17 with major depressive episode in past year; numbers in thousands, 2004-2020

| Substance | 2004 | 2005 | 2006 | 2007 | 2008 | 2009 | 2010 | 2011 | 2012 | 2013 | 2014 | 2015 | 2016 | 2017 | 2018 | 2019 | 2020 |
|---|---|---|---|---|---|---|---|---|---|---|---|---|---|---|---|---|---|
| PAST YEAR USE | | | | | | | | | | | | | | | | | |
| Illicit Drugs | nc | nc | nc | nc | nc | nc | nc | nc | nc | nc | nc | 955 | 979 | 942 | 1,138 | 1,207 | *1,183* |
| Marijuana | 601 | 553 | 483 | 473 | 485 | 472 | 481 | 523 | 547 | 664 | 664 | 675 | 751 | 724 | 878 | 930 | *908* |
| Cocaine | 66 | 73 | 64 | 69 | 61 | 43 | 46 | 54 | 53 | 28 | 41 | 34 | 35 | 37 | 35 | 29 | *38* |
| Crack | 15 | 12 | 16 | 17 | 12 | 9 | 9 | 11 | 7 | 2 | 11 | * | 4 | 2 | 0 | 10 | * |
| Heroin | 9 | 10 | 11 | 6 | 9 | 10 | 10 | 11 | 11 | 7 | 12 | 5 | 3 | 6 | 3 | * | * |
| Hallucinogens | nc | nc | nc | nc | nc | nc | nc | nc | nc | nc | nc | 129 | 127 | 145 | 112 | 147 | *152* |
| LSD | 36 | 38 | 18 | 16 | 28 | 43 | 24 | 30 | 40 | 29 | 48 | 63 | 41 | 72 | 62 | 99 | *89* |
| PCP | 21 | 16 | 11 | 8 | 20 | 12 | 8 | 12 | 9 | 6 | 11 | 2 | 6 | 12 | 6 | 7 | * |
| Ecstasy | nc | nc | nc | nc | nc | nc | nc | nc | nc | nc | nc | 45 | 59 | 47 | 46 | 60 | *34* |
| Inhalants | nc | nc | nc | nc | nc | nc | nc | nc | nc | nc | nc | 193 | 159 | 145 | 178 | 235 | *288* |
| Methamphetamine | nc | nc | nc | nc | nc | nc | nc | nc | nc | nc | nc | 14 | 6 | 14 | 8 | 10 | * |
| Misuse of Prescription Psychotherapeutics | nc | nc | nc | nc | nc | nc | nc | nc | nc | nc | nc | 370 | 411 | 369 | 375 | 355 | *229* |
| Pain Relievers | nc | nc | nc | nc | nc | nc | nc | nc | nc | nc | nc | 236 | 283 | 210 | 214 | 158 | *94* |
| Stimulants | nc | nc | nc | nc | nc | nc | nc | nc | nc | nc | nc | 166 | 142 | 158 | 126 | 184 | *115* |
| Tranquilizers or Sedatives | nc | nc | nc | nc | nc | nc | nc | nc | nc | nc | nc | 117 | 168 | 167 | 168 | 174 | *108* |
| Tranquilizers | nc | nc | nc | nc | nc | nc | nc | nc | nc | nc | nc | 103 | 149 | 164 | 153 | 155 | *96* |
| Sedatives | nc | nc | nc | nc | nc | nc | nc | nc | nc | nc | nc | 26 | 43 | 22 | 34 | 45 | *12* |
| Benzodiazepines | nc | nc | nc | nc | nc | nc | nc | nc | nc | nc | nc | 96 | 142 | 154 | 145 | 149 | *81* |
| Opioids | nc | nc | nc | nc | nc | nc | nc | nc | nc | nc | nc | 236 | 285 | 212 | 214 | 158 | *94* |
| Central Nervous System Stimulants | nc | nc | nc | nc | nc | nc | nc | nc | nc | nc | nc | 181 | 164 | 173 | 158 | 200 | *140* |
| Illicit Drugs Other Than Marijuana[1] | nc | nc | nc | nc | nc | nc | nc | nc | nc | nc | nc | 563 | 553 | 515 | 547 | 595 | *552* |
| PAST MONTH USE | | | | | | | | | | | | | | | | | |
| Alcohol | 632 | 606 | 523 | 553 | 509 | 473 | 460 | 482 | 503 | 490 | 556 | 524 | 508 | 524 | 558 | 638 | *673* |
| Binge Alcohol Use[2] | nc | nc | nc | nc | nc | nc | nc | nc | nc | nc | nc | 288 | 268 | 293 | 295 | 338 | *254* |

## **Table 11.6A.** (Continued)

| Substance | 2004 | 2005 | 2006 | 2007 | 2008 | 2009 | 2010 | 2011 | 2012 | 2013 | 2014 | 2015 | 2016 | 2017 | 2018 | 2019 | 2020 |
|---|---|---|---|---|---|---|---|---|---|---|---|---|---|---|---|---|---|
| Heavy Alcohol Use | nc | nc | nc | nc | nc | nc | nc | nc | nc | nc | nc | 51 | 52 | 39 | 22 | 53 | *49* |
| Cigarette Use | 508 | 450 | 378 | 388 | 354 | 336 | 302 | 317 | 284 | 288 | 254 | 241 | 239 | 214 | 212 | 166 | *110* |
| Daily Cigarette Use | 171 | 116 | 102 | 96 | 75 | 70 | 59 | 81 | 61 | 46 | 45 | 55 | 27 | 25 | 23 | 14 | *6* |

* = low precision; -= not available; da = does not apply; nc = not comparable due to methodological changes; nr = not reported due to measurement issues.

NOTE: Estimates in the 2020 column are italicized to indicate caution should be used when comparing estimates between 2020 and prior years because of methodological changes for 2020. Due to these changes, significance testing between 2020 and prior years was not performed. See the *2020 National Survey on Drug Use and Health: Methodological Summary and Definitions* for details.

NOTE: Some 2006 to 2010 estimates may differ from previously published estimates due to updates (see Chapter 3 of the *2020 National Survey on Drug Use and Health: Methodological Summary and Definitions*). NOTE: Respondents with unknown past year Major Depressive Episode (MDE) data were excluded.

[1]Illicit Drugs Other Than Marijuana excludes respondents who used only marijuana but includes those who used marijuana in addition to other illicit drugs.

[2]Estimates of binge alcohol use include use by those who were heavy alcohol users.

Definitions: Measures and terms are defined in Appendix A.

Source: SAMHSA, Center for Behavioral Health Statistics and Quality, National Survey on Drug Use and Health, 2004-2019, and Quarters 1 and 4, 2020.

**Table 11.6B.** Substance use in past year and past month: among people aged 12 to 17 with major depressive episode in past year; percentages, 2004-2020

| Substance | 2004 | 2005 | 2006 | 2007 | 2008 | 2009 | 2010 | 2011 | 2012 | 2013 | 2014 | 2015 | 2016 | 2017 | 2018 | 2019 | 2020 |
|---|---|---|---|---|---|---|---|---|---|---|---|---|---|---|---|---|---|
| PAST YEAR USE | | | | | | | | | | | | | | | | | |
| Illicit Drugs | nc | nc | nc | nc | nc | nc | nc | nc | nc | nc | nc | 31.5 | 31.7 | 29.3 | 32.7 | 31.9 | *28.6* |
| Marijuana | 27.0 | 25.2 | 24.5 | 23.5 | 23.9 | 24.2 | 25.2 | 26.0 | 24.7 | 25.7 | 24.1 | 22.3 | 24.3 | 22.5 | 25.2 | 24.6 | *22.0* |
| Cocaine | 3.0 | 3.4 | 3.3 | 3.4 | 3.0 | 2.2 | 2.4 | 2.7 | 2.4 | 1.1 | 1.5 | 1.1 | 1.1 | 1.1 | 1.0 | 0.8 | *0.9* |
| Crack | 0.7 | 0.6 | 0.8 | 0.9 | 0.6 | 0.5 | 0.5 | 0.5 | 0.3 | 0.1 | 0.4 | * | 0.1 | 0.1 | 0.0 | 0.3 | * |
| Heroin | 0.4 | 0.4 | 0.5 | 0.3 | 0.4 | 0.5 | 0.5 | 0.5 | 0.5 | 0.3 | 0.4 | 0.2 | 0.1 | 0.2 | 0.1 | * | * |
| Hallucinogens | nc | nc | nc | nc | nc | nc | nc | nc | nc | nc | nc | 4.2 | 4.1 | 4.5 | 3.2 | 3.9 | *3.7* |
| LSD | 1.6 | 1.7 | 0.9 | 0.8 | 1.4 | 2.2 | 1.2 | 1.5 | 1.8 | 1.1 | 1.8 | 2.1 | 1.3 | 2.2 | 1.8 | 2.6 | *2.2* |
| PCP | 0.9 | 0.7 | 0.6 | 0.4 | 1.0 | 0.6 | 0.4 | 0.6 | 0.4 | 0.2 | 0.4 | 0.1 | 0.2 | 0.4 | 0.2 | 0.2 | * |
| Ecstasy | nc | nc | nc | nc | nc | nc | nc | nc | nc | nc | nc | 1.5 | 1.9 | 1.5 | 1.3 | 1.6 | *0.8* |
| Inhalants | nc | nc | nc | nc | nc | nc | nc | nc | nc | nc | nc | 6.4 | 5.1 | 4.5 | 5.1 | 6.2 | *7.0* |
| Methamphetamine | nc | nc | nc | nc | nc | nc | nc | nc | nc | nc | nc | 0.5 | 0.2 | 0.4 | 0.2 | 0.3 | * |
| Misuse of Prescription Psychotherapeutics | nc | nc | nc | nc | nc | nc | nc | nc | nc | nc | nc | 12.2 | 13.3 | 11.5 | 10.8 | 9.4 | *5.5* |
| Pain Relievers | nc | nc | nc | nc | nc | nc | nc | nc | nc | nc | nc | 7.8 | 9.2 | 6.5 | 6.1 | 4.2 | *2.3* |
| Stimulants | nc | nc | nc | nc | nc | nc | nc | nc | nc | nc | nc | 5.5 | 4.6 | 4.9 | 3.6 | 4.9 | *2.8* |
| Tranquilizers or Sedatives | nc | nc | nc | nc | nc | nc | nc | nc | nc | nc | nc | 3.9 | 5.5 | 5.2 | 4.8 | 4.6 | *2.6* |
| Tranquilizers | nc | nc | nc | nc | nc | nc | nc | nc | nc | nc | nc | 3.4 | 4.8 | 5.1 | 4.4 | 4.1 | *2.3* |
| Sedatives | nc | nc | nc | nc | nc | nc | nc | nc | nc | nc | nc | 0.8 | 1.4 | 0.7 | 1.0 | 1.2 | *0.3* |
| Benzodiazepines | nc | nc | nc | nc | nc | nc | nc | nc | nc | nc | nc | 3.2 | 4.6 | 4.8 | 4.2 | 3.9 | *2.0* |
| Opioids | nc | nc | nc | nc | nc | nc | nc | nc | nc | nc | nc | 7.8 | 9.2 | 6.6 | 6.1 | 4.2 | *2.3* |
| Central Nervous System Stimulants | nc | nc | nc | nc | nc | nc | nc | nc | nc | nc | nc | 6.0 | 5.3 | 5.4 | 4.5 | 5.3 | *3.4* |
| Illicit Drugs Other Than Marijuana[1] | nc | nc | nc | nc | nc | nc | nc | nc | nc | nc | nc | 18.6 | 17.9 | 16.0 | 15.7 | 15.7 | *13.4* |
| PAST MONTH USE | | | | | | | | | | | | | | | | | |
| Alcohol | 28.4 | 27.6 | 26.6 | 27.4 | 25.1 | 24.2 | 24.0 | 23.9 | 22.7 | 18.9 | 20.2 | 17.3 | 16.5 | 16.3 | 16.0 | 16.9 | *16.3* |
| Binge Alcohol Use[2] | nc | nc | nc | nc | nc | nc | nc | nc | nc | nc | nc | 9.5 | 8.7 | 9.1 | 8.5 | 8.9 | *6.2* |

## **Table 11.6B.** (Continued)

| Substance | 2004 | 2005 | 2006 | 2007 | 2008 | 2009 | 2010 | 2011 | 2012 | 2013 | 2014 | 2015 | 2016 | 2017 | 2018 | 2019 | 2020 |
|---|---|---|---|---|---|---|---|---|---|---|---|---|---|---|---|---|---|
| Heavy Alcohol Use | nc | nc | nc | nc | nc | nc | nc | nc | nc | nc | nc | 1.7 | 1.7 | 1.2 | 0.6 | 1.4 | *1.2* |
| Cigarette Use | 22.8 | 20.5 | 19.2 | 19.2 | 17.4 | 17.2 | 15.8 | 15.8 | 12.8 | 11.1 | 9.2 | 8.0 | 7.8 | 6.7 | 6.1 | 4.4 | *2.7* |
| Daily Cigarette Use | 7.7 | 5.3 | 5.2 | 4.8 | 3.7 | 3.6 | 3.1 | 4.0 | 2.7 | 1.8 | 1.6 | 1.8 | 0.9 | 0.8 | 0.7 | 0.4 | *0.1* |

* = low precision; -= not available; da = does not apply; nc = not comparable due to methodological changes; nr = not reported due to measurement issues.

NOTE: Estimates in the 2020 column are italicized to indicate caution should be used when comparing estimates between 2020 and prior years because of methodological changes for 2020. Due to these changes, significance testing between 2020 and prior years was not performed. See the *2020 National Survey on Drug Use and Health: Methodological Summary and Definitions* for details.

NOTE: Some 2006 to 2010 estimates may differ from previously published estimates due to updates (see Chapter 3 of the *2020 National Survey on Drug Use and Health: Methodological Summary and Definitions*). NOTE: Respondents with unknown past year Major Depressive Episode (MDE) data were excluded.

[1] Illicit Drugs Other Than Marijuana excludes respondents who used only marijuana but includes those who used marijuana in addition to other illicit drugs.

[2] Estimates of binge alcohol use include use by those who were heavy alcohol users.

Definitions: Measures and terms are defined in Appendix A.

Source: SAMHSA, Center for Behavioral Health Statistics and Quality, National Survey on Drug Use and Health, 2004-2019, and Quarters 1 and 4, 2020.

**Table 11.7A.** Substance use in past year and past month: among people aged 12 to 17 with major depressive episode with severe impairment in past year; numbers in thousands, 2006-2020

| Substance | 2006 | 2007 | 2008 | 2009 | 2010 | 2011 | 2012 | 2013 | 2014 | 2015 | 2016 | 2017 | 2018 | 2019 | 2020 |
|---|---|---|---|---|---|---|---|---|---|---|---|---|---|---|---|
| PAST YEAR USE | | | | | | | | | | | | | | | |
| Illicit Drugs | nc | nc | nc | nc | nc | nc | nc | nc | nc | 774 | 757 | 720 | 885 | 932 | *791* |
| Marijuana | 362 | 339 | 384 | 366 | 327 | 375 | 414 | 495 | 510 | 545 | 572 | 547 | 678 | 718 | *618* |
| Cocaine | 47 | 54 | 48 | 35 | 35 | 36 | 45 | 17 | 32 | 32 | 30 | 27 | 27 | 29 | *27* |
| Crack | 10 | 17 | 5 | 6 | 7 | 11 | 7 | 2 | 6 | * | 4 | 2 | 0 | 10 | * |
| Heroin | 9 | 6 | 8 | 6 | 9 | 8 | 11 | 7 | 12 | 2 | 3 | 4 | 3 | * | * |
| Hallucinogens | nc | nc | nc | nc | nc | nc | nc | nc | nc | 116 | 102 | 122 | 96 | 133 | *126* |
| LSD | 13 | 13 | 23 | 30 | 20 | 23 | 36 | 19 | 45 | 56 | 31 | 58 | 52 | 87 | *70* |
| PCP | 10 | 5 | 16 | 6 | 4 | 7 | 8 | 6 | 11 | 2 | 6 | 11 | 6 | 7 | * |
| Ecstasy | nc | nc | nc | nc | nc | nc | nc | nc | nc | 43 | 46 | 42 | 42 | 56 | *14* |
| Inhalants | nc | nc | nc | nc | nc | nc | nc | nc | nc | 151 | 124 | 119 | 145 | 178 | *179* |
| Methamphetamine | nc | nc | nc | nc | nc | nc | nc | nc | nc | 10 | 5 | 14 | 6 | 10 | * |
| Misuse of Prescription Psychotherapeutics | nc | nc | nc | nc | nc | nc | nc | nc | nc | 325 | 349 | 285 | 301 | 301 | *188* |
| Pain Relievers | nc | nc | nc | nc | nc | nc | nc | nc | nc | 201 | 237 | 170 | 172 | 136 | *70* |
| Stimulants | nc | nc | nc | nc | nc | nc | nc | nc | nc | 148 | 130 | 122 | 106 | 157 | *100* |
| Tranquilizers or Sedatives | nc | nc | nc | nc | nc | nc | nc | nc | nc | 103 | 148 | 131 | 151 | 147 | *100* |
| Tranquilizers | nc | nc | nc | nc | nc | nc | nc | nc | nc | 89 | 131 | 127 | 136 | 129 | *88* |
| Sedatives | nc | nc | nc | nc | nc | nc | nc | nc | nc | 25 | 41 | 19 | 30 | 43 | *12* |
| Benzodiazepines | nc | nc | nc | nc | nc | nc | nc | nc | nc | 82 | 125 | 119 | 129 | 124 | *73* |
| Opioids | nc | nc | nc | nc | nc | nc | nc | nc | nc | 201 | 238 | 172 | 172 | 136 | *70* |
| Central Nervous System Stimulants | nc | nc | nc | nc | nc | nc | nc | nc | nc | 163 | 145 | 133 | 128 | 174 | *114* |
| Illicit Drugs Other Than Marijuana[1] | nc | nc | nc | nc | nc | nc | nc | nc | nc | 477 | 450 | 406 | 435 | 482 | *386* |
| PAST MONTH USE | | | | | | | | | | | | | | | |
| Alcohol | 386 | 404 | 385 | 372 | 318 | 331 | 370 | 365 | 421 | 396 | 373 | 398 | 433 | 487 | *477* |
| Binge Alcohol Use[2] | nc | nc | nc | nc | nc | nc | nc | nc | nc | 228 | 199 | 220 | 238 | 262 | *200* |

## Table 11.7A. (Continued)

| Substance | 2006 | 2007 | 2008 | 2009 | 2010 | 2011 | 2012 | 2013 | 2014 | 2015 | 2016 | 2017 | 2018 | 2019 | 2020 |
|---|---|---|---|---|---|---|---|---|---|---|---|---|---|---|---|
| Heavy Alcohol Use | nc | nc | nc | nc | nc | nc | nc | nc | nc | 49 | 40 | 29 | 17 | 43 | *45* |
| Cigarette Use | 290 | 285 | 275 | 276 | 219 | 225 | 217 | 221 | 203 | 213 | 194 | 168 | 177 | 129 | *79* |
| Daily Cigarette Use | 83 | 75 | 56 | 55 | 46 | 58 | 44 | 32 | 40 | 50 | 19 | 18 | 17 | 12 | *6* |

* = low precision; -= not available; da = does not apply; nc = not comparable due to methodological changes; nr = not reported due to measurement issues.

NOTE: Estimates in the 2020 column are italicized to indicate caution should be used when comparing estimates between 2020 and prior years because of methodological changes for 2020. Due to these changes, significance testing between 2020 and prior years was not performed. See the *2020 National Survey on Drug Use and Health: Methodological Summary and Definitions* for details.

NOTE: Some 2006 to 2010 estimates may differ from previously published estimates due to updates (see Chapter 3 of the *2020 National Survey on Drug Use and Health: Methodological Summary and Definitions*). NOTE: Respondents with unknown past year Major Depressive Episode (MDE) data were excluded.

NOTE: Respondents with unknown impairment data were excluded.

[1] Illicit Drugs Other Than Marijuana excludes respondents who used only marijuana but includes those who used marijuana in addition to other illicit drugs.

[2] Estimates of binge alcohol use include use by those who were heavy alcohol users.

Definitions: Measures and terms are defined in Appendix A.

Source: SAMHSA, Center for Behavioral Health Statistics and Quality, National Survey on Drug Use and Health, 2006-2019, and Quarters 1 and 4, 2020.

**Table 11.7B.** Substance use in past year and past month: among people aged 12 to 17 with major depressive episode with severe impairment in past year; percentages, 2006-2020

| Substance | 2006 | 2007 | 2008 | 2009 | 2010 | 2011 | 2012 | 2013 | 2014 | 2015 | 2016 | 2017 | 2018 | 2019 | 2020 |
|---|---|---|---|---|---|---|---|---|---|---|---|---|---|---|---|
| PAST YEAR USE | | | | | | | | | | | | | | | |
| Illicit Drugs | nc | nc | nc | nc | nc | nc | nc | nc | nc | 36.3 | 34.9 | 31.8 | 36.5 | 34.9 | *27.1* |
| Marijuana | 26.6 | 24.7 | 26.3 | 26.0 | 24.3 | 27.0 | 26.8 | 26.5 | 25.6 | 25.6 | 26.4 | 24.1 | 28.0 | 26.9 | *21.2* |
| Cocaine | 3.5 | 4.0 | 3.3 | 2.5 | 2.6 | 2.6 | 2.9 | 0.9 | 1.6 | 1.5 | 1.4 | 1.2 | 1.1 | 1.1 | *0.9* |
| Crack | 0.8 | 1.2 | 0.4 | 0.5 | 0.5 | 0.8 | 0.4 | 0.1 | 0.3 | * | 0.2 | 0.1 | 0.0 | 0.4 | * |
| Heroin | 0.6 | 0.5 | 0.6 | 0.4 | 0.6 | 0.6 | 0.7 | 0.4 | 0.6 | 0.1 | 0.1 | 0.2 | 0.1 | * | * |
| Hallucinogens | nc | nc | nc | nc | nc | nc | nc | nc | nc | 5.5 | 4.7 | 5.4 | 4.0 | 5.0 | *4.3* |
| LSD | 0.9 | 0.9 | 1.6 | 2.1 | 1.5 | 1.7 | 2.3 | 1.0 | 2.2 | 2.6 | 1.4 | 2.6 | 2.1 | 3.3 | *2.4* |
| PCP | 0.8 | 0.4 | 1.1 | 0.4 | 0.3 | 0.5 | 0.5 | 0.3 | 0.5 | 0.1 | 0.3 | 0.5 | 0.2 | 0.3 | * |
| Ecstasy | nc | nc | nc | nc | nc | nc | nc | nc | nc | 2.0 | 2.1 | 1.9 | 1.7 | 2.1 | *0.5* |
| Inhalants | nc | nc | nc | nc | nc | nc | nc | nc | nc | 7.1 | 5.7 | 5.2 | 6.0 | 6.7 | *6.1* |
| Methamphetamine | nc | nc | nc | nc | nc | nc | nc | nc | nc | 0.5 | 0.2 | 0.6 | 0.3 | 0.4 | * |
| Misuse of Prescription Psychotherapeutics | nc | nc | nc | nc | nc | nc | nc | nc | nc | 15.3 | 16.1 | 12.6 | 12.4 | 11.3 | *6.4* |
| Pain Relievers | nc | nc | nc | nc | nc | nc | nc | nc | nc | 9.4 | 10.9 | 7.5 | 7.1 | 5.1 | *2.4* |
| Stimulants | nc | nc | nc | nc | nc | nc | nc | nc | nc | 6.9 | 6.0 | 5.4 | 4.4 | 5.9 | *3.4* |
| Tranquilizers or Sedatives | nc | nc | nc | nc | nc | nc | nc | nc | nc | 4.8 | 6.8 | 5.8 | 6.2 | 5.5 | *3.4* |
| Tranquilizers | nc | nc | nc | nc | nc | nc | nc | nc | nc | 4.2 | 6.0 | 5.6 | 5.6 | 4.8 | *3.0* |
| Sedatives | nc | nc | nc | nc | nc | nc | nc | nc | nc | 1.2 | 1.9 | 0.8 | 1.2 | 1.6 | *0.4* |
| Benzodiazepines | nc | nc | nc | nc | nc | nc | nc | nc | nc | 3.8 | 5.8 | 5.2 | 5.3 | 4.6 | *2.5* |
| Opioids | nc | nc | nc | nc | nc | nc | nc | nc | nc | 9.4 | 11.0 | 7.6 | 7.1 | 5.1 | *2.4* |
| Central Nervous System Stimulants | nc | nc | nc | nc | nc | nc | nc | nc | nc | 7.6 | 6.7 | 5.9 | 5.3 | 6.5 | *3.9* |
| Illicit Drugs Other Than Marijuana[1] | nc | nc | nc | nc | nc | nc | nc | nc | nc | 22.4 | 20.8 | 17.9 | 18.0 | 18.0 | *13.2* |
| PAST MONTH USE | | | | | | | | | | | | | | | |
| Alcohol | 28.4 | 29.5 | 26.4 | 26.5 | 23.6 | 23.8 | 24.0 | 19.5 | 21.1 | 18.6 | 17.2 | 17.6 | 17.9 | 18.2 | *16.3* |
| Binge Alcohol Use[2] | Nc | nc | nc | nc | nc | nc | nc | nc | nc | 10.7 | 9.2 | 9.7 | 9.8 | 9.8 | *6.9* |

## **Table 11.7B.** (Continued)

| Substance | 2006 | 2007 | 2008 | 2009 | 2010 | 2011 | 2012 | 2013 | 2014 | 2015 | 2016 | 2017 | 2018 | 2019 | 2020 |
|---|---|---|---|---|---|---|---|---|---|---|---|---|---|---|---|
| Heavy Alcohol Use | nc | nc | nc | nc | nc | nc | nc | nc | nc | 2.3 | 1.8 | 1.3 | 0.7 | 1.6 | *1.5* |
| Cigarette Use | 21.3 | 20.8 | 18.8 | 19.7 | 16.2 | 16.2 | 14.1 | 11.8 | 10.2 | 10.0 | 8.9 | 7.4 | 7.3 | 4.8 | *2.7* |
| Daily Cigarette Use | 6.1 | 5.5 | 3.8 | 3.9 | 3.4 | 4.2 | 2.9 | 1.7 | 2.0 | 2.3 | 0.9 | 0.8 | 0.7 | 0.5 | *0.2* |

* = low precision; -= not available; da = does not apply; nc = not comparable due to methodological changes; nr = not reported due to measurement issues.

NOTE: Estimates in the 2020 column are italicized to indicate caution should be used when comparing estimates between 2020 and prior years because of methodological changes for 2020. Due to these changes, significance testing between 2020 and prior years was not performed. See the *2020 National Survey on Drug Use and Health: Methodological Summary and Definitions* for details.

NOTE: Some 2006 to 2010 estimates may differ from previously published estimates due to updates (see Chapter 3 of the *2020 National Survey on Drug Use and Health: Methodological Summary and Definitions*). NOTE: Respondents with unknown past year Major Depressive Episode (MDE) data were excluded.

NOTE: Respondents with unknown impairment data were excluded.

[1] Illicit Drugs Other Than Marijuana excludes respondents who used only marijuana but includes those who used marijuana in addition to other illicit drugs.

[2] Estimates of binge alcohol use include use by those who were heavy alcohol users.

Definitions: Measures and terms are defined in Appendix A.

Source: SAMHSA, Center for Behavioral Health Statistics and Quality, National Survey on Drug Use and Health, 2006-2019, and Quarters 1 and 4, 2020.

**Table 11.8A.** Substance use in past year and past month: among people aged 12 to 17 with no major depressive episode in past year; numbers in thousands, 2004-2020

| Substance | 2004 | 2005 | 2006 | 2007 | 2008 | 2009 | 2010 | 2011 | 2012 | 2013 | 2014 | 2015 | 2016 | 2017 | 2018 | 2019 | 2020 |
|---|---|---|---|---|---|---|---|---|---|---|---|---|---|---|---|---|---|
| PAST YEAR USE | | | | | | | | | | | | | | | | | |
| Illicit Drugs | nc | nc | nc | nc | nc | nc | nc | nc | nc | nc | nc | 3,251 | 2,823 | 3,010 | 2,888 | 2,926 | *2,158* |
| Marijuana | 2,998 | 2,763 | 2,803 | 2,629 | 2,693 | 2,810 | 2,836 | 2,962 | 2,746 | 2,561 | 2,479 | 2,366 | 2,136 | 2,283 | 2,164 | 2,256 | *1,582* |
| Cocaine | 335 | 335 | 337 | 302 | 238 | 196 | 178 | 165 | 123 | 93 | 115 | 115 | 91 | 87 | 66 | 67 | *46* |
| Crack | 44 | 37 | 57 | 45 | 22 | 18 | 9 | 18 | 12 | 7 | 5 | 5 | 4 | 14 | 1 | 2 | *2* |
| Heroin | 37 | 23 | 26 | 15 | 27 | 25 | 18 | 36 | 20 | 20 | 13 | 14 | 9 | 7 | 5 | * | * |
| Hallucinogens | nc | nc | nc | nc | nc | nc | nc | nc | nc | nc | nc | 371 | 308 | 346 | 254 | 279 | *212* |
| LSD | 117 | 108 | 86 | 108 | 150 | 97 | 103 | 113 | 106 | 108 | 163 | 177 | 157 | 173 | 136 | 171 | *124* |
| PCP | 47 | 64 | 47 | 48 | 40 | 35 | 26 | 26 | 36 | 20 | 22 | 29 | 12 | 10 | 7 | 14 | * |
| Ecstasy | nc | nc | nc | nc | nc | nc | nc | nc | nc | nc | nc | 151 | 111 | 121 | 80 | 78 | *50* |
| Inhalants | nc | nc | nc | nc | nc | nc | nc | nc | nc | nc | nc | 457 | 378 | 418 | 460 | 476 | *365* |
| Methamphetamine | nc | nc | nc | nc | nc | nc | nc | nc | nc | nc | nc | 22 | 23 | 31 | 32 | 28 | *11* |
| Misuse of Prescription Psychotherapeutics | nc | nc | nc | nc | nc | nc | nc | nc | nc | nc | nc | 1,044 | 851 | 824 | 767 | 643 | *427* |
| Pain Relievers | nc | nc | nc | nc | nc | nc | nc | nc | nc | nc | nc | 700 | 556 | 526 | 444 | 358 | *284* |
| Stimulants | nc | nc | nc | nc | nc | nc | nc | nc | nc | nc | nc | 305 | 275 | 280 | 231 | 230 | *153* |
| Tranquilizers or Sedatives | nc | nc | nc | nc | nc | nc | nc | nc | nc | nc | nc | 315 | 285 | 313 | 275 | 239 | *101* |
| Tranquilizers | nc | nc | nc | nc | nc | nc | nc | nc | nc | nc | nc | 277 | 260 | 282 | 253 | 214 | *85* |
| Sedatives | nc | nc | nc | nc | nc | nc | nc | nc | nc | nc | nc | 73 | 50 | 50 | 29 | 34 | *17* |
| Benzodiazepines | nc | nc | nc | nc | nc | nc | nc | nc | nc | nc | nc | 260 | 250 | 280 | 243 | 212 | *71* |
| Opioids | nc | nc | nc | nc | nc | nc | nc | nc | nc | nc | nc | 710 | 563 | 526 | 448 | 358 | *284* |
| Central Nervous System Stimulants | nc | nc | nc | nc | nc | nc | nc | nc | nc | nc | nc | 397 | 340 | 350 | 292 | 281 | *186* |
| Illicit Drugs Other Than Marijuana[1] | nc | nc | nc | nc | nc | nc | nc | nc | nc | nc | nc | 1,610 | 1,335 | 1,373 | 1,284 | 1,181 | *891* |
| PAST MONTH USE | | | | | | | | | | | | | | | | | |
| Alcohol | 3,741 | 3,515 | 3,635 | 3,413 | 3,088 | 3,114 | 2,793 | 2,759 | 2,660 | 2,316 | 2,219 | 1,823 | 1,726 | 1,862 | 1,618 | 1,658 | *1,358* |
| Binge Alcohol Use[2] | nc | nc | nc | nc | nc | nc | nc | nc | nc | nc | nc | 1,127 | 901 | 990 | 843 | 837 | *765* |

## Table 11.8A. (Continued)

| Substance | 2004 | 2005 | 2006 | 2007 | 2008 | 2009 | 2010 | 2011 | 2012 | 2013 | 2014 | 2015 | 2016 | 2017 | 2018 | 2019 | 2020 |
|---|---|---|---|---|---|---|---|---|---|---|---|---|---|---|---|---|---|
| Heavy Alcohol Use | nc | nc | nc | nc | nc | nc | nc | nc | nc | nc | nc | 165 | 132 | 129 | 105 | 146 | *89* |
| Cigarette Use | 2,420 | 2,221 | 2,214 | 2,047 | 1,858 | 1,825 | 1,659 | 1,557 | 1,294 | 1,042 | 900 | 755 | 574 | 538 | 427 | 368 | *228* |
| Daily Cigarette Use | 628 | 568 | 583 | 527 | 417 | 433 | 388 | 349 | 285 | 212 | 229 | 141 | 94 | 68 | 73 | 55 | *19* |

* = low precision; -= not available; da = does not apply; nc = not comparable due to methodological changes; nr = not reported due to measurement issues.

NOTE: Estimates in the 2020 column are italicized to indicate caution should be used when comparing estimates between 2020 and prior years because of methodological changes for 2020. Due to these changes, significance testing between 2020 and prior years was not performed. See the *2020 National Survey on Drug Use and Health: Methodological Summary and Definitions* for details.

NOTE: Some 2006 to 2010 estimates may differ from previously published estimates due to updates (see Chapter 3 of the *2020 National Survey on Drug Use and Health: Methodological Summary and Definitions*). NOTE: Respondents with unknown past year Major Depressive Episode (MDE) data were excluded.

[1] Illicit Drugs Other Than Marijuana excludes respondents who used only marijuana but includes those who used marijuana in addition to other illicit drugs.

[2] Estimates of binge alcohol use include use by those who were heavy alcohol users.

Definitions: Measures and terms are defined in Appendix A.

Source: SAMHSA, Center for Behavioral Health Statistics and Quality, National Survey on Drug Use and Health, 2004-2019, and Quarters 1 and 4, 2020.

**Table 11.8B.** Substance use in past year and past month: among people aged 12 to 17 with no major depressive episode in past year; percentages, 2004-2020

| Substance | 2004 | 2005 | 2006 | 2007 | 2008 | 2009 | 2010 | 2011 | 2012 | 2013 | 2014 | 2015 | 2016 | 2017 | 2018 | 2019 | 2020 |
|---|---|---|---|---|---|---|---|---|---|---|---|---|---|---|---|---|---|
| PAST YEAR USE | | | | | | | | | | | | | | | | | |
| Illicit Drugs | nc | nc | nc | nc | nc | nc | nc | nc | nc | nc | nc | 15.3 | 13.4 | 14.3 | 14.0 | 14.4 | *10.7* |
| Marijuana | 13.3 | 12.1 | 12.2 | 11.6 | 12.0 | 12.7 | 12.9 | 13.2 | 12.4 | 11.8 | 11.6 | 11.1 | 10.1 | 10.9 | 10.5 | 11.1 | *7.9* |
| Cocaine | 1.5 | 1.5 | 1.5 | 1.3 | 1.1 | 0.9 | 0.8 | 0.7 | 0.6 | 0.4 | 0.5 | 0.5 | 0.4 | 0.4 | 0.3 | 0.3 | *0.2* |
| Crack | 0.2 | 0.2 | 0.2 | 0.2 | 0.1 | 0.1 | 0.0 | 0.1 | 0.1 | 0.0 | 0.0 | 0.0 | 0.0 | 0.1 | 0.0 | 0.0 | *0.0* |
| Heroin | 0.2 | 0.1 | 0.1 | 0.1 | 0.1 | 0.1 | 0.1 | 0.2 | 0.1 | 0.1 | 0.1 | 0.1 | 0.0 | 0.0 | 0.0 | * | * |
| Hallucinogens | nc | nc | nc | nc | nc | nc | nc | nc | nc | nc | nc | 1.7 | 1.5 | 1.6 | 1.2 | 1.4 | *1.1* |
| LSD | 0.5 | 0.5 | 0.4 | 0.5 | 0.7 | 0.4 | 0.5 | 0.5 | 0.5 | 0.5 | 0.8 | 0.8 | 0.7 | 0.8 | 0.7 | 0.8 | *0.6* |
| PCP | 0.2 | 0.3 | 0.2 | 0.2 | 0.2 | 0.2 | 0.1 | 0.1 | 0.2 | 0.1 | 0.1 | 0.1 | 0.1 | 0.0 | 0.0 | 0.1 | * |
| Ecstasy | nc | nc | nc | nc | nc | nc | nc | nc | nc | nc | nc | 0.7 | 0.5 | 0.6 | 0.4 | 0.4 | *0.2* |
| Inhalants | nc | nc | nc | nc | nc | nc | nc | nc | nc | nc | nc | 2.2 | 1.8 | 2.0 | 2.2 | 2.3 | *1.8* |
| Methamphetamine | nc | nc | nc | nc | nc | nc | nc | nc | nc | nc | nc | 0.1 | 0.1 | 0.1 | 0.2 | 0.1 | *0.1* |
| Misuse of Prescription Psychotherapeutics | nc | nc | nc | nc | nc | nc | nc | nc | nc | nc | nc | 4.9 | 4.0 | 3.9 | 3.7 | 3.2 | *2.1* |
| Pain Relievers | nc | nc | nc | nc | nc | nc | nc | nc | nc | nc | nc | 3.3 | 2.6 | 2.5 | 2.2 | 1.8 | *1.4* |
| Stimulants | nc | nc | nc | nc | nc | nc | nc | nc | nc | nc | nc | 1.4 | 1.3 | 1.3 | 1.1 | 1.1 | *0.8* |
| Tranquilizers or Sedatives | nc | nc | nc | nc | nc | nc | nc | nc | nc | nc | nc | 1.5 | 1.3 | 1.5 | 1.3 | 1.2 | *0.5* |
| Tranquilizers | nc | nc | nc | nc | nc | nc | nc | nc | nc | nc | nc | 1.3 | 1.2 | 1.3 | 1.2 | 1.1 | *0.4* |
| Sedatives | nc | nc | nc | nc | nc | nc | nc | nc | nc | nc | nc | 0.3 | 0.2 | 0.2 | 0.1 | 0.2 | *0.1* |
| Benzodiazepines | nc | nc | nc | nc | nc | nc | nc | nc | nc | nc | nc | 1.2 | 1.2 | 1.3 | 1.2 | 1.0 | *0.4* |
| Opioids | nc | nc | nc | nc | nc | nc | nc | nc | nc | nc | nc | 3.3 | 2.7 | 2.5 | 2.2 | 1.8 | *1.4* |
| Central Nervous System Stimulants | nc | nc | nc | nc | nc | nc | nc | nc | nc | nc | nc | 1.9 | 1.6 | 1.7 | 1.4 | 1.4 | *0.9* |
| Illicit Drugs Other Than Marijuana[1] | nc | nc | nc | nc | nc | nc | nc | nc | nc | nc | nc | 7.6 | 6.3 | 6.5 | 6.2 | 5.8 | *4.4* |
| PAST MONTH USE | | | | | | | | | | | | | | | | | |
| Alcohol | 16.5 | 15.4 | 15.8 | 15.0 | 13.8 | 14.1 | 12.8 | 12.3 | 12.0 | 10.7 | 10.3 | 8.6 | 8.2 | 8.9 | 7.8 | 8.2 | *6.7* |
| Binge Alcohol Use[2] | nc | nc | nc | nc | nc | nc | nc | nc | nc | nc | nc | 5.3 | 4.3 | 4.7 | 4.1 | 4.1 | *3.8* |

## **Table 11.8B.** (Continued)

| Substance | 2004 | 2005 | 2006 | 2007 | 2008 | 2009 | 2010 | 2011 | 2012 | 2013 | 2014 | 2015 | 2016 | 2017 | 2018 | 2019 | 2020 |
|---|---|---|---|---|---|---|---|---|---|---|---|---|---|---|---|---|---|
| Heavy Alcohol Use | nc | nc | nc | nc | nc | nc | nc | nc | nc | nc | nc | 0.8 | 0.6 | 0.6 | 0.5 | 0.7 | *0.4* |
| Cigarette Use | 10.7 | 9.8 | 9.7 | 9.0 | 8.3 | 8.2 | 7.6 | 7.0 | 5.8 | 4.8 | 4.2 | 3.6 | 2.7 | 2.6 | 2.1 | 1.8 | *1.1* |
| Daily Cigarette Use | 2.8 | 2.5 | 2.5 | 2.3 | 1.9 | 2.0 | 1.8 | 1.6 | 1.3 | 1.0 | 1.1 | 0.7 | 0.4 | 0.3 | 0.4 | 0.3 | *0.1* |

* = low precision; -= not available; da = does not apply; nc = not comparable due to methodological changes; nr = not reported due to measurement issues.

NOTE: Estimates in the 2020 column are italicized to indicate caution should be used when comparing estimates between 2020 and prior years because of methodological changes for 2020. Due to these changes, significance testing between 2020 and prior years was not performed. See the *2020 National Survey on Drug Use and Health: Methodological Summary and Definitions* for details.

NOTE: Some 2006 to 2010 estimates may differ from previously published estimates due to updates (see Chapter 3 of the *2020 National Survey on Drug Use and Health: Methodological Summary and Definitions*). NOTE: Respondents with unknown past year Major Depressive Episode (MDE) data were excluded.

[1] Illicit Drugs Other Than Marijuana excludes respondents who used only marijuana but includes those who used marijuana in addition to other illicit drugs.

[2] Estimates of binge alcohol use include use by those who were heavy alcohol users.

Definitions: Measures and terms are defined in Appendix A.

Source: SAMHSA, Center for Behavioral Health Statistics and Quality, National Survey on Drug Use and Health, 2004-2019, and Quarters 1 and 4, 2020.

**Table 11.9A.** Type of treatment received in past year for depression: among people aged 12 to 17 with MAJOR Depressive Episode (MDE) in past year and among people aged 12 to 17 with MDE with severe impairment in past year; numbers in thousands, 2004-2020

| MDE/Type of Treatment | 2004 | 2005 | 2006 | 2007 | 2008 | 2009 | 2010 | 2011 | 2012 | 2013 | 2014 | 2015 | 2016 | 2017 | 2018 | 2019 | 2020 |
|---|---|---|---|---|---|---|---|---|---|---|---|---|---|---|---|---|---|
| MDE | | | | | | | | | | | | | | | | | |
| Saw or Talked to a Health Professional OR Used Prescription Medication | 856 | 778 | 700 | 739 | 731 | 638 | 682 | 724 | 791 | 944 | 1,076 | 1,139 | 1,223 | 1,286 | 1,371 | 1,577 | *1,685* |
| Saw or Talked to a Health Professional BUT Did Not Use Prescription Medication | 425 | 404 | 407 | 372 | 406 | 358 | 370 | 397 | 431 | 522 | 543 | 596 | 571 | 625 | 749 | 796 | *928* |
| Used Prescription Medication BUT Did Not See or Talk to a Health Professional | 76 | 58 | 47 | 53 | 60 | 46 | 58 | 52 | 52 | 94 | 75 | 87 | 59 | 76 | 77 | 127 | *53* |
| Saw or Talked to a Health Professional AND Used Prescription Medication | 342 | 308 | 241 | 307 | 259 | 231 | 252 | 272 | 302 | 316 | 447 | 447 | 576 | 570 | 533 | 645 | *691* |
| MDE with Severe Impairment | | | | | | | | | | | | | | | | | |
| Saw or Talked to a Health Professional OR Used Prescription Medication | -- | -- | 575 | 574 | 598 | 515 | 528 | 570 | 618 | 808 | 851 | 924 | 986 | 1,044 | 1,094 | 1,287 | *1,344* |
| Saw or Talked to a Health Professional BUT Did Not Use Prescription Medication | -- | -- | 314 | 281 | 313 | 283 | 280 | 303 | 309 | 421 | 423 | 468 | 413 | 477 | 575 | 622 | *724* |
| Used Prescription Medication BUT Did Not See or Talk to a Health Professional | -- | -- | 37 | 39 | 49 | 37 | 34 | 33 | 43 | 86 | 63 | 66 | 48 | 54 | 55 | 99 | *38* |
| Saw or Talked to a Health Professional AND Used Prescription Medication | -- | -- | 220 | 249 | 232 | 191 | 212 | 232 | 260 | 287 | 360 | 386 | 513 | 505 | 455 | 560 | *570* |

* = low precision; -= not available; da = does not apply; nc = not comparable due to methodological changes; nr = not reported due to measurement issues.

NOTE: Estimates in the 2020 column are italicized to indicate caution should be used when comparing estimates between 2020 and prior years because of methodological changes for 2020. Due to these changes, significance testing between 2020 and prior years was not performed. See the *2020 National Survey on Drug Use and Health: Methodological Summary and Definitions* for details.

NOTE: Some 2006 to 2010 estimates may differ from previously published estimates due to updates (see Chapter 3 of the *2020 National Survey on Drug Use and Health: Methodological Summary and Definitions*).

NOTE: Respondents with unknown past year treatment for depression data were excluded.

NOTE: Respondents with unknown past year Major Depressive Episode (MDE) data were excluded.

Definitions: Measures and terms are defined in Appendix A.

Source: SAMHSA, Center for Behavioral Health Statistics and Quality, National Survey on Drug Use and Health, 2004-2019, and Quarters 1 and 4, 2020.

**Table 11.9B.** Type of treatment received in past year for depression: among people aged 12 to 17 with Major Depressive Episode (MDE) in past year and among people aged 12 to 17 with MDE with severe impairment in past year; percentages, 2004-2020

| MDE/Type of Treatment | 2004 | 2005 | 2006 | 2007 | 2008 | 2009 | 2010 | 2011 | 2012 | 2013 | 2014 | 2015 | 2016 | 2017 | 2018 | 2019 | 2020 |
|---|---|---|---|---|---|---|---|---|---|---|---|---|---|---|---|---|---|
| MDE | | | | | | | | | | | | | | | | | |
| Saw or Talked to a Health Professional OR Used Prescription Medication | 38.7 | 35.9 | 35.9 | 37.0 | 36.3 | 33.0 | 35.8 | 36.3 | 36.0 | 36.9 | 39.6 | 37.9 | 40.2 | 40.3 | 40.0 | 42.2 | *41.2* |
| Saw or Talked to a Health Professional BUT Did Not Use Prescription Medication | 19.3 | 18.6 | 20.9 | 18.6 | 20.2 | 18.5 | 19.4 | 19.9 | 19.6 | 20.4 | 20.0 | 19.8 | 18.8 | 19.6 | 21.8 | 21.3 | *22.6* |
| Used Prescription Medication BUT Did Not See or Talk to a Health Professional | 3.4 | 2.7 | 2.4 | 2.7 | 3.0 | 2.4 | 3.0 | 2.6 | 2.4 | 3.7 | 2.8 | 2.9 | 1.9 | 2.4 | 2.2 | 3.4 | *1.3* |
| Saw or Talked to a Health Professional AND Used Prescription Medication | 15.5 | 14.1 | 12.3 | 15.3 | 12.8 | 11.9 | 13.2 | 13.6 | 13.7 | 12.3 | 16.4 | 14.8 | 18.9 | 17.9 | 15.4 | 17.1 | *16.8* |
| MDE with Severe Impairment | | | | | | | | | | | | | | | | | |
| Saw or Talked to a Health Professional OR Used Prescription Medication | -- | -- | 42.9 | 42.1 | 41.1 | 37.0 | 39.3 | 41.3 | 40.2 | 43.8 | 43.2 | 43.7 | 46.1 | 46.2 | 45.5 | 48.7 | *46.6* |
| Saw or Talked to a Health Professional BUT Did Not Use Prescription Medication | -- | -- | 23.4 | 20.6 | 21.5 | 20.3 | 20.8 | 21.9 | 20.1 | 22.9 | 21.5 | 22.1 | 19.3 | 21.1 | 24.0 | 23.5 | *24.9* |
| Used Prescription Medication BUT Did Not See or Talk to a Health Professional | -- | -- | 2.7 | 2.9 | 3.3 | 2.7 | 2.5 | 2.4 | 2.8 | 4.7 | 3.2 | 3.1 | 2.3 | 2.4 | 2.3 | 3.7 | *1.3* |
| Saw or Talked to a Health Professional AND Used Prescription Medication | -- | -- | 16.4 | 18.3 | 15.9 | 13.7 | 15.7 | 16.7 | 16.9 | 15.6 | 18.2 | 18.2 | 24.0 | 22.4 | 18.9 | 21.0 | *19.6* |

* = low precision; -= not available; da = does not apply; nc = not comparable due to methodological changes; nr = not reported due to measurement issues.

NOTE: Estimates in the 2020 column are italicized to indicate caution should be used when comparing estimates between 2020 and prior years because of methodological changes for 2020. Due to these changes, significance testing between 2020 and prior years was not performed. See the *2020 National Survey on Drug Use and Health: Methodological Summary and Definitions* fordetails.

NOTE: Some 2006 to 2010 estimates may differ from previously published estimates due to updates (see Chapter 3 of the *2020 National Survey on Drug Use and Health: Methodological Summary and Definitions*). NOTE: Respondents with unknown past year treatment for depression data were excluded.

NOTE: Respondents with unknown past year Major Depressive Episode (MDE) data were excluded.

Definitions: Measures and terms are defined in Appendix A.

Source: SAMHSA, Center for Behavioral Health Statistics and Quality, National Survey on Drug Use and Health, 2004-2019, and Quarters 1 and 4, 2020.

I wanted to first, before we conclude also, in addition to thanking each of our witnesses for their testimony and their presence here today, I also want to ask unanimous consent to add two statements to the record. And I will describe them.

The first is a statement from the Children's Hospital Association on the need to ensure children and adolescents receive the mental and behavioral health services they need to prepare them for healthy, young adulthood.

The second is an excerpt from the 2020 National Survey on Drug Use and Health that includes current statistics on substance use, mental health, and treatment among adolescents.

So ordered that they are made part of the record.

The CHAIRMAN. If any Senators have additional questions for the witnesses or statements to be added, the hearing record will be kept open for 7 days until next Wednesday, December the 7th.

Thank you all for participating. This concludes today's hearing.

## Childrens Hospital Association Statement for the Record

CHILDREN'S HOSPITAL ASSOCIATION

600 13th St., NW, Suite 500
Washington, DC 20005
p | 202-753-5500
f | 202-347-5147

16011 College Blvd., Suite 250
Lenexa, KS 66219
p | 913-262-1436
f | 913-262-1575

WWW.CHILDRENSHOSPITALS.ORG

### Children's Hospital Association Statement for Record

Senate Committee on Health, Education, Labor and Pensions, Subcommittee on Children and Families, "Caring for Our Kids: Supporting Mental Health in the Transition from High School to College"

November 30, 2022

On behalf of the nation's children's hospitals and the children and families we serve, thank you for holding this hearing on supporting the mental health of America's adolescents and youth, particularly during the challenging transition period into young adulthood. We appreciate the Senate HELP Committee's continued attention to the crisis in child and adolescent mental health throughout this year. We need urgent tailored action and investments for children to meaningfully address the national children's mental health emergency. Our nation's children cannot wait.

Children's Hospital Association represents more than 220 children's hospitals nationwide, dedicated to advancing the health and well-being of our nation's children through innovation in the quality, cost, and delivery of care. The mental health challenges facing our children continue to grow and our hospitals are seeing it firsthand in their emergency departments (EDs). Visits for youth suicide attempts have increased dramatically, eating disorder visits have doubled and we are seeing an increase in suicide rates for children and teens, with steeper increases among Black boys and girls under age 12. As essential providers dedicated to providing the highest quality pediatric care, addressing the children's mental health crisis is our top priority.

The periods of adolescence and early adulthood are critical for the emergence of mental health conditions, as 50% of all mental illness begins by age 14, and 75% by age 24. Yet, promoting and protecting the mental health of teens and young adults begins with a strong foundation for mental health in childhood. Improving outcomes for youth requires ensuring that children have opportunities to develop and strengthen critical social, emotional and coping skills, as well as facilitating early identification and access to developmentally appropriate treatment, including for children who are not yet diagnosed.

We encourage the HELP Committee, in partnership with your colleagues on the Senate Finance Committee and in the House of Representatives, to take steps now to safeguard children's mental health from early childhood and into young adulthood. Children's hospitals urge Congress to:

- Support the pediatric mental health workforce
- Bolster community-based systems of pediatric mental health care
- Provide dedicated resources to enhance pediatric mental health infrastructure
- Strengthen programs targeted to support mental health among teens and young adults

*Champions for Children's Health*

Children's hospitals strongly support S. 4472, the Health Capacity for Pediatric Behavioral Health Act sponsored by the Subcommittee Chair Bob Casey, D-Pa., and Ranking Member Bill Cassidy, R-La. This legislation would address these three critical facets of the children's mental health crisis, described in detail below, with dedicated grant funding through the Health Resources and Services Administration.

### Support the pediatric mental health workforce

A robust, diverse, pediatric behavioral health workforce is essential to meet children's mental, emotional and behavioral health needs with developmentally appropriate treatment delivered across the continuum care. Workforce shortages persists across pediatric behavioral health professions, which delays and too often prevents children from receiving mental health care when they need it, leaving children's conditions to worsen without intervention. Current programs not tailored and dedicated to the pediatric workforce are not meeting children's needs. We need tailored federal investments, specifically for pediatrics, to support the recruitment and retention of a diverse workforce across pediatric behavioral health professional fields, including both clinical and non-clinical roles. Additionally, growing the workforce will take time, so we must also better equip the existing workforce to meet children's mental health needs, with enhanced training and support for care coordination and integration.

### Bolster community-based systems of pediatric mental health care

Children's hospitals are continuing to see higher rates of youth presenting in mental health crisis at emergency departments, which is not the ideal place for a young person in distress and too often results in them boarding while they wait for space to become available in an appropriate treatment setting. We know the best way to prevent this is to identify children and adolescents' needs earlier and connect them to mental health care within their communities. However, many communities have a long way to go toward establishing robust, well-coordinated systems of pediatric behavioral health care, and state and federal resources are often utilized disproportionately for adult services. We encourage Congress to direct funds to strengthen pediatric community-based mental health services, allowing communities to develop new or improve existing programs and policies to fill service gaps and better meet the mental and behavioral health needs of children, teens, and young adults locally.

### Provide dedicated resources to enhance pediatric mental health infrastructure

In order to expand and sustain a full continuum of mental and behavioral health services for children and teens, which provides adequate support and connection to youth as they transition to adulthood, investments are needed to strengthen critical pediatric mental health infrastructure. There is insufficient pediatric capacity to deliver higher and intermediate levels of care, such as inpatient psychiatric treatment, for those young people who need it, contributing to a crisis in mental health boarding. We specifically urge Congress to provide resources to support efforts to scale up inpatient care capacity, including costs associated with the conversion of general beds to accommodate mental health patients. There is also a vital need to increase access to alternatives to inpatient and emergency department care including stepdown, partial hospitalization, intensive outpatient services and day programs. Children's hospitals recommend that lawmakers take additional actions this year to strengthen pediatric behavioral health infrastructure and improve access to care, both immediately and long-term.

### Strengthen programs targeted to support mental health among teens and young adults

Effectively promoting mental health among teens and youth transitioning into adulthood necessitates meeting them where they are, making schools and colleges critical connection points for screening and support. Many mental health conditions in youth can be managed, especially if identified early, through community-based outpatient treatment. Children's hospitals have long supported school-based mental health and suicide prevention programs, especially in partnerships with children's hospitals and other pediatric mental health providers to facilitate referrals to appropriate care. We have supported S. 1841/H.R. 721, the Mental Health Services for Students Act, which passed the House with bipartisan support earlier this year and would expand comprehensive school mental health programs and training for school professionals through the Substance Abuse and Mental Health Services Administration's Project AWARE program. We also support S. 4271/H.R. 7255, the Garret Lee Smith Memorial Reauthorization Act, which will increase funding for effective suicide prevention programs with teens, on college campuses and within tribal communities.

Thank you again for your commitment to improving mental and behavioral health care delivery systems for children, teens, and young adults. Children's hospitals urge you to take additional steps before the end of this year to help children and young people struggling with mental health conditions to get the care they need.

# AAFP Statement for the Record

AAFP Statement for the Record

November 30, 2022 HELP Subcommittee on Children and Families Hearing: "Caring for Our Kids: Supporting Mental Health in the Transition from High School to College"

**Background**

College students are often assuming responsibility for their health care for the first time. Although they are generally healthy, many have special health care needs such as asthma, diabetes mellitus, mental health concerns, and learning disorders. Depression, anxiety, sleep problems, and posttraumatic stress and eating disorders are common in this population and can affect school performance. As noted in AAFP policy, mental health concerns, such as non-suicidal self-injury and serious suicidal ideation, have risen among college students over the past several years.

Understanding and managing the needs of this dynamic population involve addressing the unique psychosocial stressors related to this life transition that manifest before and while attending college. Poor transitions of youth to adult care can result in declines in treatment adherence, increased emergency department use, and increased hospitalizations.

As detailed in our testimony to the Committee earlier this year, family physicians provide comprehensive mental health services and are a major source for mental health care in the US. Nearly 40% of all visits for depression, anxiety, or cases defined as "any mental illness" were with primary care physicians, and primary care physicians are more likely to be the source of physical and mental health care for patients with lower socioeconomic status and for those with co-morbidities. **Family physicians are uniquely equipped to support the transition of a youth to an adult model of health care for college students.** Family physicians are the only primary care physicians trained to care for children, adolescents, *and* adults, which enables them to care for patients across the lifespan. They have an existing relationship and established trust with the patient, as well as an understanding of a patient's medical history, including mental and behavioral health conditions, which allows them to help facilitate appropriate and continuous care.

Last year, the AAFP joined the American Academy of Pediatrics, the American Academy of Child and Adolescent Psychiatry, and the Children's Hospital Association in declaring a National State of Emergency in Children's Mental Health. We also joined a letter to Congressional leadership last month about the need for further legislation to address this issue.

As the Committee weighs the mental and behavioral health needs of college students, the AAFP strongly urges recognition of the important role primary care physicians play in the provision of mental health care services for college students. **We urge the Committee to support policies that strengthen and build upon existing patient-physician relationships.**

***Telehealth Services***

Telehealth allows patients to maintain access to their family physician and ensures continuity of care for students who are away at college. It can enhance the patient-physician relationship, increase access to care, improve health outcomes by enabling timely care interventions, and decrease costs when utilized as a component of, and coordinated with, continuous care. Mental health services, in particular, are well-suited to be delivered virtually.

A nationwide survey found that patients were most willing to see their usual physician via telemedicine and most felt it was very important that the telehealth provider have access to their complete medical record. Protecting and promoting continuity of care is essential to realizing the care quality improvements and cost reductions with the integration of telehealth. **Any permanent expansion of telehealth benefits should be structured in a way that not only increases access to care but also promotes high-quality, comprehensive, continuous care,** as outlined in our joint principles for telehealth policy. We note that tele-mental health services provided by virtual-only companies could, in some cases, be an appropriate substitute for traditional in-person care and significantly increase access to needed behavioral health services; however, such care should always include communication and coordination with the patient's usual source of primary care.

College students may experience challenges to accessing continuous mental health and other essential services. For example, many colleges only offer a few free counseling visits. Telehealth visits with a patient's usual source of care could improve timely, ongoing access to services. Unfortunately, accessing telehealth care across state lines remains a challenge for college students especially, as many pursue educational opportunities in a different state than where their primary care physician is located. Additionally, family physicians often cite state licensure requirements as a barrier to providing virtual care to their patients when they are travelling or temporarily residing in another state. Most states require physicians to obtain a license to practice medicine in the state where the patient is located, annually register with the state's board, or obtain a licensure by endorsement/telemedicine waiver. These processes are administratively burdensome, costly, and time intensive for physicians. However, **the AAFP has long supported licensure at the state level in order to ensure patient safety and necessary oversight.**

Congress could consider legislation to **allow physicians to provide telehealth services to out of state enrolled college and graduate-level students with an established physician-patient relationship to avoid emergency room and inpatient psychiatric hospitalizations.** Patients with an established relationship, who are traveling, should be allowed to be treated by their primary care physician, so long as the physician is licensed in the state in which the patient receives their usual care. In this case, as long as the student has an established relationship with their primary care physician in the student's home state, they should be able to see their primary care physician while in school, out of state. Such legislation could specify that the student's home state retains the authority to conduct oversight and enforcement activities related to the care provided to college and graduate students located in other states. This could improve access to care for college students while also guarding against fraud or patient safety concerns.

The Interstate Medical Licensure Compact (IMLC) offers an expedited pathway for physicians to apply for and receive licenses from participating states. We encourage states to engage in reciprocity compacts for physician licensing like the IMLC, especially to permit the use of telehealth. While the IMLC helps to expedite the licensure process, family physicians report that it is still burdensome and costly. Physicians must apply to participate in the IMLC, provide additional information to states to obtain licensure, and regularly renew each individual state license. According the IMLC website, physicians are required to pay a $700.00 application fee to participate in the IMLC in addition to state licensing and renewal fees for each state they wish to be licensed in. **The AAFP supports efforts to improve and streamline the IMLC to support family physicians providing virtual care to *all* their established patients across state lines. We urge Congress to consider federal policy options to:**

- Subsidize the cost of the IMLC application fee and state licensing fees;
- Improve the sharing of licensure and other relevant information between states in order to reduce the burden of application and renewal on physicians and reduce licensing wait times;
- Encourage all states to participate in the IMLC and create streamlined licensure or waiver processes for physicians in other states caring for patients with whom there is an established patient-physician relationship.

[Whereupon, at 11:34 a.m., the hearing was adjourned.]

# Chapter 4

# Bipolar Disorder in Children and Teens*


## National Institutes of Health


*Does your child go through extreme changes in mood and behavior?* Does your child get much more excited or much more irritable than other kids? Do you notice that your child goes through cycles of extreme highs and lows more often than other children? Do these mood changes affect how your child acts at school or at home?

Some children and teens with these symptoms may *have bipolar disorder,* a brain disorder that causes unusual shifts in mood, energy, activity levels, and day-to-day functioning. With treatment, children and teens with bipolar disorder can get better over time.

### What Is Bipolar Disorder?

Bipolar disorder is a mental disorder that causes people to experience noticeable, sometimes extreme, changes in mood and behavior. Sometimes children with bipolar disorder feel very happy or "up" and are much more energetic and active than usual. This is called a *manic episode.* Sometimes children with bipolar disorder feel very sad or "down" and are much less active than usual. This is called a *depressive episode.*

Bipolar disorder, which used to be called manic-depressive illness or manic depression, is not the same as the normal ups and downs every child goes through. The mood changes in bipolar disorder are more extreme, often unprovoked, and accompanied by changes in sleep, energy level, and the ability to think clearly. Bipolar symptoms can make it hard for young people to perform well in school or to get along with friends and family members. Some children and teens with bipolar disorder may try to hurt themselves or attempt suicide.

Most people are diagnosed with bipolar disorder in adolescence or adulthood, but the symptoms can appear earlier in childhood. Bipolar disorder is often episodic, but it usually lasts a lifetime.

---

* This is an edited, reformatted and augmented version of U.S. Department of Health and Human Services, National Institute of Mental Health, National Institutes of Health, Publication No. 20-MH-8081, dated 2020.


In: Understanding Youth Mental Health
Editor: Michael A. Post
ISBN: 979-8-89530-700-7

Signs and symptoms of bipolar disorder may overlap with symptoms of other disorders that are common in young people, such as attention-deficit/ hyperactivity disorder (ADHD), conduct problems, major depression, and anxiety disorders. Diagnosing bipolar disorder can be complicated and requires a careful and thorough evaluation by a trained, experienced mental health professional.

With treatment, children and teens with bipolar disorder can manage their symptoms and lead successful lives.

## What Causes Bipolar Disorder?

The exact causes of bipolar disorder are unknown, but several factors may contribute to the illness.

For example, researchers are beginning to uncover genetic mechanisms that are linked to bipolar disorder and other mental disorders. Research shows that people's chance of having bipolar disorder is higher if they have a close family member with the illness, which may be because they have the same genetic variations. However, just because one family member has bipolar disorder, it does not mean that other members of the family will have it. Many genes are involved in the disorder, and no single gene causes it.

Research also suggests that adversity, trauma, and stressful life events may increase the chances of developing bipolar disorder in people with a genetic risk of having the illness.

Some research studies have found differences in brain structure and function between people who have bipolar disorder and those who do not. Researchers are studying the disorder to learn more about its causes and effective treatments.

## What Are the Symptoms of Bipolar Disorder?

Mood episodes in bipolar disorder include intense emotions along with significant changes in sleep habits, activity levels, thoughts, or behaviors. A person with bipolar disorder may have manic episodes, depressive episodes, or "mixed" episodes. A mixed episode has both manic and depressive symptoms. These mood episodes cause symptoms that often last for several days or weeks. During an episode, the symptoms last every day for most of the day.

These mood and activity changes are very different from the child's usual behavior and from the behavior of healthy children and teens.

Children and teens having a *manic episode* may:

- Show intense happiness or silliness for long periods of time.
- Have a very short temper or seem extremely irritable.
- Talk fast about a lot of different things.
- Have trouble sleeping but not feel tired.
- Have trouble staying focused, and experience racing thoughts.
- Seem overly interested or involved in pleasurable but risky activities.
- Do risky or reckless things that show poor judgment.

Children and teens having a *depressive episode* may:

- Feel frequent and unprovoked sadness.
- Show increased irritability, anger, or hostility.
- Complain a lot about pain, such as stomachaches and headaches.
- Have a noticeable increase in amount of sleep.
- Have difficulty concentrating.
- Feel hopeless and worthless.
- Have difficulty communicating or maintaining relationships.
- Eat too much or too little.
- Have little energy and no interest in activities they usually enjoy.
- Think about death, or have thoughts of suicide.

## Can Children and Teens with Bipolar Disorder Have Other Problems?

Young people with bipolar disorder can have several problems at the same time. These include:

- *Misuse of alcohol and drugs.* Young people with bipolar disorder are at risk of misusing alcohol or drugs.
- *Attention-deficit/hyperactivity disorder (ADHD).* Children and teens who have both bipolar disorder and ADHD may have trouble staying focused.
- *Anxiety disorders.* Children and teens with bipolar disorder also may have an anxiety disorder.

Sometimes extreme behaviors go along with mood episodes. During manic episodes, young people with bipolar disorder may take extreme risks that they wouldn't usually take or that could cause them harm or injury. During depressive episodes, some young people with bipolar disorder may think about running away from home or have thoughts of suicide.

> *If your child shows signs of suicidal thinking, take these signs seriously and call your child's health care provider.*
>
> If you think your child is in crisis and needs immediate help, call 911. You also can call the National Suicide Prevention Lifeline (Lifeline) at 1-800-273-TALK (8255), or text the Crisis Text Line (text HELLO to 741741). The deaf and hard of hearing can contact the Lifeline via TTY at 1-800-799-4889. These services are confidential, free, and available 24/7.

## How Is Bipolar Disorder Diagnosed?

A health care provider will ask questions about your child's mood, sleeping patterns, energy levels, and behavior. There are no blood tests or brain scans that can diagnose bipolar disorder. However, the health care provider may use tests to see if something other than bipolar disorder is causing your child's symptoms. Sometimes health care providers need to know about medical conditions in the family, such as depression or substance use.

Other disorders have symptoms like those of bipolar disorder, including ADHD, disruptive mood regulation disorder, oppositional defiant disorder, conduct disorder, and anxiety disorders. It also can be challenging to distinguish bipolar disorder from depression that occurs without mania, which is referred to as "major depression." A health care provider who specializes in working with children and teens can make a careful and complete evaluation of your child's symptoms to provide the right diagnosis.

## How Is Bipolar Disorder Treated?

Children and teens can work with their health care provider to develop a treatment plan that will help them manage their symptoms and improve their quality of life. It is important to follow the treatment plan, even when your child is not currently experiencing a mood episode. Steady, dependable treatment works better than treatment that starts and stops.

Treatment options include:

- *Medication.* Several types of medication can help treat symptoms of bipolar disorder. Children respond to medications in different ways, so the right type of medication depends on the child. This means children may need to try different types of medication to see which one works best for them. Some children may need more than one type of medication because their symptoms are complex. Children should take the fewest number of medications and the smallest doses possible to help their symptoms. A good way to remember this is "start low, go slow." Medications can cause side effects. *Always tell your child's health care provider about any problems with side effects.* Do not stop giving your child medication without speaking to a health care provider. Stopping medication suddenly can be dangerous and can make bipolar symptoms worse.
- *Psychosocial Therapy.* Different kinds of psychosocial therapy can help children and their families manage the symptoms of bipolar disorder. Therapies that are based on scientific research—including cognitive behavioral approaches and family-focused therapy—can provide support, education, and guidance to youth and their families. These therapies teach skills that can help people manage bipolar disorder, including skills for maintaining routines, enhancing emotion regulation, and improving social interactions.

## What Can Children and Teens Expect from Treatment?

With treatment, children and teens with bipolar disorder can get better over time. Treatment is more effective when health care providers, parents, and young people work together.

Sometimes a child's symptoms may change, or disappear and then come back. When this happens, your child's health care provider may recommend changes to the treatment plan. Treatment can take time, but sticking with the treatment plan can help young people manage their symptoms and reduce the likelihood of future episodes.

Your child's health care provider may recommend keeping a daily life chart or mood chart to track your child's moods, behaviors, and sleep patterns. This may make it easier to track the illness and see whether treatment is working.

## How Can I Help My Child or Teen?

Help begins with the right diagnosis and treatment. Talk to your family health care provider about any symptoms you notice.

If your child has bipolar disorder, here are some basic things you can do:

- Be patient.
- Encourage your child to talk, and listen to your child carefully.
- Pay attention to your child's moods, and be alert to any major changes.
- Understand triggers, and learn strategies for managing intense emotions and irritability.
- Help your child have fun.
- Remember that treatment takes time: sticking with the treatment plan can help your child get better and stay better.
- Help your child understand that treatment can make life better.

## How Does Bipolar Disorder Affect Caregivers and Families?

Caring for a child or teenager with bipolar disorder can be stressful for parents and families. Coping with a child's mood episodes and other problems—such as short tempers and risky behaviors—can challenge any caregiver.

It is important that caregivers take care of themselves, too. Find someone you can talk to or consult your health care provider about support groups. Finding support and strategies for managing stress can help you and your child.

## Where Do I Go for Help?

If you're not sure where to get help, your doctor, pediatrician, or other family health care provider is a good place to start. A health care provider can refer you to a qualified mental health professional, such as a psychiatrist or psychologist, who has experience treating bipolar disorder and can evaluate your child's symptoms.

You can learn more about getting help and finding a health care provider on the National Institute of Mental Health website at www.nimh.nih.gov/findhelp. Hospital health care providers can help in an emergency. The Substance Abuse and Mental Health Services Administration (SAMHSA) has an online tool at https://findtreatment.samhsa.gov to help you find mental health services in your area.

## I Know Someone Who Is in Crisis. What Do I Do?

If you know someone who might be thinking about hurting themselves or someone else, get help quickly.

- Do not leave the person alone.
- Call 911 or go to the nearest hospital emergency room.
- Call the toll-free National Suicide Prevention Lifeline at 1-800-273-TALK (8255) or the toll-free TTY number at 1-800-799-4TTY (4889). You also can text the Crisis Text Line (text HELLO to 741741) or go to the National Suicide Prevention Lifeline website at https://suicidepreventionlifeline.org.

## What Should I Know About Clinical Trials?

Clinical trials are research studies that look at new ways to prevent, detect, or treat diseases and conditions. Although individuals may benefit from being part of a clinical trial, participants should be aware that the primary purpose of a clinical trial is to gain new scientific knowledge so that others may be better helped in the future.

Researchers at NIMH and around the country conduct clinical trials with patients and healthy volunteers. Talk to your health care provider about clinical trials, their benefits and risks, and whether one is right for you. For more information, visit www.nimh.nih.gov/clinicaltrials.

## For More Information

NIMH website
www.nimh.nih.gov
MedlinePlus (National Library of Medicine)
https://medlineplus.gov
(En español: https://medlineplus.gov/spanish)
ClinicalTrials.gov
www.clinicaltrials.gov
(En español: https://salud.nih.gov/investigacion-clinica)
National Institute of Mental Health
Office of Science Policy, Planning, and Communications
Science Writing, Press, and Dissemination Branch
6001 Executive Boulevard
Room 6200, MSC 9663
Bethesda, MD 20892-9663
Phone: 301-443-4513 or Toll-free: 1-866-615-6464
TTY: 301-443-8431 or TTY Toll-free: 1-866-415-8051
Fax: 301-443-4279
Email: nimhinfo@nih.gov
Website: www.nimh.nih.gov

## Chapter 5

# Social Media and Teen Mental Health: Guide for Parents and Caregivers to Support Healthy Social Media Use among Teens*


## Family and Youth Services Bureau


Social media is here to stay, and it's important for parents and caregivers to understand the role it plays in their teens' lives. Parents and caregivers also need to know how to support teens' mental health when it comes to social media use. If you've been wondering how to steer teens in your life toward healthy social media use, this guide is for you! It includes a quiz you can share with teens to help them discover how social media affects their lives and mental health and a discussion guide to facilitate conversations about strategies they can use to avoid the risks and maximize the benefits of social media.

> Throughout this document, the term "parents and caregivers" includes biological or adoptive parents; guardians; other relatives such as aunts, uncles, or grandparents; and other supportive adults who care for a teen.

According to a Pew Research Center survey of American teens conducted in 2022, 97% of teens aged 13–17 reported being online daily and more than a third say they use social media "almost constantly."[73] Studies have also shown that social media use is linked to anxiety, depression, and lower self-esteem among teens.[74,75,76] It can contribute to negative body

---

* This is an edited, reformatted and augmented version of This is an edited, reformatted and augmented version a Family and Youth Services Bureau Publication, dated February 2024.

[73] Vogels, E. A., Gelles-Watnick, R., & Massarat, N. (2022). Teens, social media and technology 2022. *Pew Research Center*. https://www.pewresearch.org/internet/2022/08/10/teens-social-media-and-technology-2022/.

[74] Boers, E., Afzali, M. H., Newton, N., & Conrod, P. (2019). Association of screen time and depression in adolescence. *JAMA Pediatrics, 173*(9), 853–859. https://doi.org/10.1001/jamapediatrics.2019.1759.

[75] Riehm, K. E., Feder, K. A., Tormohlen, K. N., Crum, R. M., Young, A. S., Green, K. M., Pacek, L. R., La Flair, L. N., & Mojtabai, R. (2019). Associations between time spent using social media and internalizing and externalizing problems among US youth. *JAMA Psychiatry, 76*(12), 1266–1273. https://doi.org/10.1001/jamapsychiatry.2019.2325.

[76] Zagorski, N. (2017, January 17). *Using many social media platforms linked with depression, anxiety risk.* Psychiatric News. https://psychnews.psychiatryonline.org/doi/10.1176/appi.pn.2017.1b16.


In: Understanding Youth Mental Health
Editor: Michael A. Post
ISBN: 979-8-89530-700-7

image;[77,78] interfere with sleep quality[79] and focus on schoolwork and other tasks; and put teens at risk for cyberbullying[80] and exposure to inappropriate, hate-based, violent, or other harmful or upsetting content. Social media platforms can also put teens at risk for predatory behaviors such as fraud, sexual assault, and extortion. Because of growing concerns about the effects of social media on youth mental health, the U.S. Surgeon General released an Advisory to call attention to the issue and offer recommendations about what can be done to help teens, including recommendations for parents and caregivers. These recommendations and others are provided below. Read these tips and then use the discussion guide to have a conversation with a teen you care for.

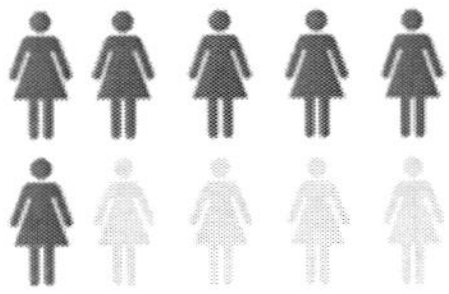

In a survey, 6 in 10 teen girls ages 13–15 and pre-teens ages 11–12 reported that they had been contacted by a stranger on certain social media platforms in ways that made them feel uncomfortable.[81]

## 1. Educate Yourself

Use the resources provided at the bottom of this guide to become familiar with the social media platforms teens commonly use, the positive and negative aspects of different online behaviors, and the ways you can help minimize risks to teens in your life. Learn about parental controls for social media and your options for monitoring for signs of potential harm.

## 2. Get on the Same Page

Despite the risks associated with social media use, teens experience many benefits, including connections with friends and family, opportunities to share ideas and information with people who share their interests, and an opportunity for self-expression and creativity. To help teens

---

[77] Bickham, D., Hunt, E., Bediou, B., Rich, M. (2022). *Adolescent media use: Attitudes, effects, and online experiences.* Boston Children's Hospital Digital Wellness Lab. https://digitalwellnesslab.org/wp-content/uploads/Pulse-Survey_Adolescent-Attitudes-Effects-and-Experiences.pdf.

[78] Holland, G., & Tiggemann, M. (2016). A systematic review of the impact of the use of social networking sites on body image and disordered eating outcomes. *Body Image, 17*, 100–110. https://doi.org/10.1016/j.bodyim.2016.02.008.

[79] Alonzo, R., Hussain, J., Stranges, S., & Anderson, K. K. (2021). Interplay between social media use, sleep quality, and mental health in youth: A systematic review. *Sleep Medicine Reviews, 56*, 101414. https://doi.org/10.1016/j.smrv.2020.101414.

[80] Alhajji, M., Bass, S., & Dai, T. (2019). Cyberbullying, mental health, and violence in adolescents and associations with sex and race: Data from the 2015 Youth Risk Behavior Survey. *Global Pediatric Health, 6.* https://doi.org/10.1177/2333794X19868887.

[81] Nesi, J., Mann, S. & Robb, M. B. (2023). *Teens and mental health: How girls really feel about social media.* Common Sense. https://www.commonsensemedia.org/sites/default/files/research/report/how-girls-really-feel-about-social-media-researchreport_final_1.pdf.

find the right balance, it's especially important to begin your conversation with an open mind and non-judgmental approach. The teens in your life may have experienced many of the following benefits of social media use. Which ones are you aware of?

- Strengthened friendships/connecting with friends
- Connections with others who have shared interests
- Motivation to participate in worthwhile endeavors
- Interactions with others across geographic barriers
- Reduced feelings of isolation
- Increased sense of belonging
- Strengthened social support (especially for LGBTQIA2S+ teens, other teens who might face exclusion in their regular social circles, or teens with disabilities)
- Increased outlets for personal or artistic expression
- Greater access to information about topics of interest

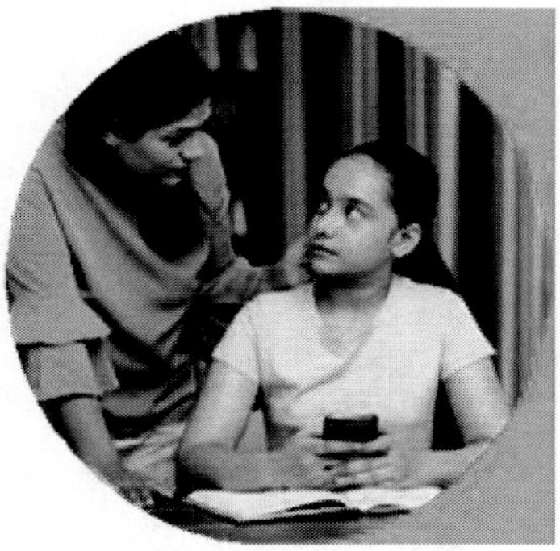

When you talk with the teens in your life, make a point to acknowledge the positive sides and see what you can learn about the positive ways they are using social media. Then, open the door to discussing the potential harms and how to minimize them. They may be more open to talking if they know you aren't trying to take away their use of social media altogether.

## 3. Establish Rules About Privacy and Security and Help Them Set Their Own Boundaries for Screen Time

They might not say so, but teens need and appreciate clear limits from their parents and caregivers:

- *Rules about privacy and security.* Make sure they use appropriate privacy settings to control what others can see. They should restrict posts with personal information to people they know and trust in real life and should disable location services for all social media apps on their phone to minimize the risk that someone could use that information to harm them. Make sure they know there are serious lifelong consequences for sharing sexually explicit photos, videos, or messages through phones or online. Such images can be easily shared, which can cause significant emotional trauma and have legal consequences. You can also help them set their own boundaries about what is appropriate to post by talking with them about oversharing highly personal or sensitive information in a public space. Remind them that anything they post could be shared and therefore become extremely difficult to remove from the internet. It's best to assume that anything posted could stay on the internet forever. Make sure they consider who might see a post in the future (employers, teachers, family members).

- *Screen time limits*. Talk about your expectations regarding how much, where and when they can use social media. There are ways teens can manage screen time on both iPhone and Android that help them become more aware of their social media use, and you can find many other apps that let you set time limits. Some parents and caregivers even create a written agreement that can serve as a reminder about expectations. To encourage healthy sleep, you may want to designate appropriate hours for social media and restrict use entirely during the hour before bedtime. Having screen-free zones (like the bedroom or dinner table) can help. Encourage them to learn how to recognize when they need boundaries and to set their own. For example, some teens decide to turn off notifications or delete certain apps from their phone when they know they need a break.

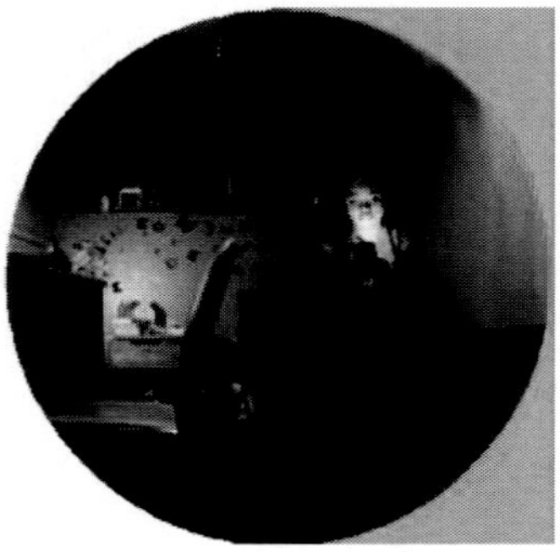

## 4. Model Healthy Social Media Use

Show the teen you care for what it looks like to have mindful use of social media. You could even take a "social media cleanse" or do a "digital detox" to completely disconnect for a period of time and ask other family members to join you. The U.S. Surgeon General's Advisory on Social Media and Youth Mental Health cited a randomized controlled trial among young adults and adults showing that deactivating a social media platform for 4 weeks improved their sense of well-being by about 25%–40% of the effect of psychological interventions like self-help therapy, group training, and individual therapy.[82] That's a huge benefit for a simple behavior change! Be sure you also model empathy and kindness toward others in your own use of social media.

---

[82] Allcott, H., Braghieri, L., Eichmeyer, S., & Gentzkow, M. (2020). The welfare effects of social media. *American Economic Review, 110*(3), 629–676. http://dx.doi.org/10.1257/aer.20190658.

## 5. Encourage Balance

Help the teens in your life find hobbies, sports, and other activities to keep them busy offline. Foster their in-person social skills by facilitating opportunities for face-to-face interactions with peers. Work with other parents and caregivers to provide opportunities for social interaction and establish shared norms around social media use.

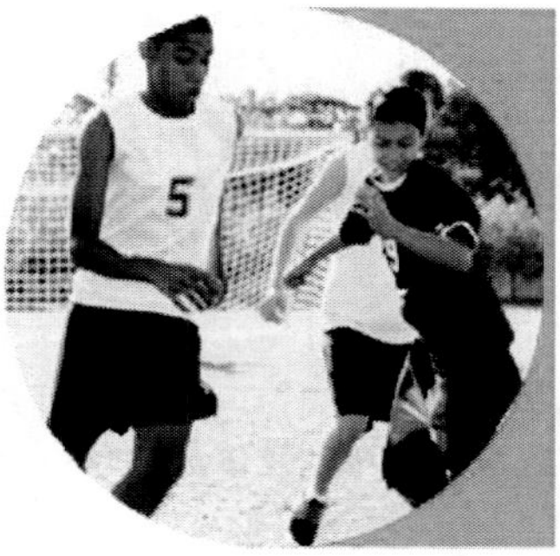


## 6. Help Teens Develop Critical Thinking Skills and Media Literacy

Talk with them about how what they see online isn't usually a complete or accurate picture. Remind them that most people try to project an image of perfection on their social media accounts, leaving out the difficulties, failures, and mundane parts of their lives, which can make others think their own lives aren't as good in comparison. Help them focus on all the positive things they have going on and encourage them to mute or unfollow accounts that make them feel bad. Help them to learn how to identify misinformation and avoid spreading it.

## 7. Make Sure Teens Know They Can Come to You or Another Trusted Adult for Support

Sometimes teens feel like they need to handle difficult issues—like cyberbullying, identity theft, or sextortion—alone. They need to know they have a trusted adult who can help them manage the situation and seek out the appropriate resources if they are a victim of cyberbullying or another online attack. Visit CyberTipline or Take it Down or contact your local law enforcement to report any instances of online exploitation.

## 8. Learn How to Identify Warning Signs of Excessive or Problematic Social Media Use and Seek Professional Help if Needed

Social media may be causing problems if it interferes with teens' responsibilities at school or work or with extracurricular activities, if it prevents them from getting enough sleep or physical activity, if it keeps them from participating in in-person activities, or if they want to stop or cut down on using social media but don't seem to be able to. If you notice signs that teens in your life are struggling with their mental health or engaging in harmful social media practices that you can't address on your own, seek professional help. The Family & Youth Services Bureau's Supporting Your Teen's Mental Health tip sheet helps identify warning signs that teens might be experiencing challenges with mental health and provides suggestions on locating an appropriate mental health specialist when needed. It also includes hotlines for teens in distress.

By recognizing that social media will likely continue to play an important role in teens' lives, and by keeping the lines of communication open, you can teach the teens you care for how to navigate the digital landscape independently, safely, and productively.

## Activity: Mental Health and Social Media Quiz and Discussion Guide

Discover how teens in your life are using social media and start a conversation with them about the topic using the discussion guide that accompanies this resource, *Mental Health and Social Media: Discussion Guide for Teens and Their Parents/Caregivers*. Have them complete the Mental Health and Social Media Quiz to discover ways social media might be affecting their mental health. Their results will give you both a starting point for a constructive discussion. The quiz is from *We Think Twice*™, a movement designed *with* teens, *for* teens, which provides tools and resources to equip and empower teens to form healthy relationships, set goals for the future, make smart decisions, and look out for their mental health.

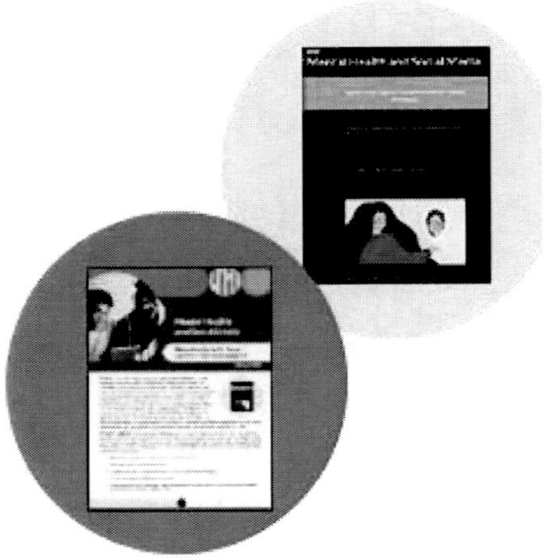

## Additional Resources

For parents/caregivers:

- Social Media and Youth Mental Health: The U.S. Surgeon General's Advisory
- Social Media Can…Help Connect: Research-Based Tips from Pediatricians for Families:
- American Academy of Pediatrics, Center of Excellence on Social Media and Youth
- Mental Health
- Family Media Plan: American Academy of Pediatrics

- Keeping Teens Safe on Social Media: What Parents Should Know to Protect their Kids: American Psychological Association
- Health Advisory on Social Media Use in Adolescence: American Psychological Association
- Teens, Social Media and Technology 2022: Pew Research Center

To share with the teens in your life:

- Mental Health Resources for Teens: *We Think Twice*™
- Teen Sexting—Think Twice Before You Hit "Send": Administration for Children and Families,
- Family and Youth Services Bureau
- Tip Sheet on Social Media Use and Mental Health: Youth Engaged 4 Change
- Grades 9–12 Student Tip Card: U.S. Department of Homeland Security, Stop.Think.Connect.™
- Social Media Safety for Teens: National Center for Missing and Exploited Children
- General Tips and Advice: U.S. Department of Homeland Security, Stop.Think.Connect.™
- CyberTipline: National center for Missing and Exploited Children

This guide was created by the *We Think Twice*™ campaign with support from the Family and Youth Services Bureau. It is one of several valuable resources designed for youth-serving professionals as well as parents/caregivers. It is intended to encourage positive youth development by strengthening prevention education and other youth development programs.



This resource was developed by RTI International under contract GS-00F-354-CA/75ACF122F80038 with the U.S. Department of Health and Human Services, Administration on Children, Youth and Families, Family and Youth Services Bureau.

# Chapter 6

# Social Media and Youth Mental Health, 2023*

## U.S. Surgeon General's Advisory

### About the Advisory

A Surgeon General's Advisory is a public statement that calls the American people's attention to an urgent public health issue and provides recommendations for how it should be addressed. Advisories are reserved for significant public health challenges that require the nation's immediate awareness and action.

This Advisory calls attention to the growing concerns about the effects of social media on youth mental health. It explores and describes the current evidence on the positive and negative impacts of social media on children and adolescents, some of the primary areas for mental health and well-being concerns, and opportunities for additional research to help understand the full scope and scale of social media's impact. This document is not an exhaustive review of the literature. Rather, it was developed through a substantial review of the available evidence, primarily found via electronic searches of research articles published in English and resources suggested by a wide range of subject matter experts, with priority given to, but not limited to, meta-analyses and systematic literature reviews. It also offers actionable recommendations for the institutions that can shape online environments—policymakers and technology companies—as well as for what parents and caregivers, young people, and researchers can do.

For additional background and to read other Surgeon General's Advisories, visit SurgeonGeneral.gov

* * *

Social media[83] use by youth is nearly universal. Up to 95% of youth ages 13–17 report using a social media platform, with more than a third saying they use social media "almost

---

* This is an edited, reformatted and augmented version of The U.S. Surgeon General's Advisory, dated 2023.

83 The definition of social media has been highly debated over the past few decades. As a result, there isn't a single, widely-accepted scholarly definition of social media. (Aichner et al., 2021) The definition may vary from the cited research in this document based on the methods used in each study. In making conclusions and recommendations, this document regards social media as "internet-based channels that allow users to opportunistically interact and selectively self-present, either in real-time or asynchronously, with both broad and narrow audiences who derive

In: Understanding Youth Mental Health
Editor: Michael A. Post
ISBN: 979-8-89530-700-7

constantly."[84] Although age 13 is commonly the required minimum age used by social media platforms in the U.S.,[85] nearly 40% of children ages 8–12 use social media.[86] Despite this widespread use among children and adolescents, robust independent safety analyses on the impact of social media on youth have not yet been conducted. There are increasing concerns among researchers, parents and caregivers, young people, healthcare experts, and others about the impact of social media on youth mental health.[87,88]

More research is needed to fully understand the impact of social media; however, the current body of evidence indicates that while social media may have benefits for some children and adolescents, there are ample indicators that social media can also have a profound risk of harm to the mental health and well-being of children and adolescents. At this time, we do not yet have enough evidence to determine if social media is sufficiently safe for children and adolescents. We must acknowledge the growing body of research about potential harms, increase our collective understanding of the risks associated with social media use, and urgently take action to create safe and healthy digital environments that minimize harm and safeguard children's and adolescents' mental health and well-being during critical stages of development.

> Up to 95% of youth ages 13–17 report using a social media platform, with more than a third saying they use social media "almost constantly."

## Social Media Has Both Positive and Negative Impacts on Children and Adolescents

The influence of social media on youth mental health is shaped by many complex factors, including, but not limited to, the amount of time children and adolescents spend on platforms,

---

value from user-generated content and the perception of interaction with others." (Carr & Hayes, 2015) For the purposes of this product, we did not include studies specific to online gaming or e-sports. Source: Aichner, T., Grünfelder, M., Maurer, O., & Jegeni, D. (2021). Twenty-Five Years of Social Media: A Review of Social Media Applications and Definitions from 1994 to 2019. *Cyberpsychology, Behavior And Social Networking*, 24(4), 215–222. https://doi.org/10.1089/cyber.2020.0134 Source: Carr, C. T., & Hayes, R. A. (2015). Social Media: Defining, Developing, and Divining. *Atlantic Journal of Communication*, 23:1, 46-65. https://doi.org/10.1080/15456870.2015.972282.

84 Vogels, E., Gelles-Watnick, R. & Massarat, N. (2022). Teens, Social Media and Technology 2022. Pew Research Center: Internet, Science & Tech. United States of America. Retrieved from https://www.pewresearch.org/internet/2022/08/10/teens-social-media-and-technology-2022/.

85 The minimum required age set by social media platforms is informed by the Children's Online Privacy Protection Act that requires social media platforms to collect verifiable parental consent before collecting, storing, and sharing data from children under age 13. Source: Federal Trade Commission. (n.d.). Children's Online Privacy Protection Act ("COPPA"). Federal Trade Commission. Retrieved from https://www.ftc.gov/legal- library/browse/statutes/childrens-online-privacy-protection-act.

86 Rideout, V., Peebles, A., Mann, S., & Robb, M. B. (2022). Common Sense Census: Media use by tweens and teens, 2021. San Francisco, CA: Common Sense. Retrieved from https://www. commonsensemedia.org/sites/default/files/research/report/8-18-census-integrated-report-final-web_0.pdf.

87 It is important to note that many factors can shape mental health, and a comprehensive approach, including prevention strategies, will be needed to support and protect the mental health of children and adolescents. Source: Office of the Surgeon General (OSG). (2021). Protecting Youth Mental Health: The U.S. Surgeon General's Advisory. US Department of Health and Human Services. Retrieved from https://www.hhs.gov/sites/default/files/surgeon-general-youth-mental-health-advisory.pdf.

88 American Psychological Association. (2023). Health Advisory on Social Media Use in Adolescence. American Psychological Association. Retrieved from https://www.apa.org/topics/social- media-internet/health-advisory-adolescent-social-media-use. pdf.

the type of content they consume or are otherwise exposed to, the activities and interactions social media affords, and the degree to which it disrupts activities that are essential for health like sleep and physical activity.[6] Importantly, different children and adolescents are affected by social media in different ways, based on their individual strengths and vulnerabilities, and based on cultural, historical, and socio-economic factors.[89,90] There is broad agreement among the scientific community that social media has the potential to both benefit and harm children and adolescents.[6,91]

Brain development is a critical factor to consider when assessing the risk for harm. Adolescents, ages 10 to 19, are undergoing a highly sensitive period of brain development.[92,93] This is a period when risk-taking behaviors reach their peak, when well-being experiences the greatest fluctuations, and when mental health challenges such as depression typically emerge.[94,95,96] Furthermore, in early adolescence, when identities and sense of self-worth are forming, brain development is especially susceptible to social pressures, peer opinions, and peer comparison.[11,13] Frequent social media use may be associated with distinct changes in the developing brain in the amygdala (important for emotional learning and behavior) and the prefrontal cortex (important for impulse control, emotional regulation, and moderating social behavior), and could increase sensitivity to social rewards and punishments.[97,98] As such, adolescents may experience heightened emotional sensitivity to the communicative and interactive nature of social media.[16] Adolescent social media use is predictive of a subsequent decrease in life satisfaction for certain developmental stages including for girls 11–13 years old and boys 14–15 years old.[99] Because adolescence is a vulnerable period of brain development, social media exposure during this period warrants additional scrutiny.

---

[89] Beyens, I., Pouwels, J. L., van Driel, I. I., Keijsers, L., & Valkenburg, P. M. (2020). The effect of social media on well- being differs from adolescent to adolescent. *Scientific reports*, 10(1), 10763. https://doi.org/10.1038/s41598-020-67727-7.

[90] Hollis, C., Livingstone, S., & Sonuga-Barke, E. (2020). Editorial: The role of digital technology in children and young people's mental health -a triple-edged sword?. *Journal of child psychology and psychiatry, and allied disciplines*, 61(8), 837–841. https://doi.org/10.1111/jcpp.13302.

[91] Uhls, Y. T., Ellison, N. B., & Subrahmanyam, K. (2017). Benefits and Costs of Social Media in Adolescence. *Pediatrics*, 140(Suppl 2), S67–S70. https://doi.org/10.1542/peds.2016-1758E.

[92] Fuhrmann, D., Knoll, L. J., & Blakemore, S. J. (2015). Adolescence as a Sensitive Period of Brain Development. *Trends in cognitive sciences*, 19(10), 558–566. https://doi.org/10.1016/j. tics.2015.07.008.

[93] Blakemore, S. J., & Mills, K. L. (2014). Is adolescence a sensitive period for sociocultural processing?. *Annual review of psychology*, 65, 187–207. https://doi.org/10.1146/annurev- psych-010213-115202.

[94] Romer D. (2010). Adolescent risk taking, impulsivity, and brain development: implications for prevention. *Developmental psychobiology*, 52(3), 263–276. https://doi.org/10.1002/dev.20442.

[95] National Academies of Sciences, Engineering, and Medicine (NASEM). (2019). The Promise of Adolescence: Realizing Opportunity for All Youth. Washington, DC: The National Academies Press. https://doi.org/10.17226/25388.

[96] Kessler, R. C., Amminger, G. P., Aguilar-Gaxiola, S., Alonso, J., Lee, S., & Ustün, T. B. (2007). Age of onset of mental disorders: a review of recent literature. *Current opinion in psychiatry*, 20(4), 359–364. https://doi.org/10.1097/YCO.0b013e32816ebc8c.

[97] Maza, M. T., Fox, K. A., Kwon, S. J., Flannery, J. E., Lindquist, K. A., Prinstein, M. J., & Telzer, E. H. (2023). Association of Habitual Checking Behaviors on Social Media With Longitudinal Functional Brain Development. *JAMA pediatrics*, 177(2), 160–167. https://doi.org/10.1001/jamapediatrics.2022.4924.

[98] Crone, E. A., & Konijn, E. A. (2018). Media use and brain development during adolescence. *Nature communications*, 9(1), 588. https://doi.org/10.1038/s41467-018-03126-x.

[99] Orben, A., Przybylski, A. K., Blakemore, S. J., & Kievit, R. A. (2022). Windows of developmental sensitivity to social media. *Nature communications*, 13(1), 1649. https://doi.org/10.1038/ s41467-022-29296-3.

## The Potential Benefits of Social Media Use among Children and Adolescents

Social media can provide benefits for some youth by providing positive community and connection with others who share identities, abilities, and interests. It can provide access to important information and create a space for self-expression.[9] The ability to form and maintain friendships online and develop social connections are among the positive effects of social media use for youth.[100,101] These relationships can afford opportunities to have positive interactions with more diverse peer groups than are available to them offline and can provide important social support to youth.[18] The buffering effects against stress that online social support from peers may provide can be especially important for youth who are often marginalized, including racial, ethnic, and sexual and gender minorities.[102,103,104] For example, studies have shown that social media may support the mental health and well-being of lesbian, gay, bisexual, asexual, transgender, queer, intersex and other youths by enabling peer connection, identity development and management, and social support.[105] Seven out of ten adolescent girls of color report encountering positive or identity-affirming content related to race across social media platforms.[106] A majority of adolescents report that social media helps them feel more accepted (58%), like they have people who can support them through tough times (67%), like they have a place to show their creative side (71%), and more connected to what's going on in their friends' lives (80%).[107] In addition, research suggests that social media-based and other digitally-based mental health interventions may also be helpful for some children and

---

[100] Anderson, M. & Jiang, J. (2018). Teens' Social Media Habits and Experiences. Pew Research Center: Internet, Science & Tech. United States of America. Retrieved from https://www. pewresearch.org/internet/2018/11/28/ teens-social-media-habits-and-experiences/.

[101] Seabrook, E. M., Kern, M. L., & Rickard, N. S. (2016). Social Networking Sites, Depression, and Anxiety: A Systematic Review. *JMIR mental health*, 3(4), e50. https://doi.org/10.2196/ mental.5842.

[102] According to the National Institutes of Health, sexual and gender minority (SGM) populations include, but are not limited to, individuals who identify as lesbian, gay, bisexual, asexual, transgender, Two-Spirit, queer, and/or intersex. Individuals with same-sex or -gender attractions or behaviors and those with a difference in sex development are also included. These populations also encompass those who do not self-identify with one of these terms but whose sexual orientation, gender identity or expression, or reproductive development is characterized by non-binary constructs of sexual orientation, gender, and/or sex. Source: U.S. Department of Health and Human Services. National Institutes of Health. (2022, December 8). Sex, gender, and Sexuality. National Institutes of Health. https://www.nih. gov/nih-style-guide/sex-gender-sexuality.

[103] Charmaraman, L., Hernandez, J., & Hodes, R. (2022). Marginalized and Understudied Populations Using Digital Media. In J. Nesi, E. Telzer, & M. Prinstein (Eds.), Handbook of Adolescent Digital Media Use and Mental Health (pp. 188-214). Cambridge: Cambridge University Press. https://doi. org/10.1017/9781108976237.011.

[104] Ybarra, M. L., Mitchell, K. J., Palmer, N. A., & Reisner, S. L. (2015). Online social support as a buffer against online and offline peer and sexual victimization among U.S. LGBT and non-LGBT youth. *Child abuse & neglect*, 39, 123–136. https://doi. org/10.1016/j.chiabu.2014.08.006.

[105] Berger, M. N., Taba, M., Marino, J. L., Lim, M. S. C., & Skinner, S. R. (2022). Social Media Use and Health and Well-being of Lesbian, Gay, Bisexual, Transgender, and Queer Youth: Systematic Review. *Journal of medical Internet research*, 24(9), e38449. https://doi.org/10.2196/38449.

[106] Nesi, J., Mann, S. and Robb, M. B. (2023). Teens and mental health: How girls really feel about social media. San Francisco, CA: Common Sense. Retrieved from https://www. commonsensemedia.org/sites/default/files/ research/report/how-girls-really-feel-about-social-media-researchreport_ final_1.pdf.

[107] Vogels, E., & Gelles-Watnick, R. (2023). Teens and social media: Key findings from Pew Research Center surveys. Pew Research Center: Internet, Science & Tech. United States of America. Retrieved from https://www.pewresearch.org/short-reads/2023/04/24/teens-and-social-media-key-findings-from-pew-research-center-surveys/.

adolescents by promoting help-seeking behaviors and serving as a gateway to initiating mental health care.[8,108,109,110,111]

## The Potential Harms of Social Media Use Among Children and Adolescents

Over the last decade, evidence has emerged identifying reasons for concern about the potential negative impact of social media on children and adolescents.

A longitudinal cohort study of U.S. adolescents aged 12–15 (n=6,595) that adjusted for baseline mental health status found that adolescents who spent more than 3 hours per day on social media faced double the risk of experiencing poor mental health outcomes including symptoms of depression and anxiety.[112]

As of 2021, 8th and 10th graders now spend an average of 3.5 hours per day on social media.[113] In a unique natural experiment that leveraged the staggered introduction of a social media platform across U.S. colleges, the roll-out of the platform was associated with an increase in depression (9% over baseline) and anxiety (12% over baseline) among college-aged youth (n = 359,827 observations).[114] The study's co-author also noted that when applied across the entirety of the U.S. college population, the introduction of the social media platform may have contributed to more than 300,000 new cases of depression.[32,115] If such sizable effects occurred in college-aged youth, these findings raise serious concerns about the risk of harm from social media exposure for children and adolescents who are at a more vulnerable stage of brain development.

Limits on the use of social media have resulted in mental health benefits for young adults and adults. A small, randomized controlled trial in college-aged youth found that limiting social media use to 30 minutes daily over three weeks led to significant improvements in depression

---

[108] Kauer, S. D., Mangan, C., & Sanci, L. (2014). Do online mental health services improve help-seeking for young people? A systematic review. *Journal of medical Internet research*, *16*(3), e66. https://doi.org/10.2196/jmir.3103.

[109] Rice, S. M., Goodall, J., Hetrick, S. E., Parker, A. G., Gilbertson, T., Amminger, G. P., Davey, C. G., McGorry, P. D., Gleeson, J., & Alvarez-Jimenez, M. (2014). Online and social networking interventions for the treatment of depression in young people: a systematic review. *Journal of medical Internet research*, 16(9), e206. https://doi.org/10.2196/jmir.3304.

[110] Ridout, B., & Campbell, A. (2018). The Use of Social Networking Sites in Mental Health Interventions for Young People: Systematic Review. *Journal of medical Internet research*, 20(12), e12244. https://doi.org/10.2196/12244.

[111] Kruzan, K. P., Williams, K. D. A., Meyerhoff, J., Yoo, D. W., O'Dwyer, L. C., De Choudhury, M., & Mohr, D. C. (2022). Social media-based interventions for adolescent and young adult mental health: A scoping review. *Internet interventions*, 30, 100578. https://doi.org/10.1016/j.invent.2022.100578.

[112] Riehm, K. E., Feder, K. A., Tormohlen, K. N., Crum, R. M., Young, A. S., Green, K. M., Pacek, L. R., La Flair, L. N., & Mojtabai, R. (2019). Associations Between Time Spent Using Social Media and Internalizing and Externalizing Problems Among US Youth. *JAMA psychiatry*, 76(12), 1266–1273. https://doi.org/10.1001/jamapsychiatry.2019.2325.

[113] Miech, R. A., Johnston, L. D., Bachman, J. G., O'Malley, P. M., Schulenberg, J. E., and Patrick, M. E. (2022). Monitoring the Future: A Continuing Study of American Youth (8th-and 10th-Grade Surveys), 2021. Inter-university Consortium for Political and Social Research [distributor]. https://doi.org/10.3886/ ICPSR38502.v1.

[114] Braghieri, L., Levy, R., & Makarin, A. (2022). Social Media and Mental Health. *American Economic Review*, 112(11), 3660-3693. https://pubs.aeaweb.org/doi/abs/10.1257/aer.20211218.

[115] Doucleff, M. (2023, April 25). The Truth About Teens, Social Media and the Mental Health Crisis. NPR. Retrieved May 2, 2023, from https://www.npr.org/sections/health-shots/2023/04/25/1171773181/social-media-teens-mental-health.

severity.[116] This effect was particularly large for those with high baseline levels of depression who saw an improvement in depression scores by more than 35%.[117] Another randomized controlled trial among young adults and adults found that deactivation of a social media platform for four weeks improved subjective well-being (i.e., self-reported happiness, life satisfaction, depression, and anxiety) by about 25–40% of the effect of psychological interventions like self-help therapy, group training, and individual therapy.[118]

In addition to these recent studies, correlational research on associations between social media use and mental health has indicated reason for concern and further investigation. These studies point to a higher relative concern of harm in adolescent girls and those already experiencing poor mental health,[119,120,121] as well as for particular health outcomes like cyberbullying-related depression,[122] body image and disordered eating behaviors,[123] and poor sleep quality linked to social media use.[124] For example, a study conducted among 14-year-olds (n = 10,904) found that greater social media use predicted poor sleep, online harassment, poor body image, low self-esteem, and higher depressive symptom scores with a larger association for girls than boys.[125] A majority of parents of adolescents say they are somewhat, very, or extremely worried that their child's use of social media could lead to problems with anxiety or depression (53%), lower self-esteem (54%), being harassed or bullied by others (54%), feeling pressured to act a certain way (59%), and exposure to explicit content (71%).[126]

---

[116] Hunt, M. G., Marx, R., Lipson, C., & Young, J. (2018). No more FOMO: Limiting social media decreases loneliness and depression. *Journal of Social and Clinical Psychology, 37*(10), 751–768. https://doi.org/10.1521/jscp.2018.37.10.751.

[117] From a mean Beck Depression Inventory (BDI) of 23 at baseline to a mean BDI of 14.5 at Week 4.

[118] Allcott, H., Braghieri, L., Eichmeyer, S., & Gentzkow, M. (2020). The Welfare Effects of Social Media. *American Economic Review*, 110(3), 629-76. DOI: 10.1257/aer.20190658.

[119] Abi-Jaoude, E., Naylor, K. T., & Pignatiello, A. (2020). Smartphones, social media use and youth mental health. *Canadian Medical Association journal*, 192(6), E136–E141. https:// doi.org/10.1503/cmaj.190434.

[120] Orben, A., & Przybylski, A. K. (2020). Reply to: Underestimating digital media harm. *Nature human behaviour*, 4(4), 349–351. https://doi.org/10.1038/s41562-020-0840-y.

[121] Twenge, J. M., Haidt, J., Lozano, J., & Cummins, K. M. (2022). Specification curve analysis shows that social media use is linked to poor mental health, especially among girls. *Acta psychologica*, 224, 103512. https://doi.org/10.1016/j. actpsy.2022.103512.

[122] Hamm, M. P., Newton, A. S., Chisholm, A., Shulhan, J., Milne, A., Sundar, P., Ennis, H., Scott, S. D., & Hartling, L. (2015). Prevalence and Effect of Cyberbullying on Children and Young People: A Scoping Review of Social Media Studies. *JAMA pediatrics*, 169(8), 770–777. https://doi.org/10.1001/ jamapediatrics.2015.0944.

[123] Holland, G., & Tiggemann, M. (2016). A systematic review of the impact of the use of social networking sites on body image and disordered eating outcomes. *Body image*, 17, 100–110. https:// doi.org/10.1016/j.bodyim.2016.02.008.

[124] Alonzo, R., Hussain, J., Stranges, S., & Anderson, K. K. (2021). Interplay between social media use, sleep quality, and mental health in youth: A systematic review. *Sleep medicine reviews*, 56, 101414. https://doi.org/10.1016/j.smrv.2020.101414.

[125] Kelly, Y., Zilanawala, A., Booker, C., & Sacker, A. (2019). Social Media Use and Adolescent Mental Health: Findings From the UK Millennium Cohort Study. *EClinicalMedicine*, 6, 59–68. https://doi.org/10.1016/j.eclinm.2018.12.005.

[126] Gelles-Watnick, R. (2022). Explicit Content, Time-wasting Are Key Social Media Worries For Parents Of U.S. Teens. Pew Research Center. United States of America. Retrieved from https://www.pewresearch.org/fact-tank/2022/12/15/explicit-content-time-wasting-are-key-social-media-worries-for-parents-of-u-s-teens/.

## What Drives Mental Health and Well-Being Concerns: A Snapshot of the Scientific Evidence

Scientific evidence suggests that harmful content exposure as well as excessive and problematic social media use are primary areas for concern.

### Potential Risk of Harm from Content Exposure

Extreme, inappropriate, and harmful content continues to be easily and widely accessible by children and adolescents. This can be spread through direct pushes, unwanted content exchanges, and algorithmic designs. In certain tragic cases, childhood deaths have been linked to suicide- and self-harm-related content and risk-taking challenges on social media platforms.[127,128] This content may be especially risky for children and adolescents who are already experiencing mental health difficulties.[129] Despite social media providing a sense of community for some, a systematic review of more than two dozen studies found that some social media platforms show live depictions of self-harm acts like partial asphyxiation, leading to seizures, and cutting, leading to significant bleeding.[130] Further, these studies found that discussing or showing this content can normalize such behaviors, including through the formation of suicide pacts and posting of self-harm models for others to follow.

Social media may also perpetuate body dissatisfaction, disordered eating behaviors, social comparison, and low self-esteem, especially among adolescent girls.[131,132,133,134] A synthesis of 20 studies demonstrated a significant relationship between social media use and body image concerns and eating disorders, with social comparison as a potential contributing factor.[41] Social comparison driven by social media is associated with body dissatisfaction, disordered

---

[127] Dyer C. (2022). Social media content contributed to teenager's death "in more than a minimal way," says coroner. *BMJ* (Clinical research ed.), 379, o2374. https://doi.org/10.1136/ bmj.o2374.

[128] Carville, O. (2022, November 30). TikTok's Viral Challenges Keep Luring Young Kids to Their Deaths. Bloomberg. Retrieved from https://www.bloomberg.com/news/features/2022-11-30/is-tiktok-responsible-if-kids-die-doing-dangerous-viral-challenges.

[129] Sumner, S. A., Ferguson, B., Bason, B., Dink, J., Yard, E., Hertz, M., Hilkert, B., Holland, K., Mercado-Crespo, M., Tang, S., & Jones, C. M. (2021). Association of Online Risk Factors With Subsequent Youth Suicide-Related Behaviors in the US. *JAMA network open*, 4(9), e2125860. https://doi.org/10.1001/ jamanetworkopen.2021.25860.

[130] Dyson, M. P., Hartling, L., Shulhan, J., Chisholm, A., Milne, A., Sundar, P., Scott, S. D., & Newton, A. S. (2016). A Systematic Review of Social Media Use to Discuss and View Deliberate Self-Harm Acts. *PloS one*, 11(5), e0155813. https://doi.org/10.1371/ journal.pone.0155813.

[131] Lonergan, A. R., Bussey, K., Fardouly, J., Griffiths, S., Murray, S. B., Hay, P., Mond, J., Trompeter, N., & Mitchison, D. (2020). Protect me from my selfie: Examining the association between photo-based social media behaviors and self-reported eating disorders in adolescence. *The International journal of eating disorders*, 53(5), 485–496. https://doi.org/10.1002/eat.23256.

[132] Meier, E. P., & Gray, J. (2014). Facebook photo activity associated with body image disturbance in adolescent girls. *Cyberpsychology, behavior and social networking*, 17(4), 199–206. https://doi.org/10.1089/cyber. 2013.0305.

[133] Thai, H., Davis, C. G., Mahboob, W., Perry, S., Adams, A., & Goldfield, G. S. (2023). Reducing Social Media Use Improves Appearance and Weight Esteem in Youth With Emotional Distress. *Psychology of Popular Media*. 10.1037/ppm0000460.

[134] Vogel, E. A., Rose, J. P., Roberts, L. R., & Eckles, K. (2014). Social comparison, social media, and self-esteem. *Psychology of Popular Media Culture*, 3(4), 206–222. https://doi.org/10.1037/ ppm0000047.

eating, and depressive symptoms.[135,136,137,138] When asked about the impact of social media on their body image, nearly half (46%) of adolescents aged 13–17 said social media makes them feel worse, 40% said it makes them feel neither better nor worse, and only 14% said it makes them feel better.[139]

Additionally, roughly two-thirds (64%) of adolescents are "often" or "sometimes" exposed to hate-based content.[140] Among adolescent girls of color, one-third or more report exposure to racist content or language on social media platforms at least monthly.[24] In a review of 36 studies, a consistent relationship was found between cyberbullying via social media and depression among children and adolescents,[40] with adolescent females and sexual minority youth more likely to report experiencing incidents of cyberbullying.[141,142] Nearly 75% of adolescents say social media sites are only doing a fair to poor job of addressing online harassment and cyberbullying.[143]

In addition, social media platforms can be sites for predatory behaviors and interactions with malicious actors who target children and adolescents (e.g., adults seeking to sexually exploit children, to financially extort them through the threat or actual distribution of intimate images, or to sell illicitly manufactured fentanyl).[144,145,146] Adolescent girls and transgender youth are disproportionately impacted by online harassment and abuse, which is associated

---

[135] Nesi, J., & Prinstein, M. J. (2015). Using Social Media for Social Comparison and Feedback-Seeking: Gender and Popularity Moderate Associations with Depressive Symptoms. *Journal of abnormal child psychology*, 43(8), 1427–1438. https:// doi.org/10.1007/s10802-015-0020-0.

[136] Appel, H., Gerlach, A. L., & Crusius, J. (2016). The Interplay Between Facebook Use, Social Comparison, Envy, And Depression. *Current Opinion in Psychology*, 9, 44–49. https://doi. org/10.1016/j.copsyc.2015.10.006.

[137] Kleemans, M., Daalmans, S., Carbaat, I., & Anschütz, D. (2018). Picture Perfect: The Direct Effect Of Manipulated Instagram Photos On Body Image In Adolescent Girls. *Media Psychology*, 21(1), 93–110. https://doi. org/10.1080/15213269.2016.1257392.

[138] Mabe, A. G., Forney, K. J., & Keel, P. K. (2014). Do You "Like" My Photo? Facebook Use Maintains Eating Disorder Risk. *The International journal of eating disorders*, 47(5), 516–523. https:// doi.org/10.1002/eat.22254.

[139] Bickham, D.S., Hunt, E., Bediou, B., & Rich, M. (2022). Adolescent Media Use: Attitudes, Effects, and Online Experiences. Boston, MA: Boston Children's Hospital Digital Wellness Lab. Retrieved from https://digitalwellnesslab.org/wp-content/uploads/Pulse-Survey_Adolescent-Attitudes-Effects-and-Experiences.pdf.

[140] Rideout, V., & Robb, M. B. (2018). Social media, social life: Teens reveal their experiences. San Francisco, CA: Common Sense Media. Retrieved from https://www.commonsensemedia.org/sites/default/files/research/report/2018-social-media-social-life-executive-summary-web.pdf.

[141] Alhajji, M., Bass, S., & Dai, T. (2019). Cyberbullying, Mental Health, and Violence in Adolescents and Associations With Sex and Race: Data From the 2015 Youth Risk Behavior Survey. *Global pediatric health*, 6, 2333794X19868887. https://doi. org/10.1177/2333794X19868887.

[142] Rice, E., Petering, R., Rhoades, H., Winetrobe, H., Goldbach, J., Plant, A., Montoya, J., & Kordic, T. (2015). Cyberbullying perpetration and victimization among middle-school students. *American journal of public health*, 105(3), e66–e72. https://doi. org/10.2105/AJPH.2014.302393.

[143] Vogels, E. (2022). Teens and Cyberbullying 2022. Pew Research Center: Internet, Science & Tech. United States of America. Retrieved from https://www.pewresearch.org/ internet/2022/12/15/teens-and-cyberbullying-2022/.

[144] Wolak, J., Finkelhor, D., Walsh, W., & Treitman, L. (2018). Sextortion of Minors: Characteristics and Dynamics. *The Journal of adolescent health,* 62(1), 72–79. https://doi.org/10.1016/j. jadohealth.2017.08.014.

[145] Federal Bureau of Investigations. (2022, December 19). FBI and Partners Issue National Public Safety Alert on Financial Sextortion Schemes. FBI. Retrieved from https://www.fbi.gov/ news/press-releases/fbi-and-partners-issue-national-public-safety-alert-on-financial-sextortion-schemes.

[146] U.S. Drug Enforcement Administration. (2021, July 23). DEA Washington warns of deadly counterfeit drugs on social media. DEA. Retrieved from https://www.dea.gov/stories/2021/2021-07/2021-07-23/counterfeit-drugs-social-media.

with negative emotional impacts (e.g., feeling sad, anxious or worried).[147,148] Nearly 6-in-10 adolescent girls say they've been contacted by a stranger on certain social media platforms in ways that make them feel uncomfortable.[24]

## Potential Risk of Harm from Excessive and Problematic Use

Excessive and problematic use of social media can harm children and adolescents by disrupting important healthy behaviors. Social media platforms are often designed to maximize user engagement, which has the potential to encourage excessive use and behavioral dysregulation.[149,150,151,152] Push notifications, autoplay, infinite scroll, quantifying and displaying popularity (i.e., 'likes'), and algorithms that leverage user data to serve content recommendations are some examples of these features that maximize engagement. According to one recent model, nearly a third (31%) of social media use may be attributable to self-control challenges magnified by habit formation.[153] Further, some researchers believe that social media exposure can overstimulate the reward center in the brain and, when the stimulation becomes excessive, can trigger pathways comparable to addiction.[68,154] Small studies have shown that people with frequent and problematic social media use can experience changes in brain structure similar to changes seen in individuals with substance use or gambling addictions.[155,156] In a nationally representative survey of girls aged 11–15, one-third or more say they feel "addicted" to a social media platform.[24] Over half of teenagers report that it would be hard to give up social media.[2] Nearly 3-in-4 teenagers believe that technology companies manipulate users to spend more time on their devices.[68] In addition, according to a survey of 8th and 10th

---

147 Finkelhor, D., Turner, H.A., & Colburn, D. (2023). Which dynamics make online child sexual abuse and cyberstalking more emotionally impactful: Perpetrator identity and images? *Child Abuse & Neglect*, 137, 106020. https://doi.org/10.1016/j. chiabu.2023.106020.

148 Finkelhor, D., Turner, H., & Colburn, D. (2022). Prevalence of Online Sexual Offenses Against Children in the US. *JAMA network open*, 5(10), e2234471. https://doi.org/10.1001/ jamanetworkopen.2022.34471.

149 5Rights Foundation. (2021). Pathways: How Digital Design Puts Children At Risk. Retrieved from https://5rightsfoundation. com/uploads/Pathways-how-digital-design-puts-children-at-risk.pdf.

150 Kuss, D. J., & Griffiths, M. D. (2011). Online social networking and addiction--a review of the psychological literature. *International journal of environmental research and public health*, 8(9), 3528–3552. https://doi.org/10.3390/ijerph8093528.

151 Griffiths, M.D. (2018). Adolescent social networking: How do social media operators facilitate habitual use? *Education and Health*, 36(3), 66-69. Retrieved from https://sheu.org.uk/sheux/EH/eh363mdg.pdf.

152 Marino, C., Gini, G., Vieno, A., & Spada, M. M. (2018). The associations between problematic Facebook use, psychological distress and well-being among adolescents and young adults: A systematic review and meta-analysis. *Journal of affective disorders*, 226, 274–281. https://doi.org/10.1016/j. ypmed.2020.106270.

153 Allcott, H., Gentzkow, M., & Song, L. (2022). Digital Addiction. *American Economic Review*, 112 (7): 2424-63. https://doi. org/10.1257/aer.20210867.

154 Andreassen, C. S. (2015). Online Social Network Site Addiction: A Comprehensive Review. *Current Addiction Reports*, 2, 175–184. https://doi.org/10.1007/s40429-015-0056-9.

155 He, Q., Turel, O., & Bechara, A. (2017). Brain anatomy alterations associated with Social Networking Site (SNS) addiction. *Scientific reports*, 7, 45064. https://doi.org/10.1038/ srep45064.

156 Montag, C., Markowetz, A., Blaszkiewicz, K., Andone, I., Lachmann, B., Sariyska, R., Trendafilov, B., Eibes, M., Kolb, J., Reuter, M., Weber, B., & Markett, S. (2017). Facebook Usage On Smartphones And Gray Matter Volume Of The Nucleus Accumbens. *Behavioural Brain Research*, 329, 221–228. https:// doi.org/10.1016/j.bbr.2017.04.035.

graders, the average time spent on social media is 3.5 hours per day, 1-in-4 spend 5+ hours per day and 1-in-7 spend 7+ hours per day on social media.[31]

Excessive and problematic social media use, such as compulsive or uncontrollable use, has been linked to sleep problems, attention problems, and feelings of exclusion among adolescents.[43,157,158,159] Sleep is essential for the healthy development of adolescents. A systematic review of 42 studies on the effects of excessive social media use found a consistent relationship between social media use and poor sleep quality, reduced sleep duration, sleep difficulties, and depression among youth.[42] Poor sleep has been linked to altered neurological development in adolescent brains, depressive symptoms, and suicidal thoughts and behaviors.[160,161,162] On a typical weekday, nearly 1-in-3 adolescents report using screen media until midnight or later.[58] While screen media use encompasses various digital activities, social media applications are the most commonly used applications by adolescents.[58]

In a recent narrative review of multiple studies, problematic social media use has also been linked to both self-reported and diagnosed attention-deficit/ hyperactivity disorder (ADHD) in adolescents, although more research is necessary to understand whether one causes the other.[163] A longitudinal prospective study of adolescents without ADHD symptoms at the beginning of the study found that, over a 2-year follow-up, high-frequency use of digital media, with social media as one of the most common activities, was associated with a modest yet statistically significant increased odds of developing ADHD symptoms (OR 1.10; 95% CI, 1.05-1.15).[164] Additionally, social media-induced fear of missing out, or "the pervasive apprehension that others might be having rewarding experiences from which one is absent,"[165] has been associated with depression, anxiety, and neuroticism.[166]

---

[157] Shannon, H., Bush, K., Villeneuve, P. J., Hellemans, K. G., & Guimond, S. (2022). Problematic Social Media Use in Adolescents and Young Adults: Systematic Review and Meta-analysis. *JMIR mental health*, 9(4), e33450. https://doi. org/10.2196/33450.

[158] Boer, M., Stevens, G., Finkenauer, C., & van den Eijnden, R. (2020). Attention deficit hyperactivity disorder-symptoms, social media use intensity, and social media use problems in adolescents: Investigating directionality. *Child Development*, 91(4), e853-e865. https://doi. org/10.1111/cdev.13334.

[159] Franchina, V., Vanden Abeele, M., van Rooij, A. J., Lo Coco, G., & De Marez, L. (2018). Fear of Missing Out as a Predictor of Problematic Social Media Use and Phubbing Behavior among Flemish Adolescents. *International Journal Of Environmental Research And Public Health*, 15(10), 2319. https://doi. org/10.3390/ijerph15102319.

[160] Telzer, E. H., Goldenberg, D., Fuligni, A. J., Lieberman, M. D., & Gálvan, A. (2015). Sleep variability in adolescence is associated with altered brain development. *Developmental cognitive neuroscience*, 14, 16–22. https://doi.org/10.1016/j. dcn.2015.05.007.

[161] Liu, R. T., Steele, S. J., Hamilton, J. L., Do, Q. B. P., Furbish, K., Burke, T. A., Martinez, A. P., & Gerlus, N. (2020). Sleep and suicide: A systematic review and meta-analysis of longitudinal studies. *Clinical psychology review*, 81, 101895. https://doi. org/10.1016/j.cpr.2020.101895.

[162] Shochat, T., Cohen-Zion, M., & Tzischinsky, O. (2014). Functional consequences of inadequate sleep in adolescents: a systematic review. *Sleep medicine reviews*, 18(1), 75–87. https:// doi.org/10.1016/j.smrv. 2013.03.005.

[163] Dekkers, T. J., & van Hoorn, J. (2022). Understanding Problematic Social Media Use in Adolescents with Attention-Deficit/Hyperactivity Disorder (ADHD): A Narrative Review and Clinical Recommendations. *Brain Sciences*, 12(12), 1625. https:// doi.org/10.3390/brainsci12121625.

[164] Ra, C. K., Cho, J., Stone, M. D., De La Cerda, J., Goldenson, N. I., Moroney, E., Tung, I., Lee, S. S., & Leventhal, A. M. (2018). Association of Digital Media Use With Subsequent Symptoms of Attention-Deficit/Hyperactivity Disorder Among Adolescents. *JAMA*, 320(3), 255–263. https://doi.org/10.1001/jama.2018.8931.

[165] Przybylski A. K., Murayama K., DeHaan C.R., & Gladwell V. (2013). Motivational, emotional, and behavioral correlates of fear of missing out. *Computers in Human Behavior*; 29:1841–1848.

[166] Fioravanti, G., Casale, S., Benucci, S.B., Prostamo, A., Falone, A., Ricca, V., & Rotella, F. (2021). Fear of missing out and social networking sites use and abuse: A meta-analysis. *Computers in Human Behavior*, 122, 106839. https://doi.org/10.1016/j. chb.2021.106839.

## Critical Questions Remain Unanswered

Nearly every teenager in America uses social media, and yet we do not have enough evidence to conclude that it is sufficiently safe for them. Our children have become unknowing participants in a decades-long experiment. It is critical that independent researchers and technology companies work together to rapidly advance our understanding of the impact of social media on children and adolescents. This section describes the known gaps and proposes additional areas for research that warrant urgent consideration.

### Known Evidence Gaps

The relationship between social media and youth mental health is complex and potentially bidirectional.[19] There is broad concern among the scientific community that a lack of access to data and lack of transparency from technology companies have been barriers to understanding the full scope and scale of the impact of social media on mental health and well-being. Most prior research to date has been correlational, focused on young adults or adults, and generated a range of results.[167] Critical areas of research have been proposed to fill knowledge gaps and create evidence-based interventions, resources, and tools to support youth mental health.[168] Thus, there is an urgent need for additional research including on, but not limited to, the following questions:

- How do in-person vs. digital social interactions differ in terms of the impact on health, and what are the unique contributions of social media behavior to social connectedness, social isolation, and mental health symptoms?
- What are the potential pathways through which social media may cause harm to children's and adolescents' mental health and well-being? For example:
  - How does social comparison affect one's sense of life satisfaction and in-person relationships?
  - How does the use of social media, including specific designs and features, relate to dopamine pathways involved in motivation, reward, and addiction?
- What type of content, and at what frequency and intensity, generates the most harm? Through which modes of social media access (e.g., smartphone, computer) and design features? For which users and why?
- What are the beneficial effects of social media? For whom are the benefits greatest? In what ways, and under what circumstances?
- What individual-, community-, and societal-level factors may protect youth from the negative effects of social media?

---

[167] Odgers, C. L., & Jensen, M. R. (2020). Annual Research Review: Adolescent mental health in the digital age: facts, fears, and future directions. *Journal of Child Psychology and Psychiatry*, and Allied Disciplines, 61(3), 336–348. https://doi.org/10.1111/ jcpp.13190.

[168] Office of the Surgeon General (OSG). (2021). Protecting Youth Mental Health: The U.S. Surgeon General's Advisory. U.S. Department of Health and Human Services. Retrieved from https://www.hhs.gov/sites/default/files/surgeon-general-youth-mental-health-advisory.pdf.

- What types of strategies and approaches are effective in protecting the mental health and well-being of children and adolescents on social media (e.g., programs, policies, design features, interventions, norms)?
- How does social media use interact with a person's developmental stage for measuring risk of mental health impact?

> It is critical that independent researchers and technology companies work together to rapidly advance our understanding of the impact of social media on children and adolescents.

## We Must Take Action: A Way Forward

Our children and adolescents don't have the luxury of waiting years until we know the full extent of social media's impact. Their childhoods and development are happening now. While social media use can have positive impacts for some children, the evidence noted throughout this Surgeon General's Advisory necessitates significant concern with the way it is currently designed, deployed, and utilized. Child and adolescent use of platforms designed for adults places them at high risk of "unsupervised, developmentally inappropriate, and potentially harmful" use according to the National Scientific Council on Adolescence.[169] At a moment when we are experiencing a national youth mental health crisis, now is the time to act swiftly and decisively to protect children and adolescents from risk of harm.

To date, the burden of protecting youth has fallen predominantly on children, adolescents, and their families. Parents face significant challenges in managing children and adolescents' use of social media applications, and youth are using social media at increasingly earlier ages.[4,170] Nearly 70% of parents say parenting is now more difficult than it was 20 years ago, with technology and social media as the top two cited reasons.[171] While nearly all parents believe they have a responsibility to protect their children from inappropriate content online,[89] the entire burden of mitigating the risk of harm of social media cannot be placed on the shoulders of children and parents. Nearly 80% of parents believe technology companies have a responsibility to protect children from inappropriate content as well.[89]

We must provide children and their families with the information and tools to navigate the changing digital environment, but this burden to support our children must be further shared. There are actions technology companies can take to make their platforms safer for children and adolescents. There are actions researchers can take to develop the necessary research base to support further safeguards. And there is a role for local, state, and federal policy to implement protections for our children and adolescents.

---

169 Odgers, C.L., Allen, N.B., Pfeifer, J.H., Dahl, R.E., Nesi, J., Schueller, S.M., Williams, J. L., & the National Scientific Council on Adolescence (2022). Engaging, safe, and evidence-based: What science tells us about how to promote positive development and decrease risk in online spaces, Council Report No 2. doi: 10.31234/osf.io/rvn8q.

170 Clark, S. J., Schultz, S. L., Gebremariam, A., Singer, D. C., & Freed, G. L. (2021). Sharing too soon? Children and social media apps. C.S. Mott Children's Hospital National Poll on Children's Health, University of Michigan, 39(4). Retrieved from https://mottpoll.org/sites/default/files/documents/101821_ SocialMedia.pdf.

171 Auxier, B., Anderson, M., Perrin, A., & Turner, E. (2020). Parenting Children in the Age of Screens. Pew Research Center: Internet, Science & Tech. Retrieved from https://www. pewresearch.org/internet/2020/07/28/parenting-children-in-the-age-of-screens/.

The U.S. has a strong history of taking action in such circumstances. In the case of toys, transportation, and medications—among other sectors that have widespread adoption and impact on children—the U.S. has often adopted a safety-first approach to mitigate the risk of harm to consumers. According to this principle, a basic threshold for safety must be met, and until safety is demonstrated with rigorous evidence and independent evaluation, protections are put in place to minimize the risk of harm from products, services, or goods. For example, the Consumer Product Safety Commission requires toy manufacturers to undergo third-party testing and be certified through a Children's Product Certificate as compliant with the federal toy safety standard for toys intended for use by children.[172] To reduce the risk of injury from motor vehicle accidents, the National Highway Traffic Safety Administration requires manufacturers to fit new motor vehicles with standard airbags and seat belts, among other safety features, and conduct crash tests to be compliant with the Federal Motor Vehicle Safety Standards.[173] Medications must demonstrate safety to the Food and Drug Administration before being made available and marketed for use.[174] Given the mounting evidence for the risk of harm to some children and adolescents from social media use, a safety-first approach should be applied in the context of social media products.

To better safeguard the mental health and well-being of children and adolescents, policymakers, technology companies, researchers, families, and young people must all engage in a proactive and multifaceted approach. Through the recommendations below, we can provide more resources and tools to children and families, we can gain a better understanding of the full impact of social media, and we can maximize the benefits and minimize the harms of social media platforms to create safer, healthier online environments for children.

We can maximize the benefits and minimize the harms of social media platforms to create safer, healthier online environments for children.

## What Policymakers Can Do

Policymakers play an important role in addressing the complex and multifaceted issues related to social media use and in protecting youth from harm.

- Strengthen protections to ensure greater safety for children interacting with all social media platforms, in collaboration with governments, academic organizations, public health experts, and technology companies.
    - Develop age-appropriate health and safety standards for technology platforms. Such standards may include designing technology that is appropriate and safe for a child's developmental stage; protecting children and adolescents from accessing harmful content (e.g., content that encourages eating disorders, violence,

---

[172] U.S. Consumer Product Safety Commission. (n.d.). Toy Safety Business Guidance & Small Entity Compliance Guide. U.S. Consumer Product Safety Commission. Retrieved from https://www.cpsc.gov/Business--Manufacturing/Business-Education/Toy-Safety-Business-Guidance-and-Small-Entity-Compliance-Guide.

[173] Unites States Department of Transportation. (n.d.). National Highway Traffic Safety Administration. Retrieved from https:// www.nhtsa.gov/.

[174] U.S. Food and Drug Administration. (n.d.). Center for Drug Evaluation and Research. U.S. Food and Drug Administration. Retrieved from https://www.fda.gov/drugs.

substance abuse, sexual exploitation, and suicide or discusses suicide means); limiting the use of features that attempt to maximize time, attention, and engagement; developing tools that protect activities that are essential for healthy development like sleep; and regularly assessing and mitigating risks to children and adolescents.

  - Require a higher standard of data privacy for children to protect them from potential harms like exploitation and abuse. Six-in-ten adolescents say they think they have little or no control over the personal information that social media companies collect about them.[32]
  - Pursue policies that further limit access—in ways that minimize the risk of harm—to social media for all children, including strengthening and enforcing age minimums.
- Ensure technology companies share data relevant to the health impact of their platforms with independent researchers and the public in a manner that is timely, sufficiently detailed, and protects privacy.
- Support the development, implementation, and evaluation of digital and media literacy curricula in schools and within academic standards. Digital and media literacy provides children and educators with digital skills to strengthen digital resilience, or the ability to recognize, manage, and recover from online risks (e.g., cyberbullying and other forms of online harassment and abuse, as well as excessive social media use).
- Support increased funding for future research on both the benefits and harms of social media use and other technology and digital media use for children, adolescents, and families.
- Engage with international partners working to protect children and adolescents against online harm to their health and safety.

## What Technology Companies Can Do

Technology companies play a central role and have a fundamental responsibility in designing safe online environments and in preventing, minimizing, and addressing the risks associated with social media.

- Conduct and facilitate transparent and independent assessments of the impact of social media products and services on children and adolescents. Assume responsibility for the impact of products on different subgroups and ages of children and adolescents, regardless of the intent behind them.
  - Be transparent and share assessment findings and underlying data with independent researchers and the public in a privacy protecting manner.
  - Assess the potential risks of online interactions and take active steps to prevent potential misuse, reducing exposure to harms. When proactive responses fail, take immediate action to mitigate unintended negative effects.
  - Establish scientific advisory committees to inform approaches and policies aimed at creating safe online environments for children. Scientific advisory committees

should be comprised of independent experts and members of user subgroups, including youth.

- Prioritize user health and safety in the design and development of social media products and services.[175,176,177,178] Prioritize and leverage expertise in developmental psychology and user mental health and well-being in product teams to minimize risks of harm to children and adolescents.
    - Ensure default settings for children are set to highest safety and privacy standards. Provide easy-to-read and highly visible information about policies regarding use by children.
    - Adhere to and enforce age minimums in ways that respect the privacy of youth users.
- Design, develop, and evaluate platforms, products, and tools that foster safe and healthy online environments for youth, keeping in mind the needs of girls, racial, ethnic, and sexual and gender minorities. The platform design and algorithms should prioritize health and safety as the first principle, seek to maximize the potential benefits, and avoid design features that attempt to maximize time, attention, and engagement.
- Share data relevant to the health impact of platforms and strategies employed to ensure safety and well-being with independent researchers and the public in a manner that is timely and protects privacy.
- Create effective and timely systems and processes to adjudicate requests and complaints from young people, families, educators, and others to address online abuse, harmful content and interactions, and other threats to children's health and safety. Social media platforms should take these complaints seriously, thoroughly investigate and consider them, and respond in a timely and transparent manner.

## What Parents and Caregivers Can Do

The onus of mitigating the potential harms of social media should not be placed solely on the shoulders of parents and caregivers, but there are steps they can take to help protect and support children and adolescents against the risk of harm.

- Create a family media plan.[179] Agreed-upon expectations can help establish healthy technology boundaries at home –including social media use. A family media plan can

[175] Australian Government, eSafety Commissioner. (nd). Safety by Design. Retrieved from https://www.esafety.gov.au/industry/ safety-by-design.

[176] Information Commissioner's Office. (nd). Introduction To The Age Appropriate Design Code. Retrieved from https://ico.org.uk/ for-organisations/childrens-code-hub/.

[177] Perrino, J. (2022, July 27). Using "Safety By Design" To Address Online Harms. Brookings Institute. https://www.brookings.edu/techstream/using-safety-by-design-to-address-online-harms/.

[178] Lenhart, A., & Owens, K. (2021). The Unseen Teen: The Challenges of Building Healthy Tech for Young People. Data & Society. Retrieved from https://datasociety.net/library/the-unseen-teen/.

[179] American Academy of Pediatrics (AAP). (2018, October 8). Kids & Tech: Tips for parents in the Digital age. HealthyChildren. org. Retrieved from https://www.healthychildren.org/English/family-life/Media/Pages/Tips-for-Parents-Digital-Age.aspx.

promote open family discussion and rules about media use and include topics such as balancing screen/online time, content boundaries, and not disclosing personal information. For information on creating a family media plan, visit www.healthychildren. org/MediaUsePlan.

- Create tech-free zones and encourage children to foster in-person friendships.[180] Since electronics can be a potential distraction after bedtime and can interfere with sleep, consider restricting the use of phones, tablets, and computers for at least 1 hour before bedtime and through the night. Consider keeping family mealtimes and in-person gatherings device-free to build social bonds and engage in a two-way conversation. Help your child develop social skills and nurture his or her in-person relationships by encouraging unstructured and offline connections with others and making unplugged interactions a daily priority. See the American Academy of Pediatrics (AAP) guidelines for media use.
- Model responsible social media behavior. As children often learn behaviors and habits from what they see around them, try to model the behavior you want to see.[97,181] Parents can set a good example of what responsible and healthy social media use looks like by limiting their own use, being mindful of social media habits (including when and how parents share information or content about their child), and modeling positive behavior on your social media accounts.
- Teach kids about technology and empower them to be responsible online participants at the appropriate age.[182] Discuss with children the benefits and risks of social media as well as the importance of respecting privacy and protecting personal information in age-appropriate ways. Have conversations with children about who they are connecting with, their privacy settings, their online experiences, and how they are spending their time online. Empower and encourage them to seek help should they need it. Learn more about the benefits and risks of social media use and get guidance from experts at AAP's Center of Excellence on Social Media and Youth Mental Health and from the American Psychological Association's Health Advisory on Social Media Use in Adolescence.
- Report cyberbullying and online abuse and exploitation. Talk to your child about their reporting options, and provide support, without judgment, if he or she tells or shows you that they (a) are being harassed through email, text message, online games, or social media or (b) have been contacted by an adult seeking private images or asking them to perform intimate or sexual acts. You or your child can report cyberbullying to the school and/or the online platform, or your local law enforcement.[183] Visit

---

[180] Morgan Stanley Alliance For Children's Mental Health & Child Mind Institute. (2022, May). How to set limits on screen time and internet use. Retrieved from https://www.morganstanley.com/assets/pdfs/setting-limits-on-screen-time-tip-sheet.pdf.

[181] Ehmke, R. (2023, March 13). How using social media affects teenagers. Child Mind Institute. Retrieved from https://childmind.org/article/how-using-social-media-affects-teenagers/.

[182] American Psychological Association. (2019, December 12). Digital Guidelines: Promoting healthy technology use for children. American Psychological Association. Retrieved from https://www.apa.org/topics/social-media-internet/technology-use-children.

[183] US Department of Health and Human Services, Assistant Secretary for Public Affairs (ASPA). (2021, November 10). Prevent cyberbullying. StopBullying.gov. Retrieved from https:// www.stopbullying.gov/cyberbullying/prevention https://www.stopbullying.gov/cyberbullying/how-to-report.

CyberTipline, Take it Down, or contact your local law enforcement to report any instances of online exploitation.

- Work with other parents to help establish shared norms and practices and to support programs and policies around healthy social media use. Such norms and practices among parents facilitate collective action and can make it easier to set and implement boundaries on social media use for children.

## What Children and Adolescents Can Do

The burden of mitigating the potential harms of social media does not rest solely on the shoulders of children and adolescents, but there are measures they can take to navigate social media in a safe and healthy way.

- Reach out for help. If you or someone you know is being negatively affected by social media, reach out to a trusted friend or adult for help. For information from experts, visit AAP's Center of Excellence on Social Media and Youth Mental Health. If you or someone you know is experiencing a mental health crisis, contact the 988 Suicide and Crisis Lifeline by calling or texting 988 for immediate help.
- Create boundaries to help balance online and offline activities. Limit the use of phones, tablets, and computers for at least 1 hour before bedtime and through the night to enable sufficient and quality sleep. Keep mealtimes and in-person gatherings device-free to help build social bonds and engage in two-way conversations with others. Nurture your in-person relationships by connecting with others and making unplugged interactions a daily priority.
- Develop protective strategies and healthy practices such as tracking the amount of time you spend online, blocking unwanted contacts and content, learning about and using available privacy and safety settings, learning and utilizing digital media literacy skills to help tell the difference between fact and opinion, and ensuring you are connecting with peers in-person. See this Tip Sheet on Social Media Use and Mental Health for healthy social media use created for and by young people.
- Be cautious about what you share. Personal information about you has value. Be selective with what you post and share online and with whom, as it is often public and can be stored permanently. If you aren't sure if you should post something, it's usually best if you don't. Talk to a family member or trusted adult to see if you should.
- Protect yourself and others. Harassment that happens in email, text messaging, direct messaging, online games, or on social media is harmful and can be cyberbullying. It might involve trolling, rumors, or photos passed around for others to see –and it can leave people feeling angry, sad, ashamed, or hurt. If you or someone you know is the victim of cyberbullying or other forms of online harassment and abuse:
- Don't keep online harassment or abuse a secret. Reach out to at least one person you trust, such as a close friend, family member, counselor, or teacher, who can give you the help and support you deserve. Visit stopbullying.gov for helpful tips on how to report cyberbullying. If you have experienced online harassment and abuse by a dating partner, contact an expert at Love is Respect for support or if your private images have

been taken and shared online without your permission, visit Take it Down to help get them removed.

- Don't take part in online harassment or abuse. Avoid forwarding or sharing messages or images and tell others to stop. Another way is to report offensive content to the site or network where you saw it.

## What Researchers Can Do

Researchers play a critical role in helping to gain a better understanding of the full impact of social media on mental health and well-being and informing policy, best practices, and effective interventions.

- Establish the impact of social media on youth mental health as a research priority and develop a shared research agenda.[184] Research should include but not be limited to:
  - Rigorous evaluation of social media's impact on youth mental health and well-being, including longitudinal and experimental studies. This could also include research on specific outcomes and clinical diagnoses (e.g., sleep duration and quality, attention, depression, anxiety, and body image), among specific populations (e.g., racial, ethnic, and sexual and gender minorities), and based on specific aspects of social media (e.g., designs, features, and algorithms).
  - Role of age, developmental stage, cohort processes, and the in-person environment in influencing the onset and progression of poor mental health outcomes among social media users.
  - Benefits and risks associated with specific social media designs, features, and content.
  - Long-term effects on adults of social media use during childhood and adolescence.
- Develop and establish standardized definitions and measures for social media and mental health outcomes that are regularly evaluated and can be applied across basic research, population surveillance, intervention evaluation, and other contexts.
- Evaluate best practices for healthy social media use in collaboration with experts including healthcare providers, parents, and youth.[94,185],[186]
- Enhance research coordination and collaboration. Example opportunities include developing an accessible evidence database and forming a consortium of researchers focused on examining the positive and negative effects of social media on mental

---

[184] National Academies of Sciences, Engineering, and Medicine (NASEM). (n.d.). Assessment of the Impact of Social Media on the Health and Wellbeing of Adolescents and Children. Retrieved from https://www.nationalacademies.org/our-work/assessment-of-the-impact-of-social-media-on-the-health-and-wellbeing-of-adolescents-and-children.

[185] American Academy of Pediatrics. (2023, February 7). Center of Excellence on Social Media and Youth Mental Health. Retrieved from https://www.aap.org/en/patient-care/media-and-children/center-of-excellence-on-social-media-and-youth-mental-health/#:~:text=What%20We%20Do,protect%20youth%20mental%20health%20online.

[186] American Academy of Pediatrics. (2017). *Bright Futures Guidelines for Health Supervision of Infants, Children, and Adolescents* (4th ed., pp. 229-234). American Academy of Pediatrics. https://downloads.aap.org/AAP/PDF/Bright%20 Futures/BF4_HealthySocialMedia.pdf.

health and well-being. Researchers should work with community partners to make research findings publicly accessible and digestible.

## Acknowledgments

We are grateful to all of the experts, academic researchers, associations, and community-based organizations across the country who shared their insights.

The U.S. Surgeon General's Advisory on Social Media and Youth Mental Health was prepared by the Office of the Surgeon General with valuable contributions from partners across the U.S. Government, including but not limited to:

Office of the Assistant Secretary for Health (OASH)
Office of the General Counsel (OGC)
Office of the Assistant Secretary for Planning and Evaluation (ASPE)
Centers for Disease Control and Prevention (CDC)
Office of the Director
National Center for Injury Prevention and Control (NCIPC)
National Center for HIV, Viral Hepatitis, STD, and TB Prevention, Division of Adolescent and School Health (DASH)
Health Resources and Services Administration (HRSA)
National Institutes of Health (NIH)
*Eunice Kennedy Shriver* National Institute of Child Health and Human Development (NICHD)
National Institute of Mental Health (NIMH)
Substance Abuse and Mental Health Services Administration (SAMHSA)

## Chapter 7

# Protecting Youth Mental Health*

## U.S. Surgeon General's Advisory

### Introduction from the Surgeon General

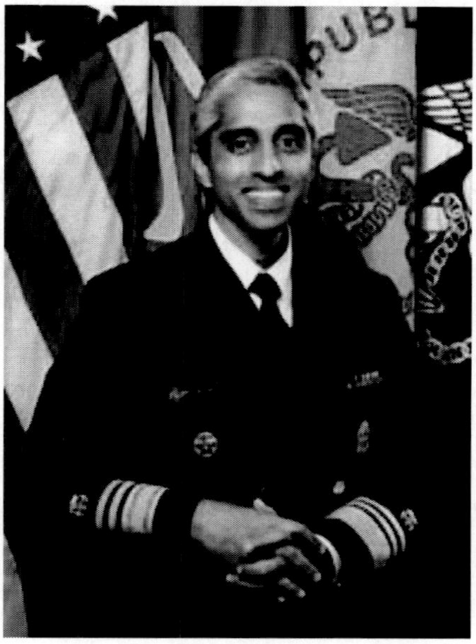

Every child's path to adulthood—reaching developmental and emotional milestones, learning healthy social skills, and dealing with problems—is different and difficult. Many face added challenges along the way, often beyond their control. There's no map, and the road is never straight.

But the challenges today's generation of young people face are unprecedented and uniquely hard to navigate. And the effect these challenges have had on their mental health is devastating.

Recent national surveys of young people have shown alarming increases in the prevalence of certain mental health challenges— in 2019, one in three high school students and half of

* This is an edited, reformatted and augmented version of The U.S. Surgeon General's Advisory, dated 2021.

In: Understanding Youth Mental Health
Editor: Michael A. Post
ISBN: 979-8-89530-700-7

female students reported persistent feelings of sadness or hopelessness, an overall increase of 40% from 2009. We know that mental health is shaped by many factors, from our genes and brain chemistry to our relationships with family and friends, neighborhood conditions, and larger social forces and policies. We also know that, too often, young people are bombarded with messages through the media and popular culture that erode their sense of self-worth—telling them they are not good looking enough, popular enough, smart enough, or rich enough. That comes as progress on legitimate, and distressing, issues like climate change, income inequality, racial injustice, the opioid epidemic, and gun violence feels too slow.

And while technology platforms have improved our lives in important ways, increasing our ability to build new communities, deliver resources, and access information, we know that, for many people, they can also have adverse effects. When not deployed responsibly and safely, these tools can pit us against each other, reinforce negative behaviors like bullying and exclusion, and undermine the safe and supportive environments young people need and deserve.

All of that was true even before the COVID-19 pandemic dramatically altered young peoples' experiences at home, at school, and in the community. The pandemic era's unfathomable number of deaths, pervasive sense of fear, economic instability, and forced physical distancing from loved ones, friends, and communities have exacerbated the unprecedented stresses young people already faced.

It would be a tragedy if we beat back one public health crisis only to allow another to grow in its place. That's why I am issuing this Surgeon General's Advisory. Mental health challenges in children, adolescents, and young adults are real, and they are widespread. But most importantly, they are treatable, and often preventable. This Advisory shows us how.

To be sure, this isn't an issue we can fix overnight or with a single prescription. Ensuring healthy children and families will take an all-of-society effort, including policy, institutional, and individual changes in how we view and prioritize mental health. This Advisory provides actionable recommendations for young people and their families, schools and health care systems, technology and media companies, employers, community organizations, and governments alike.

Our obligation to act is not just medical—it's moral. I believe that, coming out of the COVID-19 pandemic, we have an unprecedented opportunity as a country to rebuild in a way that refocuses our identity and common values, puts people first, and strengthens our connections to each other.

If we seize this moment, step up for our children and their families in their moment of need, and lead with inclusion, kindness, and respect, we can lay the foundation for a healthier, more resilient, and more fulfilled nation.

Vivek H. Murthy, M.D., M.B.A.
Vice Admiral, U.S. Public Health Service
Surgeon General of the United States

## About the Advisory

A Surgeon General's Advisory is a public statement that calls the American people's attention to an urgent public health issue and provides recommendations for how it should be addressed.

Advisories are reserved for significant public health challenges that need the nation's immediate awareness and action.

This Advisory offers recommendations for supporting the mental health of children, adolescents, and young adults. While many of these recommendations apply to *individuals,* the reality is that people have widely varying degrees of control over their circumstances. As a result, not all recommendations will be feasible for everyone.

That's why systemic change is essential. The Advisory includes essential recommendations for the *institutions* that surround young people and shape their day-to-day lives—schools, community organizations, health care systems, technology companies, media, funders and foundations, employers, and government. They all have an important role to play in supporting the mental health of children and youth.

For additional background and to read other Surgeon General's Advisories, visit SurgeonGeneral.gov.

## Background

### Youth Mental Health Prior to the COVID-19 Pandemic

Mental health affects every aspect of our lives: how we feel about ourselves and the world; solve problems, cope with stress, and overcome challenges; build relationships and connect with others; and perform in school, at work, and throughout life. Mental health encompasses our emotional, psychological, and social wellbeing, and is an essential component of overall health.[187] As described in the 1999 Surgeon General's Report on Mental Health, it is the "springboard of thinking and communication skills, learning, emotional growth, resilience and self-esteem."[188]

Mental health challenges can be difficult to define, diagnose, and address, partly because it isn't always clear when an issue is serious enough to warrant intervention.[2] All of us, at all ages, occasionally experience fear, worry, sadness, or distress. In most cases, these symptoms are short-lived and don't affect our ability to function. But, at other times, symptoms can cause serious difficulties with daily functioning and affect our relationships with others, as in the case of conditions such as anxiety disorders, major depressive disorder, schizophrenia, bipolar disorder, and eating disorders, among others.[189]

Mental health conditions can be shaped by biological factors, including genes and brain chemistry, and environmental factors, including life experiences. Some mental health disorders seem to cluster in families, but they are often shaped by multiple genes, and whether an individual develops symptoms can be further modified by their experiences and surrounding

---

187 U.S. Department of Health & Human Services. (2020 May 28). What is Mental Health. MentalHealth.gov. Accessed on November 10, 2021. Retrieved from https://www.mentalhealth.gov/basics/what-is-mental-health.

188 U.S. Department of Health and Human Services. (1999) Mental health: A report of the Surgeon General, Rockville, MD. U.S. Department of Health and Human Services, Substance Abuse and Mental Health Services Administration, Center for Mental Health Services, National Institutes of Health, National Institute of Mental Health. Retrieved from https://profiles.nlm. nih.gov/101584932X120.

189 U.S. National Library of Medicine. (2021 October 12). Mental Disorders. MedlinePlus. Accessed on November 10, 2021. Retrieved from https://medlineplus.gov/mentaldisorders.html.

environment.[190,191] Environmental factors can range from exposure to alcohol or drugs during pregnancy, to birth complications, to discrimination and racism, to adverse childhood experiences (ACEs) such as abuse, neglect, exposure to community violence, and living in under-resourced or racially segregated neighborhoods.[192,193,194,195,196,197,198] ACEs can undermine a child's sense of safety, stability, bonding, and wellbeing.[199] Moreover, ACEs may lead to the development of toxic stress. Toxic stress can cause long lasting changes, including disrupting brain development and increasing the risk for mental health conditions and other health problems such as obesity, heart disease, and diabetes, both during and beyond childhood as well as for future generations.[12,200]

Biological and environmental factors can also be interrelated, making it difficult to isolate unique "causes" of mental health challenges. For example, if a child is genetically predisposed to depression, they might be more affected by experiences such as bullying than other children.[201,202]

---

[190] Cross-Disorder Group of the Psychiatric Genomics Consortium (2013). Identification of risk loci with shared effects on five major psychiatric disorders: a genome-wide analysis. *Lancet* (London, England), 381(9875), 1371–1379. https://doi. org/10.1016/S0140-6736(12)62129-1.

[191] Marshall M. (2020). The hidden links between mental disorders. *Nature*, 581(7806), 19–21. https://doi.org/10.1038/ d41586-020-00922-8.

[192] Williams D. R. (2018). Stress and the Mental Health of Populations of Color: Advancing Our Understanding of Race-related Stressors. *Journal of Health and Social Behavior*, 59(4), 466–485. https://doi.org/10.1177/ 0022146518814251.

[193] Kalin N. H. (2021). Impacts of Structural Racism, Socioeconomic Deprivation, and Stigmatization on Mental Health. *The American Journal of Psychiatry*, 178(7), 575–578. https://doi.org/10.1176/appi.ajp.2021.21050524.

[194] Doom, J. R., Seok, D., Narayan, A. J., & Fox, K. R. (2021). Adverse and Benevolent Childhood Experiences Predict Mental Health During the COVID-19 Pandemic. *Adversity and resilience science*, 1–12. Advance online publication. https://doi. org/10.1007/s42844-021-00038-6.

[195] Hughes, K., Bellis, M. A., Hardcastle, K. A., Sethi, D., Butchart, A., Mikton, C., Jones, L., Dunne, M. P. (2017). The effect of multiple adverse childhood experiences on health: A systematic review and meta-analysis. *The Lancet Public Health*, 2(8), e356–e366.

[196] U.S. Department of Health and Human Services, Substance Abuse and Mental Health Services Administration. (2009). Risk and Protective Factors for Mental, Emotional and Behavioral Disorders Across the Life Cycle. https://www.csifdl.org/wp-content/uploads/2018/07/Risk-and-Protective-Factors-Study.pdf.

[197] Trent, M., Dooley, D. G., Dougé, J., Section on Adolescent Health, Council on Community Pediatrics, & Committee on Adolescence. (2019). The Impact of Racism on Child and Adolescent Health. *Pediatrics*, 144(2), e20191765. https://doi. org/10.1542/peds.2019-1765.

[198] Bhushan D, Kotz K, McCall J, Wirtz S, Gilgoff R, Dube SR, Powers C, Olson-Morgan J, Galeste M, Patterson K, Harris L, Mills A, Bethell C, Burke Harris N, Office of the California Surgeon General. (2020). Roadmap for Resilience: The California Surgeon General's Report on Adverse Childhood Experiences, Toxic Stress, and Health. Office of the California Surgeon General. DOI: 10.48019/PEAM8812.

[199] Centers for Disease Control and Prevention. (2021 April 6). What are adverse childhood experiences? Retrieved from https:// www.cdc.gov/violenceprevention/aces/fastfact.html.

[200] Shonkoff, J. P., Garner, A. S., & Committee on Psychosocial Aspects of Child and Family Health, Committee `on Early Childhood, Adoption, and Dependent Care and Section on Developmental and Behavioral Pediatrics. (2012). The lifelong effects of early childhood adversity and toxic stress. *Pediatrics*, 129(1), e232-e246.

[201] Arango, C., Díaz-Caneja, C. M., McGorry, P. D., Rapoport, J., Sommer, I. E., Vorstman, J. A., McDaid, D., Marín, O., Serrano-Drozdowskyj, E., Freedman, R., & Carpenter, W. (2018). Preventive strategies for mental health. *The Lancet*. Psychiatry, 5(7), 591–604. https://doi.org/10.1016/S2215-0366(18)30057-9.

[202] Schmidt C. W. (2007). Environmental connections: a deeper look into mental illness. *Environmental Health Perspectives*, 115(8), A404–A410. https://doi.org/10.1289/ehp.115-a404.

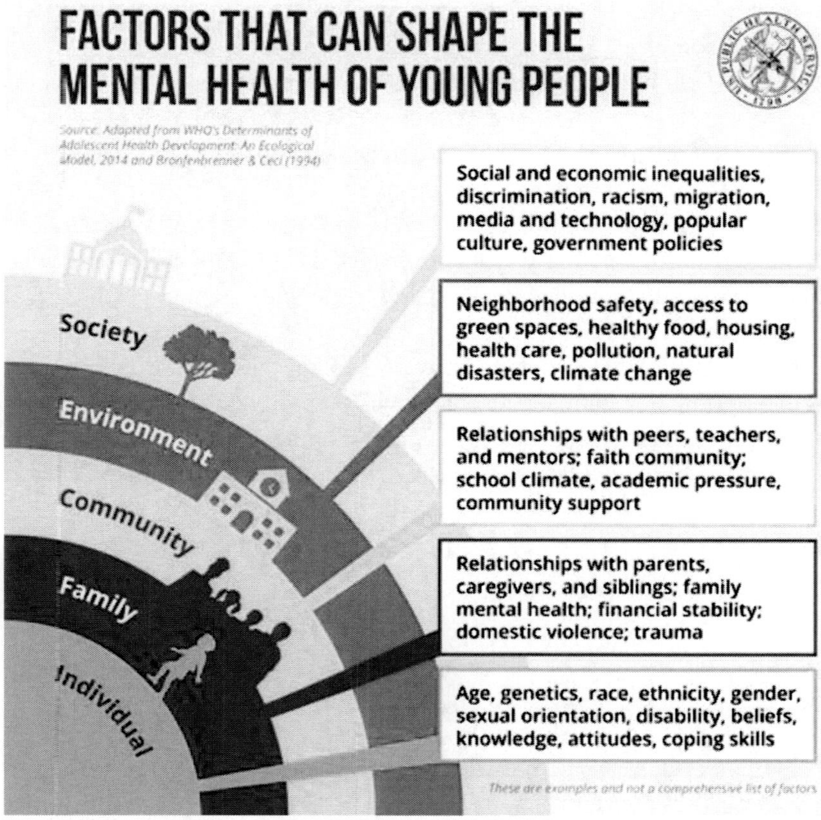
FACTORS THAT CAN SHAPE THE
MENTAL HEALTH OF YOUNG PEOPLE
Source: Adapted from WHO's Determinants of Adolescent Health Development: An Ecological Model, 2014 and Bronfenbrenner & Ceci (1994)
Social and economic inequalities, discrimination, racism, migration, media and technology, popular culture, government policies
Society
Neighborhood safety, access to green spaces, healthy food, housing, health care, pollution, natural disasters, climate change
Environment
Relationships with peers, teachers, and mentors; faith community; school climate, academic pressure, community support
Community
Relationships with parents, caregivers, and siblings; family mental health; financial stability; domestic violence; trauma
Family
Age, genetics, race, ethnicity, gender, sexual orientation, disability, beliefs, knowledge, attitudes, coping skills
Individual
These are examples and not a comprehensive list of factors

Sources: World Health Organization. (2014). *Health for the World's Adolescents: A second chance in the second decade*. WHO Press, World Health Organization. https://apps.who.int/adolescent/second-decade/files/1612_MNCAH_HWA_Executive_ Summary.pdf.

Bronfenbrenner, U., & Ceci, S. J. (1994). Nature-nurture reconceptualized in developmental perspective: A bioecological model. *Psychological Review*, 101(4), 568-586. doi:10.1037/0033-295X.101.4.568.

**Figure 1.**

Figure 1 includes a longer list of factors that shape the mental health of young people.

Even before the COVID-19 pandemic, mental health challenges were the leading cause of disability and poor life outcomes in young people, with up to 1 in 5 children ages 3 to 17 in the US with a reported mental, emotional, developmental, or behavioral disorder.[203] In 2016, of the 7.7 million children with treatable mental health disorder, about half did not receive adequate treatment.[204]

---

[203] Perou, R., Bitsko, R. H., Blumberg, S. J., Pastor, P., Ghandour, R. M., Gfroerer, J. C., Hedden, S. L., Crosby, A. E., Visser, S. N., Schieve, L. A., Parks, S. E., Hall, J. E., Brody, D., Simile, C. M., Thompson, W. W., Baio, J., Avenevoli, S., Kogan, M. D., Huang, L. N., & Centers for Disease Control and Prevention (CDC) (2013). Mental health surveillance among children--United States, 2005-2011. *MMWR. Morbidity and Mortality Weekly Report Supplements*, 62(2), 1–35.

[204] Whitney, D.G. & Peterson, M. (2019). US national and state-level prevalence of mental health disorders and disparities of mental health care use in children. *JAMA Pediatrics*, 173(4), 389-391. doi:10.1001/jamapediatrics.2018.5399.

Unfortunately, in recent years, national surveys of youth have shown major increases in certain mental health symptoms, including depressive symptoms and suicidal ideation. From 2009 to 2019, the proportion of high school students reporting persistent feelings of sadness or hopelessness increased by 40%; the share seriously considering attempting suicide increased by 36%; and the share creating a suicide plan increased by 44%.[205] Between 2011 and 2015, youth psychiatric visits to emergency departments for depression, anxiety, and behavioral challenges increased by 28%.[206] Between 2007 and 2018, suicide rates among youth ages 10-24 in the US increased by 57%.[207] Early estimates from the National Center for Health Statistics suggest there were tragically more than 6,600 deaths by suicide among the 10-24 age group in 2020.[208]

Scientists have proposed various hypotheses to explain these trends. While some believe that the trends in reporting of mental health challenges are partly due to young people becoming more willing to openly discuss mental health concerns,[209] other researchers point to the growing use of digital media,[210,211,212] increasing academic pressure,[213,214,215] limited access to mental

---

[205] Centers for Disease Control and Prevention. (2020). Youth Risk Behavior Surveillance Data Summary & Trends Report: 2009-2019. Retrieved from https://www.cdc.gov/nchhstp/dear_colleague/2020/dcl-102320-YRBS-2009-2019-report.html.

[206] Kalb, L. G., Stapp, E. K., Ballard, E. D., Holingue, C., Keefer, A., & Riley, A. (2019). Trends in Psychiatric Emergency Department Visits Among Youth and Young Adults in the US. *Pediatrics*, 143(4), e20182192. https://doi.org/10.1542/ peds.2018-2192.

[207] Curtin, S. C. (2020). State suicide rates among adolescents and young adults aged 10–24: United States, 2000–2018. *National Vital Statistics Reports;* vol 69 no 11. Hyattsville, MD: National Center for Health Statistics.

[208] Curtin, S. C., Hedegaard, H., Ahmad, F. B. (2021). Provisional numbers and rates of suicide by month and demographic characteristics: United States, 2020. *Vital Statistics Rapid Release*; no 16. Hyattsville, MD: National Center for Health Statistics.

[209] Armstrong, K. (2020 September 30). Technology in Context: The Surprising Social Upsides of Constant Connectivity. *Association for Psychological Science*. Accessed on November 30, 2021. Retrieved from https://www.psychologicalscience.org/ observer/technology-social-context.

[210] Hagan, J. F., Shaw, J. S., & Duncan, M. P. (2017). Bright Futures: Guidelines for Health Supervision of Infants, Children, and Adolescents. 4th ed. Elk Grove Village, IL: American Academy of Pediatrics. https://brightfutures.aap.org/materials-and-tools/guidelines-and-pocket-guide/Pages/default.aspx.

[211] Twenge, J. M., Joiner, T. E., Rogers, M. L., & Martin, G. N. (2018). Increases in Depressive Symptoms, Suicide-Related Outcomes, and Suicide Rates Among U.S. Adolescents After 2010 and Links to Increased New Media Screen Time. Clinical Psychological Science, 6(1), 3–17. https://doi. org/10.1177/2167702617723376.

[212] Riehm, K. E., Feder, K. A., Tormohlen, K. N., Crum, R. M., Young, A. S., Green, K. M., Pacek, L. R., La Flair, L. N., & Mojtabai, R. (2019). Associations Between Time Spent Using Social Media and Internalizing and Externalizing Problems Among US Youth. JAMA psychiatry, 76(12), 1266–1273. https://doi.org/10.1001/jamapsychiatry.2019.2325.

[213] Kasser, T., & Ryan, R. M. (1996). Further Examining the American Dream: Differential Correlates of Intrinsic and Extrinsic Goals. *Personality and Social Psychology Bulletin*, 22(3), 280–287. https://doi.org/10.1177/0146167296223006.

[214] Eckersley, R., & Dear, K. (2002). Cultural correlates of youth suicide. *Social science & medicine* (1982), 55(11), 1891–1904. https://doi.org/10.1016/s0277-9536(01)00319-7.

[215] Twenge, J. M., Gentile, B., DeWall, C. N., Ma, D., Lacefield, K., & Schurtz, D. R. (2010). Birth cohort increases in psychopathology among young Americans, 1938-2007: A cross-temporal meta-analysis of the MMPI. *Clinical Psychology Review*, 30(2), 145–154. https://doi.org/10.1016/j.cpr.2009.10.005.

health care,[18,216] health risk behaviors such as alcohol and drug use,[217] and broader stressors such as the 2008 financial crisis, rising income inequality, racism, gun violence, and climate change.[218,219,220,221]

It's also important to acknowledge that the prevalence of mental health challenges varies across subpopulations. For instance, girls are much more likely to be diagnosed with anxiety, depression, or an eating disorder, while boys are more likely to die by suicide or be diagnosed with a behavior disorder, such as attention deficit hyperactivity disorder (ADHD).[222,223,224] In recent years, suicide rates among Black children (below age 13) have been increasing rapidly, with Black children nearly twice as likely to die by suicide than White children.[225] Moreover, socioeconomically disadvantaged children and adolescents— for instance, those growing up in poverty—are two to three times more likely to develop mental health conditions than peers with higher socioeconomic status.[226]

## The COVID-19 Pandemic's Impact on the Mental Health of Children and Youth

During the pandemic, children, adolescents, and young adults have faced unprecedented challenges. The COVID-19 pandemic has dramatically changed their world, including how they attend school, interact with friends, and receive health care. They missed first days of school, months or even years of in-person schooling, graduation ceremonies, sports competitions, playdates, and time with relatives. They and their family may have lost access to

---

[216] Fairbrother, G., Stuber, J., Galea, S., Pfefferbaum, B., & Fleischman, A. R. (2004). Unmet need for counseling services by children in New York City after the September 11th attacks on the World Trade Center: implications for pediatricians. *Pediatrics*, 113(5), 1367–1374. https://doi.org/10.1542/peds.113.5.1367.

[217] Rodway, C., Tham, S. G., Ibrahim, S., Turnbull, P., Windfuhr, K., Shaw, J., Kapur, N., & Appleby, L. (2016). Suicide in children and young people in England: a consecutive case series. *The Lancet Psychiatry*, 3(8), 751–759. https://doi. org/10.1016/S2215-0366(16)30094-3.

[218] Golberstein, E., Gonzales, G., & Meara, E. (2019). How do economic downturns affect the mental health of children? Evidence from the National Health Interview Survey. *Health Economics*, 28(8), 955–970. https://doi.org/10.1002/hec.3885.

[219] Doepke, M., & Zilibotti, F. (2019). Love, money & parenting: How economics explains the way we raise our kids. Princeton, NJ: Princeton University Press.

[220] Marks, E., Hickman, C., Pihkala, P., Clayton, S., Lewandowski, ER., Mayall, EE., Wray, B., Mellor, C., & van Susteren, L. (2021). Young People's Voices on Climate Anxiety, Government Betrayal and Moral Injury: A Global Phenomenon. The Lancet. Preprint. http://dx.doi.org/10.2139/ssrn.3918955.

[221] Clayton, S., Manning, C. M., Speiser, M., & Hill, A. N. (2021). Mental Health and Our Changing Climate: Impacts, Inequities, Responses. Washington, D.C.: American Psychological Association, and ecoAmerica.

[222] McLean, C. P., Asnaani, A., Litz, B. T., & Hofmann, S. G. (2011). Gender differences in anxiety disorders: prevalence, course of illness, comorbidity and burden of illness. *Journal of Psychiatric Research*, 45(8), 1027–1035. https://doi. org/10.1016/j.jpsychires.2011.03.006.

[223] Salk, R. H., Hyde, J. S., & Abramson, L. Y. (2017). Gender differences in depression in representative national samples: Meta-analyses of diagnoses and symptoms. *Psychological Bulletin*, 143(8), 783–822. https://doi.org/10.1037/bul0000102.

[224] Hedegaard, H., Curtin, S. C., & Warner, M. (2020). Increase in suicide mortality in the United States, 1999–2018. NCHS Data Brief, (362), 1-8. Hyattsville, MD: National Center for Health Statistics.

[225] Bridge JA, Horowitz LM, Fontanella CA, et al. (2018). Age-Related Racial Disparity in Suicide Rates Among US Youths From 2001 Through 2015. *JAMA Pediatrics*, 172(7):697–699. doi:10.1001/jamapediatrics.2018.0399.

[226] Reiss F. (2013). Socioeconomic inequalities and mental health problems in children and adolescents: a systematic review. *Social Science & Medicine* (1982), 90, 24–31. https://doi. org/10.1016/j.socscimed.2013.04.026.

mental health care, social services, income, food, or housing.[227] They may have had COVID-19 themselves, suffered from long COVID symptoms, or lost a loved one to the disease—it's estimated that as of June 2021, more than 140,000 children in the US had lost a parent or grandparent caregiver to COVID-19.[228]

Since the pandemic began, rates of psychological distress among young people, including symptoms of anxiety, depression, and other mental health disorders, have increased. Recent research covering 80,000 youth globally found that depressive and anxiety symptoms doubled during the pandemic, with 25% of youth experiencing depressive symptoms and 20% experiencing anxiety symptoms.[229] Negative emotions or behaviors such as impulsivity and irritability—associated with conditions such as ADHD— appear to have moderately increased.[230] Early clinical data are also concerning: In early 2021, emergency department visits in the United States for suspected suicide attempts were 51% higher for adolescent girls and 4% higher for adolescent boys compared to the same time period in early 2019.[231] Moreover, pandemic-related measures reduced in-person interactions among children, friends, social supports, and professionals such as teachers, school counselors, pediatricians, and child welfare workers. This made it harder to recognize signs of child abuse, mental health concerns, and other challenges.[232]

During the pandemic, young people also experienced other challenges that may have affected their mental and emotional wellbeing: the national reckoning over the deaths of Black Americans at the hands of police officers, including the murder of George Floyd; COVID-related violence against Asian Americans; gun violence; an increasingly polarized political

---

[227] Substance Abuse and Mental Health Services Administration. (2021). Key substance use and mental health indicators in the United States: Results from the 2020 National Survey on Drug Use and Health (HHS Publication No. PEP21-07-01-003, NSDUH Series H-56). Rockville, MD: Center for Behavioral Health Statistics and Quality, Substance Abuse and Mental Health Services Administration. Retrieved from https://www. samhsa.gov/data/.

[228] Hillis, S. D., Blenkinsop A., Villaveces A., Annor F. B., Liburd, L., Massetti, G. M., Demissie, Z., Mercy, J. A., Nelson, C. A., Cluver, L., Flaxman, S., Sherr, L., Donelly, C. A., Ratmann, O., & Unwin, J. T. (2021). Covid-19-Associated Orphanhood and Caregiver Death in the United States. *Pediatrics*. DOI: 10.1542/peds.2021-053760.

[229] Racine, N., McArthur, B. A., Cooke, J. E., Eirich, R., Zhu, J., & Madigan, S. (2021). Global Prevalence of Depressive and Anxiety Symptoms in Children and Adolescents During COVID-19: A Meta-analysis. *JAMA Pediatrics*, 175(11), 1142– 1150. https://doi.org/10.1001/jamapediatrics.2021.2482.

[230] Sharma, M., Idele, P., Manzini, A., Aladro, CP., Ipince, A., Olsson, G., Banati, P., Anthony, D. (2021). Life in Lockdown: Child and adolescent mental health and well-being in the time of COVID-19, UNICEF Office of Research – Innocenti, Florence; pages 43-46, https://www.unicef-irc.org/publications/pdf/Life-in-Lockdown.pdf.

[231] Yard, E., Radhakrishnan, L., Ballesteros, M. F., Sheppard, M., Gates, A., Stein, Z., Hartnett, K., Kite-Powell, A., Rodgers, L., Adjemian, J., Ehlman, D. C., Holland, K., Idaikkadar, N., Ivey-Stephenson, A., Martinez, P., Law, R., & Stone, D. M. (2021). Emergency Department Visits for Suspected Suicide Attempts Among Persons Aged 12-25 Years Before and During the COVID-19 Pandemic - United States, January 2019-May 2021. *MMWR. Morbidity and Mortality Weekly Report*, 70(24), 888–894. https://doi.org/10.15585/mmwr.mm7024e1.

[232] The New York Times. (2020 June 9). Child Abuse Cases Drop 51 Percent. The Authorities Are Very Worried. Accessed on November 23, 2021. Retrieved from https://www.nytimes. com/2020/06/09/nyregion/coronavirus-nyc-child-abuse.html.

dialogue; growing concerns about climate change; and emotionally-charged misinformation.[233,234,235,236,237]

Although the pandemic's long-term impact on children and young people is not fully understood, there is some cause for optimism. According to more than 50 years of research, increases in distress symptoms are common during disasters, but most people cope well and do not go on to develop mental health disorders.[238] Several measures of distress that increased early in the pandemic appear to have returned to pre-pandemic levels by mid-2020.[239,240] Some other measures of wellbeing, such as rates of life satisfaction and loneliness, remained largely unchanged throughout the first year of the pandemic.[241],[242] And while data on youth suicide rates are limited, early evidence does not show significant increases.[56,243]

In addition, some young people thrived during the pandemic: They got more sleep, spent more quality time with family, experienced less academic stress and bullying, had more flexible

---

[233] Ssentongo, P., Fronterre, C., Ssentongo, A. E., Advani, S., Heilbrunn, E. S., Hazelton, J. P., Oh, J. S., McCall-Hosenfeld, J. S , & Chinchilli, V. M. (2021). Gun violence incidence during the COVID-19 pandemic is higher than before the pandemic in the United States. *Scientific Reports*, 11(1), 20654. https://doi. org/10.1038/s41598-021-98813-z.

[234] Office of the Surgeon General (OSG). (2021). Confronting Health Misinformation: The U.S. Surgeon General's Advisory on Building a Healthy Information Environment. US Department of Health and Human Services. https://www.hhs.gov/sites/ default/files/surgeon-general-misinformation-advisory.pdf.

[235] WHO, UN, UNICEF, UNDP, UNESCO, UNAIDS, ITU, UN Global Pulse, & IFRC. (2020, September 23). Managing the COVID-19 infodemic: Promoting healthy behaviours and mitigating the harm from misinformation and disinformation. World Health Organization. https://www.who.int/news/item/23-09-2020-managing-the-covid-19-infodemic-promoting-healthy-behaviours-andmitigating-the-harm-from-misinformation-and-disinformation.

[236] Johnston, W. M., & Davey, G. C. (2011). The psychological impact of negative TV news bulletins: the catastrophizing of personal worries. *British Journal of Psychology* (London, England: 1953), 88 (Pt 1), 85-91. https://doi. org/10.1111/j.2044-8295.1997.tb02622.x.

[237] Duan, L., Shao, X., Wang, Y., Huang, Y., Miao, J., Yang, X., & Zhu, G. (2020). An investigation of mental health status of children and adolescents in china during the outbreak of COVID-19. *Journal of Affective Disorders*, 275, 112–118. https:// doi.org/10.1016/j.jad.2020.06.029.

[238] Goldmann, E., & Galea, S. (2014). Mental health consequences of disasters. *Annual Review of Public Health*, 35, 169–183. https://doi.org/10.1146/annurev-publhealth-032013-182435.

[239] Aknin, L. B., De Neve, J. E., Dunn, E. W., Fancourt, D., Goldberg, E., Helliwell, J., Jones, S.P., Karam, E., Layard, R., Lyubomirsky, S., Rzepa, A., Saxena, S., Thornton, E., VanderWeele, T., Whillans, A., Zaki, J., Caman, O. K., Ben Amor, Y. (2021, February 19). Mental health during the first year of the COVID-19 pandemic: A review and recommendations for moving forward. https://doi.org/10.31234/osf.io/zw93g.

[240] Brülhart, M., Klotzbücher, V., Lalive, R., & Reich, S. K. (2021). Mental health concerns during the COVID-19 pandemic as revealed by helpline calls. *Nature*, 10.1038/s41586-021-04099-6. Advance online publication. https://doi.org/10.1038/ s41586-021-04099-6.

[241] Luchetti, M., Lee, J. H., Aschwanden, D., Sesker, A., Strickhouser, J. E., Terracciano, A., & Sutin, A. R. (2020). The trajectory of loneliness in response to COVID-19. *American Psychologist*, 75(7), 897–908. https://doi.org/10.1037/ amp0000690.

[242] Appleby, L., Richards, N., Ibrahim, S., Turnbull, P., Rodway, C., & Kapur, N. (2021). Suicide in England in the COVID-19 pandemic: Early observational data from real time surveillance. *The Lancet Regional Health*. Europe, 4, 100110. https://doi. org/10.1016/j.lanepe.2021.100110.

[243] Ahmad, F. B., & Cisewski, J. A. (2021). Quarterly provisional estimates for selected indicators of mortality, 2019-Quarter 1, 2021. National Center for Health Statistics. National Vital Statistics System, Vital Statistics Rapid Release Program. Retrieved from https://www.cdc.gov/nchs/nvss/vsrr/ mortality-dashboard.htm#.

schedules, and improved their coping skills.[44,244,245,246] Many young people are resilient, able to bounce back from difficult experiences such as stress, adversity, and trauma.[247]

That said, the pandemic is ongoing, with nearly 1,000 Americans dying per day as of early December 2021.[248] And many millions of children and youth have faced and continue to face major challenges. Importantly, the pandemic's negative impacts, such as illness and death in families and disruptions in school and social life, disproportionately impacted those who were vulnerable to begin with and widened disparities.[249]

**Box 1.** Risk factors contributing to youth mental health symptoms during the pandemic

Having mental health challenges before the pandemic[61,250]
Living in an urban area or an area with more severe COVID-19 outbreaks[251]
Having parents or caregivers who were frontline workers[252]
Having parents or caregivers at elevated risk of burnout (for example, due to parenting demands)[253,254]
Being worried about COVID-19[64]

---

[244] Roy, A., Breaux, R., Sciberras, E., Patel, P., Ferrara, E., Shroff, D., Cash, A., Dvorsky, M., Langberg, J., Quach, J., Melvin, G. A., Jackson, A., & Becker, S. P. (2021). A Preliminary Examination of Key Strategies, Challenges, and Benefits of Remote Learning Expressed by Parents During the COVID-19 Pandemic. https://doi.org/10.31234/osf.io/5ca4v.

[245] Wright, K. P., Jr, Linton, S. K., Withrow, D., Casiraghi, L., Lanza, S. M., Iglesia, H., Vetter, C., & Depner, C. M. (2020). Sleep in university students prior to and during COVID-19 Stay-at-Home orders. *Current Biology*: CB, 30(14), R797–R798. https://doi.org/10.1016/j.cub.2020.06.022.

[246] Vaillancourt, T., Brittain, H., Krygsman, A., Farrell, A. H., Landon, S., & Pepler, D. (2021). School bullying before and during COVID-19: Results from a population-based randomized design. *Aggressive Behavior*, 47, 557–569. https:// doi.org/10.1002/ab.21986.

[247] Osgood, K., Sheldon-Dean, H., & Kimball, H. (2021). 2021 Children's Mental Health Report: What we know about the COVID-19 pandemic's impact on children's mental health — and what we don't know. Child Mind Institute.

[248] Centers for Disease Control and Prevention. COVID Data Tracker. Trends in Number of COVID-19 Cases and Deaths in the US Reported to CDC, by State/Territory. Accessed on November 29, 2021. Retrieved from https://covid.cdc.gov/covid-data-tracker/#trends_dailydeaths.

[249] Jones, K. (2021). The Initial Impact of COVID-19 on Children and Youth (Birth to 24 years): Literature Review in Brief. Retrieved from https://aspe.hhs.gov/reports/impact-covid-19-children-youth.

[250] Nikolaidis, A., DeRosa, J., Kass, M., Droney, I., Alexander, L., Di Martino, A., Bromet, E., Merikangas, K., Milham, M. P., & Paksarian, D. (2021). Heterogeneity in COVID-19 Pandemic-Induced Lifestyle Stressors and Predicts Future Mental Health in Adults and Children in the US and UK. medRxiv: the preprint server for health sciences, 2021.08.10.21261860. https://doi.org/ 10.1101/2021.08.10.21261860.

[251] Fitzpatrick, K. M., Harris, C., & Drawve, G. (2020). Fear of COVID-19 and the mental health consequences in America. *Psychological Trauma: Theory, Research, Practice, and Policy*. 12(S1), S17-S21. https://doi.org/10.1037/tra0000924.

[252] Sugg, M. M., Runkle, J. D., Andersen, L., Weiser, J., & Michael, K. D. (2021). Crisis response among essential workers and their children during the COVID-19 pandemic. *Preventive Medicine*, 153, 106852. Advance online publication. https://doi. org/10.1016/j.ypmed.2021.106852.

[253] Griffith A. K. (2020). Parental Burnout and Child Maltreatment During the COVID-19 Pandemic. *Journal of Family Violence*, 1–7. Advance online publication. https://doi. org/10.1007/s10896-020-00172-2.

[254] Sinko, L., He, Y., Kishton, R. et al. (2021). "The Stay at Home Order is Causing Things to Get Heated Up": Family Conflict Dynamics During COVID-19 From The Perspectives of Youth Calling a National Child Abuse Hotline. *J Fam Viol*. https://doi.org/10.1007/s10896-021-00290-5.

| |
|---|
| Experiencing disruptions in routine, such as not seeing friends or going to school in person[255,256,257] |
| Experiencing more adverse childhood experiences (ACEs) such as abuse, neglect, community violence, and discrimination[258,259,260] |
| Experiencing more financial instability, food shortages, or housing instability[261,262] |
| Experiencing trauma, such as losing a family member or caregiver to COVID-19[263] |

Note: Not a comprehensive list of risk factors.

For additional details, see Boxes 1 and 2. Box 1 discusses risk factors contributing to children's mental health symptoms during the pandemic. Box 2 discusses demographic groups at greater risk of developing mental health problems during the pandemic.

---

[255] Esposito, S., Giannitto, N., Squarcia, A., Neglia, C., Argentiero, A., Minichetti, P., Cotugno, N. & Principi, N. (2021). Development of Psychological Problems Among Adolescents During School Closures Because of the COVID-19 Lockdown Phase in Italy: A Cross-Sectional Survey. *Frontiers in Pediatrics*, 8:628072. https://doi.org/10.3389/fped.2020.628072.

[256] Verlenden, J. V., Pampati, S., Rasberry, C. N., Liddon, N., Hertz, M., Kilmer, G., Viox, M. H., Lee, S., Cramer, N. K., Barrios, L. C., & Ethier, K. A. (2021). Association of Children's Mode of School Instruction with Child and Parent Experiences and Well-Being During the COVID-19 Pandemic - COVID Experiences Survey, United States, October 8-November 13, 2020. *MMWR. Morbidity and mortality weekly report*, 70(11), 369–376. https://doi.org/10.15585/mmwr.mm7011a1.

[257] Hawrilenko M, Kroshus E, Tandon P, Christakis D. The Association Between School Closures and Child Mental Health During COVID-19. *JAMA Netw Open*. 2021;4(9):e2124092. doi:10.1001/jamanetworkopen.2021.24092.

[258] Stinson, E. A., Sullivan, R. M., Peteet, B. J., Tapert, S. F., Baker, F. C., Breslin, F. J., Dick, A. S., Gonzalez, M. R., Guillaume, M., Marshall, A. T., McCabe, C. J., Pelham, W. E., 3rd, Van Rinsveld, A. M., Sheth, C. S., Sowell, E. R., Wade, N. E., Wallace, A. L., & Lisdahl, K. M. (2021). Longitudinal Impact of Childhood Adversity on Early Adolescent Mental Health During the COVID-19 Pandemic in the ABCD Study® Cohort: Does Race or Ethnicity Moderate Findings?. *Biological Psychiatry Global Open Science*, 10.1016/j.bpsgos.2021.08.007. Advance online publication. https://doi.org/10.1016/j. bpsgos.2021.08.007.

[259] Henderson MD, Schmus CJ, McDonald C, Irving SY. (2020). The COVID-19 pandemic and the impact on child mental health: a socio-ecological perspective. *Pediatric Nursing*. 46(6). https://www.pediatricnursing.net/issues/20novdec/267.pdf.

[260] [Pediatrics publication not currently available] Hernandez, J. (2021, November 8). A study links facing discrimination at a young age with future mental health issues. NPR. Retrieved November 9, 2021, from https://www.npr.org/2021/11/08/1053632912/study-discrimination-young-age-future-mental-health-issue.

[261] Westrupp, E. M., Bennett, C., Berkowitz, T., Youssef, G. J., Toumbourou, J. W., Tucker, R., Andrews, F. J., Evans, S., Teague, S. J., Karantzas, G. C., Melvin, G. M., Olsson, C., Macdonald, J. A., Greenwood, C. J., Mikocka-Walus, A., Hutchinson, D., Fuller-Tyszkiewicz, M., Stokes, M. A., Olive, L., Wood, A. G., … Sciberras, E. (2021). Child, parent, and family mental health and functioning in Australia during COVID-19: comparison to pre-pandemic data. *European child & adolescent psychiatry*, 1–14. Advance online publication. https://doi.org/10.1007/s00787-021-01861-z.

[262] Patrick, S. W., Henkhaus, L. E., Zickafoose, J. S., Lovell, K., Halvorson, A., Loch, S., Letterie, M., & Davis, M. M. (2020). Well-being of Parents and Children During the COVID-19 Pandemic: A National Survey. *Pediatrics*, 146(4), e2020016824. https://doi.org/10.1542/peds.2020-016824.

[263] Bergman, A. S., Axberg, U., & Hanson, E. (2017). When a parent dies - a systematic review of the effects of support programs for parentally bereaved children and their caregivers. *BMC palliative care*, 16(1), 39. https://doi.org/10.1186/s12904-017-0223-y.

**BOX 2.** Groups at higher risk of mental health challenges during the pandemic

**Youth with intellectual and developmental disabilities (IDDs)**, who found it especially difficult to manage disruptions to school and services such as special education, counseling, occupational, and speech therapies[264,265,266,267,268]

Racial and ethnic minority youth,[269] including:

- *American Indian and Alaska Native youth,* many of whom faced challenges staying connected with friends and attending school due to limited internet access[270]
- *Black youth,* who were more likely than other youth to lose a parent or caregiver to COVID-1942
- *Latino youth,* who reported high rates of loneliness and poor or decreased mental health during the pandemic[271],[272]
- *Asian American, Native Hawaiian, and Pacific Islander youth,* who reported increased stress due to COVID-19-related hate and harassment[273,274]

---

[264] White, L. C., Law, J. K., Daniels, A. M., Toroney, J., Vernoia, B., Xiao, S., The SPARK Consortium, Feliciano, P., & Chung, W. K. (2020). Brief Report: Impact of COVID-19 on individuals with ASD and their caregivers: A perspective form the SPARK cohort. *Journal of Autism and Developmental Disorders*. https://doi.org/10.1007/s10803-020-04816-6.

[265] Jeste, S., Hyde, C., Distefano, C., Halladay, A., Ray, S., Porath, M., Wilson, R. B., & Thurm, A. (2020). Changes in access to educational and healthcare services for individuals with intellectual and developmental disabilities during COVID-19 restrictions. *Journal of intellectual disability research: JIDR*, 10.1111/jir.12776. Advance online publication. https://doi. org/10.1111/jir.12776.

[266] Neece, C., McIntyre, L. L., & Fenning, R. (2020). Examining the impact of COVID-19 in ethnically diverse families with young children with intellectual and developmental disabilities. *Journal of intellectual disability research: JIDR*, 64(10), 739–749. https://doi.org/10.1111/jir.12769.

[267] Patel K. (2020). Mental health implications of COVID-19 on children with disabilities. *Asian journal of psychiatry*, 54, 102273. https://doi.org/10.1016/j.ajp.2020.102273.

[268] National Council on Disability. (2021). 2021 Progress Report: The Impact of COVID-19 on People with Disabilities. https://ncd.gov/sites/default/files/NCD_COVID-19_Progress_ Report_508.pdf.

[269] Racial and ethnic disparities in pediatric mental health. *Child and adolescent psychiatric clinics of North America*, 19(4), 759–774. https://doi.org/10.1016/j.chc.2010.07.001).

[270] American Indian Policy Institute. (2021). Tribal Digital Divide: Policy Brief and Recommendations. Accessed on November 10, 2021. Retrieved from https://aipi.asu.edu/ sites/default/files/tribal_digital_divide_stimulus_bill_ advocacy_04032020.pdf.

[271] Rogers, A. A., Ha, T., & Ockey, S. (2021). Adolescents' Perceived Socio-Emotional Impact of COVID-19 and Implications for Mental Health: Results From a U.S.-Based Mixed-Methods Study. *The Journal of adolescent health*, 68(1), 43–52. https://doi.org/10.1016/j.jadohealth.2020.09.039.

[272] Flanagan, S., Margolius, M., Pileggi, M., Glaser L., Burkander, K., Kincheloe, M., &Freeman, J. (2021). Where Do We Go Next? Youth Insights on the High School Experience During a Year of Historic Upheaval. America's Promise Alliance and Research for Action. https://www.researchforaction.org/wp-content/uploads/2021/07/where-do-we-go-next.pdf.

[273] Cheah, C., Wang, C., Ren, H., Zong, X., Cho, H. S., & Xue, X. (2020). COVID-19 Racism and Mental Health in Chinese American Families. *Pediatrics*, 146(5), e2020021816. https://doi. org/10.1542/peds.2020-021816.

[274] Wakabayashi, K., Cheah, C. S. L., Chang, T., Lai, G., Subrahmanyam, K., Chaudhary, N., Hyun, S., & Patel P. (2020). Addressing Inequities in Education: Considerations for Asian American Children and Youth in the Era of COVID-19. Society for Research in Child Development. https://www.srcd.org/research/addressing-inequities-education-considerations-asian-american-children-and-youth-era-covid.

**LGBTQ+ youth**, who lost access to school-based services and were sometimes confined to homes where they were not supported or accepted[275],[276]

**Low-income youth**, who faced economic, educational, and social disruptions (for example, losing access to free school lunches)[277]

**Youth in rural areas**, who faced additional challenges in participating in school or accessing mental health services (for example, due to limited internet connectivity)[278]

**Youth in immigrant households**, who faced language and technology barriers to accessing health care services and education[279]

**Special youth populations**, including youth involved with the juvenile justice, or child welfare systems, as well as runaway youth and youth experiencing homelessness[61,280,281,282]

Additional considerations:

- *Youth with multiple risk factors.* Many young people are part of more than one at-risk group, which can put at them at even higher risk of mental health challenges. For example, children with IDDs who lost a parent to COVID-19, or Black children from low-income families, may require additional support to address multiple risk factors.[283]
- *Discrimination in the health care system.* Some groups of youth and their families, such as people of color, immigrants, LGBTQ+ people, and people with disabilities, may be

[275] Panchal, N., Kamal, R., Cox, C., Garfield, R., & Chidambaram, P. (2021, May 26). Mental health and substance use considerations among children during the COVID-19 pandemic. Kaiser Family Foundation. https://www.kff.org/coronavirus-covid-19/issue-brief/mental-healthand-substance-use-considerations-among-children-during-the-covid19-pandemic/.

[276] Department of Education Office of Civil Rights. (2021). *Education in a Pandemic: The Disparate Impacts of COVID-19 on America's Students*. https://www2.ed.gov/about/offices/list/ocr/ docs/20210608-impacts-of-covid19.pdf.

[277] Dooley, D., Bandealy, A., & Tschudy, M. (2020). Low-income children and coronavirus disease 2019 (COVID-19) in the US. *JAMA Pediatrics*, 174(10), 922-923.

[278] Lai, J., & Widmar, N. O. (2020). Revisiting the Digital Divide in the COVID-19 Era. *Applied economic perspectives and policy*, 10.1002/aepp.13104. Advance online publication. https://doi.org/10.1002/aepp.13104.

[279] Endale, T., St Jean, N., & Birman, D. (2020). COVID-19 and refugee and immigrant youth: A community-based mental health perspective. *Psychological trauma: theory, research, practice and policy*, 12(S1), S225–S227. https://doi.org/10.1037/ tra0000875.

[280] Robinson, L. R., Holbrook, J. R., Bitsko, R. H., Hartwig, S. A., Kaminski, J. W., Ghandour, R. M., Peacock, G., Heggs, A., & Boyle, C. A. (2017). Differences in Health Care, Family, and Community Factors Associated with Mental, Behavioral, and Developmental Disorders Among Children Aged 2-8 Years in Rural and Urban Areas - United States, 2011-2012. *Morbidity and mortality weekly report. Surveillance summaries* (Washington, D.C.: 2002), 66(8), 1–11. https://doi.org/10.15585/mmwr.ss6608a1.

[281] Lawrence, H. R., Burke, T. A., Sheehan, A. E., Pastro, B., Levin, R. Y., Walsh, R., Bettis, A. H., & Liu, R. T. (2021). Prevalence and correlates of suicidal ideation and suicide attempts in preadolescent children: A US population-based study. *Translational psychiatry*, 11(1), 489. https://doi.org/10.1038/ s41398-021-01593-3.

[282] Development Services Group, Inc. (2017). "Intersection Between Mental Health and the Juvenile Justice System." Literature review. Washington, D.C.: Office of Juvenile Justice and Delinquency Prevention. https://www.ojjdp.gov/mpg/litreviews/Intersection-Mental-Health-Juvenile-Justice.pdf.

[283] Houtrow, A., Harris, D., Molinero, A., Levin-Decanini, T., & Robichaud, C. (2020). Children with disabilities in the United States and the COVID-19 pandemic. *Journal of pediatric rehabilitation medicine*, 13(3), 415–424. https://doi.org/10.3233/ PRM-200769.

more hesitant to engage with the health care system (including mental health services) due to current and past experiences with discrimination.[97,284,285]

- *Risks of COVID-19 to children with mental health conditions.* Children with mood disorders, such as depression and bipolar disorder, as well as schizophrenia spectrum disorders, are at elevated risk of severe COVID-19 illness.[286,287,288]

Note: Not a comprehensive list of groups or risk factors.

## We Can Take Action

The good news is that, throughout the pandemic, many people have recognized the unprecedented need to support youth mental health and wellbeing and have taken action to do so. Many young people found ways to cope with disruption and stay connected.[289] Families helped children adjust to remote learning.[290] Educators and school staff supported their students while facing unprecedented challenges themselves.[291] Health care professionals rapidly shifted to telehealth.[292] Community organizations stepped in to protect at-risk youth.[293] Employers helped employees adapt to remote work environments.[294] And governments invested trillions of dollars to mitigate financial hardship for families, support COVID-19 testing and

---

[284] Kugelmass H. (2016). "Sorry, I'm Not Accepting New Patients": An Audit Study of Access to Mental Health Care. *Journal of health and social behavior*, 57(2), 168–183. https://doi. org/10.1177/0022146516647098.

[285] Drescher J. (2015). Out of DSM: Depathologizing Homosexuality. *Behavioral sciences* (Basel, Switzerland), 5(4), 565–575. https://doi.org/10.3390/bs5040565.

[286] Centers for Disease Control and Prevention. (2021 October 14). Medical Conditions. Accessed on November 10, 2021. Retrieved from https://www.cdc.gov/coronavirus/2019-ncov/need-extra-precautions/people-with-medical-conditions.html.

[287] Fond, G., Nemani, K., Etchecopar-Etchart, D., Loundou, A., Goff, D. C., Lee, S. W., Lancon, C., Auquier, P., Baumstarck, K., Llorca, P. M., Yon, D. K., & Boyer, L. (2021). Association Between Mental Health Disorders and Mortality Among Patients With COVID-19 in 7 Countries: A Systematic Review and Meta-analysis. *JAMA psychiatry*, 78(11), 1208–1217. https://doi. org/10.1001/jamapsychiatry.2021.2274.

[288] Ceban, F., Nogo, D., Carvalho, I. P., Lee, Y., Nasri, F., Xiong, J., Lui, L., Subramaniapillai, M., Gill, H., Liu, R. N., Joseph, P., Teopiz, K. M., Cao, B., Mansur, R. B., Lin, K., Rosenblat, J. D., Ho, R. C., & McIntyre, R. S. (2021). Association Between Mood Disorders and Risk of COVID-19 Infection, Hospitalization, and Death: A Systematic Review and Meta-analysis. *JAMA psychiatry*, 78(10), 1079–1091. https://doi. org/10.1001/jamapsychiatry.2021.1818.

[289] World Economic Forum. (2020 October 9). 7 ways young people are making a difference in mental health. Accessed on November 10, 2021. Retrieved from https://www.weforum.org/ agenda/2020/10/7-ways-young-people-making-a-difference-mental-health/.

[290] Packman, K.J. (2020 October 15). The pandemic has shown us that parents have a bigger role to play in education. Accessed on November 10, 2021. Retrieved from: https://www.involve.org.uk/resources/blog/opinion/pandemic-has-shown-us-parents-have-bigger-role-play-education.

[291] Edsource. (2021 March 19). Teachers reflect on a year of Covid: students struggling, others thriving. Accessed on November 10, 2021. Retrieved from: https://edsource.org/2021/teachers-reflect-on-a-year-of-covid-students-struggling-others-thriving/649705.

[292] Children's Hospital Colorado. (2021). Providing Mental Health Care During the COVID-19 Pandemic. Accessed on November 10, 2021. Retrieved from https://www.childrenscolorado.org/health-professionals/coronavirus-professional-resources/clinical-guidance-practice-resources/providing-care-during-covid-19-pandemic/.

[293] Boys and Girls Club of America. (2020 March 19). Clubs Offer Critical Care During COVID-19. Accessed on November 10, 2021. Retrieved from https://www.bgca.org/news-stories/2020/ March/Clubs-Offer-Critical-Care-During-COVID-19.

[294] Mental Health America. (2020 May 5). 8 Employers Supporting Employee Mental Health During COVID-19. Accessed on November 10, 2021. Retrieved from https:// mhanational.org/blog/8-employers-supporting-employee-mental-health-during-covid-19.

vaccination, provide health care and other social services, and support the safe reopening of schools, among other policies.[295,296,297]

*But there is much more to be done, and each of us has a role to play. Supporting the mental health of children and youth will require a whole-of-society effort* to address longstanding challenges, strengthen the resilience of young people, support their families and communities, and mitigate the pandemic's mental health impacts. Here is what we must do:

- *Recognize that mental health is an essential part of overall health.* Mental health conditions are real, common, and treatable, and people experiencing mental health challenges deserve support, compassion, and care, not stigma and shame. Mental health is no less important than physical health. And that must be reflected in our how we communicate about and prioritize mental health.
- *Empower youth and their families to recognize, manage, and learn from difficult emotions.* For youth, this includes building strong relationships with peers and supportive adults, practicing techniques to manage emotions, taking care of body and mind, being attentive to use of social media and technology, and seeking help when needed. For families and caregivers, this means addressing their own mental health and substance use conditions, being positive role models for children, promoting positive relationships between children and others as well as with social media and technology, and learning to identify and address challenges early. Youth and families should know that asking for help is a sign of strength.
- *Ensure that every child has access to high-quality, affordable, and culturally competent mental health care.* Care should be tailored to children's developmental stages and health needs, and available in primary care practices, schools, and other community-based settings. It's particularly important to intervene early, so that emerging symptoms don't turn into crises.
- *Support the mental health of children and youth in educational, community, and childcare settings.* This includes creating positive, safe, and affirming educational environments, expanding programming that promotes healthy development (such as social and emotional learning), and providing a continuum of supports to meet the social, emotional, behavioral, and mental health needs of children and youth. To achieve this, we must also expand and support the early childhood and education workforce.
- *Address the economic and social barriers that contribute to poor mental health for young people, families, and caregivers.* Priorities should include reducing child poverty and ensuring access to quality childcare, early childhood services, and

---

[295] National Conference of State Legislatures. (2021 April 17). Bridging the gap to youth mental health during COVID-19. Accessed on November 10, 2021. Retrieved from https://www. ncsl.org/blog/2020/04/17/bridging-the-gap-to-youth-mental-health-during-covid-19.aspx.

[296] The White House. (2021 October 29). Fact Sheet: Biden Administration Announces Additional Actions to Increase COVID-19 Screening Testing in Schools and Keep Students Safe. https://www.whitehouse.gov/briefing-room/statements-releases/2021/10/29/fact-sheet-biden-administration-announces-additional-actions-to-increase-covid-19-screening-testing-in-schools-and-keep-students-safe/.

[297] The White House. (2021 July 15). FACT SHEET: Biden-Harris Administration Distributes First Monthly Payments of the Expanded Child Tax Credit. https://www.whitehouse.gov/briefing-room/statements-releases/2021/07/15/fact-sheet-biden-harris-administration-distributes-first-monthly-payments-of-the-expanded-child-tax-credit/.

education; healthy food; affordable health care; stable housing; and safe neighborhoods.[298],[299]

- *Increase timely data collection and research to identify and respond to youth mental health needs more rapidly.* The country needs an integrated, real-time data infrastructure for understanding youth mental health trends. More research is also needed on the relationship between technology and mental health, and technology companies should be more transparent with their data and algorithmic processes to enable this research. We also need to better understand the needs of at-risk youth, including youth facing multiple risk factors. Governments and other stakeholders should engage directly with young people to understand trends and design effective solutions.

## We Can Take Action

### What Young People Can Do

Since many of the challenges young people face are outside of their control, we need a whole-of-society effort to support children's mental health and wellbeing from birth to adulthood. That said, below are important steps children and young people themselves can take to protect, improve, and advocate for their mental health and that of their family, friends, and neighbors:

- *Remember that mental health challenges are real, common, and treatable.* Struggling with your mental health does not mean you are broken or that you did something wrong. Mental health is shaped by many factors, including biology and life experiences, and there are many ways mental health challenges can be addressed.
- *Ask for help.* Find trusted adults, friends, or family members to talk to about stressful situations. For example, if you or someone you know is being bullied, tell a trusted adult. If you are struggling to manage negative emotions, reach out to a school nurse or counselor, a teacher, a parent or caregiver, a coach, a faith leader, or someone else you look up to and trust. Look into therapy or counseling resources to get support when something causes distress and interferes with your life. Reaching out to others can be hard and takes courage, but it is worth the effort and reminds us we are not alone.
- *Invest in healthy relationships.* Social connection is a powerful buffer to stress and a source of wellbeing. But too often in our fast-paced lives, quality time with people gets crowded out. Make space in your life for the people you love. Spend time with others

[298] Department of Health and Human Services, Office of Disease Prevention and Health Promotion. (nd). Social Determinants of Health. Accessed on November 10, 2021. Retrieved from https://health.gov/healthypeople/objectives-and-data/social-determinants-health.

[299] Parolin, Zachary, Sophie Collyer, Megan A. Curran, and Christopher Wimer. 2021. "Monthly Poverty Rates among Children after Expansion of the Child Tax Credit." Poverty and Social Policy Brief. *Center on Poverty and Social Policy*, Columbia University. Vol. 5, no. 4. https://www.povertycenter.columbia.edu/news-internal/monthly-poverty-july-2021.

regularly, in-person and virtually.[300] Find people who support and care about you and have open and honest conversations with them about your feelings. Get involved in group activities, such as recreation and outdoor activities, after-school programs, and mentorship programs.[301]

- *Find ways to serve.* Volunteering in your community and helping others can be a great way to connect with people, build a sense of purpose, and develop your own sense of self-worth.[302] Helping others when you are the one struggling can seem counterintuitive. But service is a powerful antidote to isolation, and it reminds us that we have value to add to the world.
- *Learn and practice techniques to manage stress and other difficult emotions.* Try to recognize situations that may be emotionally challenging for you, and come up with strategies to manage those emotions. For example, if you find it stressful to look at COVID-related news, try to check the news less often, take a break for a day or a week at a time, keep notifications off throughout the day, and avoid looking at negative stories before bed.[51]
- *Take care of your body and mind.* Stick to a schedule, eat well, stay physically active, get quality sleep, stay hydrated, and spend time outside.[303,304,305] And avoid substances that can ultimately make you feel tired, down, or depressed, such as alcohol, marijuana, vaping, and tobacco.[306]
- *Be intentional about your use of social media, video games, and other technologies.* Here are some questions to help guide your technology use: How much time are you spending online? Is it taking away from healthy offline activities, like exercising, seeing friends, reading, and sleeping? What content are you consuming, and how does it make you feel? Are you online because you want to be, or because you feel like you have to be?

---

300 Roehlkepartain, E. C., Pekel, K., Syvertsen, A. K., Sethi, J., Sullivan, T. K., & Scales, P. C. (2017). Relationships First: Creating Connections that Help Young People Thrive. Minneapolis, MN: Search Institute. https://www.search-institute.org/wp-content/ uploads/2017/12/2017-Relationships-First-final.pdf.

301 Oberle, E., Guhn, M., Gadermann, A. M., Thomson, K., & Schonert-Reichl, K. A. (2018). Positive mental health and supportive school environments: A population-level longitudinal study of dispositional optimism and school relationships in early adolescence. *Social science & medicine* (1982), 214, 154–161. https://doi.org/10.1016/ j.socscimed.2018.06.041.

302 Ballard, P. J., Hoyt, L. T., & Pachucki, M. C. (2019). Impacts of Adolescent and Young Adult Civic Engagement on Health and Socioeconomic Status in Adulthood. *Child development*, 90(4), 1138–1154. https://doi.org/10.1111/cdev.12998.

303 Spagnola, M., & Fiese, B. (2007). Family routines and rituals. *Infants and Young Children*, 20(4), 284-299. https://doi. org/10.1097/01.IYC.0000290352.32170.5A.

304 Glynn, L. M., Davis, E. P., Luby, J. L., Baram, T. Z., & Sandman, C. A. (2021). A predictable home environment may protect child mental health during the COVID-19 pandemic. *Neurobiology of stress*, 14, 100291. https://doi.org/10.1016/j. ynstr.2020.100291.

305 National Academies of Sciences, Engineering, and Medicine; Health and Medicine Division; Division of Behavioral and Social Sciences and Education; Board on Children, Youth, and Families; Committee on Applying Lessons of Optimal Adolescent Health to Improve Behavioral Outcomes for Youth, Kahn, N. F., & Graham, R. (Eds.). (2019). Promoting Positive Adolescent Health Behaviors and Outcomes: Thriving in the 21st Century. *National Academies Press* (US).

306 Centers for Disease Control and Prevention. (2021). Coping with Stress. Accessed on November 10, 2021. Retrieved from: https://www.cdc.gov/mentalhealth/stress-coping/cope-with-stress/index.html.

- *Be a source of support for others.* Talk to your family and friends about mental health, listen and be a source of support to them, and connect them to the right resources.[307] Advocate for and contribute your ideas at the local, state, or national levels. For example, look into joining Youth Advisory Councils or mental health peer support programs in your community.[308]

**Resources for Young People**

*If you're in crisis, get immediate help:* Call the National Suicide Prevention Lifeline at 1-800-273-8255, chat with trained counselors 24/7, or get help in other ways through the Lifeline

*How Right Now* (Centers for Disease Control and Prevention): Resources for coping with negative emotions and stress, talking to loved ones, and finding inspiration

*Youth Engaged 4 Change:* Opportunities for youth to make a difference in their lives and in the world around them

*Supporting Emotional Wellbeing in Children and Youth* (National Academies of Medicine): Tools for children, teens, and parents to learn how to cope with challenges

*Mental Health Resource Center* (JED Foundation): Information about common emotional health issues and how to overcome challenges

*Youth Wellbeing Initiatives* (National Council for Mental Wellbeing): Collection of initiatives to improve mental wellbeing in youth and young adults

*Kids, Teens, and Young Adults* (National Alliance on Mental Illness): Resources for young people to get mental health support

*One Mind PsyberGuide:* A guide to navigating mental health apps and digital technologies

*FindTreatment.gov* (SAMHSA): Information on substance use and mental health treatment

*Trevor Project:* Suicide prevention and crisis intervention resources for LGBTQ+ young people

*AAKOMA Mental Health Resources* (The AAKOMA Project): Resources to support the mental health of youth of color and their caregivers

*Mental Health for Immigrants* (Informed Immigrant): Tips for managing the mental health of yourself and others

---

307 The National Institute of Mental Health Information Resource Center. (2021). 5 Action Steps for Helping Someone in Emotional Pain. Accessed on November 10, 2021. Retrieved from: https://www.nimh.nih.gov/health/publications/5-action-steps-for-helping-someone-in-emotional-pain?utm_campaign=shareNIMH&utm_medium=Portal&utm_source=NIMHwebsite.

308 Substance Abuse and Mental Health Administration. (2016). Creating a Youth Advisory Board. Accessed on November 12, 2021. Retrieved from https://youthmovenational.org/wp-content/uploads/2019/05/T2C_3-Final_Youth_Advisory_Boards.pdf.

## What Family Members and Caregivers Can Do

Families and caregivers play a critical role in providing the safe, stable, and nurturing environments and relationships young people need to thrive. Below are recommendations for how families and caregivers can engage with children and youth on mental health topics, help them become more resilient, and address emerging mental health challenges:

- *Be the best role model you can be for young people by taking care of your own mental and physical health.* Young people often learn behaviors and habits from what they see around them. You can model good habits by talking to children about the importance of mental health, seeking help when you need it, and showing positive ways you deal with stress so children learn from you. Additional ways to take care of your own mental health include taking breaks, getting enough sleep, exercising, eating balanced meals, maintaining regular routines, obtaining health insurance coverage, staying connected with family and friends, and taking time to unplug from technology or social media.[309]
- *Help children and youth develop strong, safe, and stable relationships with you and other supportive adults.* Research shows that the most important thing a child needs to be resilient is a stable and committed relationship with a supportive adult.[310] Spend time with children on activities that are meaningful to them, show them love and acceptance, praise them for the things they do well, listen to them, and communicate openly about their feelings. Encourage children to ask for help and connect them with other adults who can serve as mentors.[311]
- *Encourage children and youth to build healthy social relationships with peers.* This can be done through self-directed play and structured activities such as school, after school programs, sports, and volunteering.[312] Since peers can play a major role (both positive and negative) in children's development, it's important to help children learn how to deal with peer pressure. Have open conversations with your child about their values and teach them to be confident and comfortable in expressing their needs and boundaries.
- *Do your best to provide children and youth with a supportive, stable, and predictable home and neighborhood environment.* A lot may be outside of your control, and there will be trial and error as you figure out what works best for your child. That said, try to help children stick to a regular and predictable daily schedule, such as regular dinnertime and bedtime.[117,126,313] Be thoughtful about whether and how to discuss

---

[309] Centers for Disease Control and Prevention. (2021). Care for Yourself. Accessed on November 12, 2021. Retrieved from: https://www.cdc.gov/mentalhealth/stress-coping/care-for-yourself/index.html.

[310] National Scientific Council on the Developing Child (2015). *Supportive Relationships and Active Skill-Building Strengthen the Foundations of Resilience: Working Paper No. 13.* Retrieved from www.developingchild.harvard.edu.

[311] U.S. Department of Justice, Office of Juvenile Justice and Delinquency Prevention. (nd). Mentoring. Accessed on November 12, 2021. Retrieved from https://ojjdp.ojp.gov/ programs/mentoring.

[312] Whitebread D. (2017). Free play and children's mental health. *The Lancet. Child & adolescent health*, 1(3), 167–169. https://doi.org/10.1016/S2352-4642(17)30092-5.

[313] Masten, A. S. (2014). *Ordinary magic: Resilience in development*. New York, NY: Guilford Press. https://doi.org/10.1002/imhj.21625.

stressful topics such as financial and marital problems. The American Psychological Association offers tips on how to talk with your child about difficult topics.[314] It's also important to minimize children's exposure to violence, which puts them at risk of mental health and substance use challenges.[315]

- *Try to minimize negative influences and behaviors in young people's lives.*[316] Talk to children early about the risks of alcohol and other drugs, both short-term (such as car crashes and other accidents) and long-term (such as reduced cognitive abilities). The earlier a child or adolescent begins using substances, the greater their chances of developing substance use problems.[317] Mental health and substance use problems can also occur at the same time. For example, some young people struggling with stress or difficult feelings turn to alcohol or drug use.[318] And alcohol and other drugs can also affect mental health, for example by altering mood or energy levels.[319]
- *Ensure children and youth have regular check-ups with a pediatrician, family doctor, or other health care professional.* Health care professionals can help you monitor your children's health, give you advice on how to prevent problems, and diagnose and treat physical and mental illnesses.
- Obtaining health insurance coverage for your children can help. To learn more about enrolling in Medicaid, the Children's Health Insurance Program (CHIP), or a Marketplace plan, go to HealthCare.gov or InsureKidsNow.gov.
- *Look out for warning signs of distress, and seek help when needed.* Signs of distress in children can show up in a number of ways, such as irritability, anger, withdrawal, and other changes in their thoughts, appearance, performance at school, sleeping or eating patterns, or other behaviors.)[320] If you notice concerning changes in your child, let them know you're there and ready to support them however they need. Don't be afraid to ask for help by talking to a doctor, nurse, or other professional or looking into other available resources in your community. For example, schools often have counseling services and additional accommodations (e.g., for students enrolled in special education programs).
- *Minimize children's access to means of self-harm, including firearms and prescription medications.* Dispose of unused or expired prescriptions and keep medications out of reach for children and youth. If you choose to keep firearms in the home, ensure that

---

[314] American Psychological Association. (2021 January 14). How to talk to children about difficult news. Accessed on November 29, 2021. Retrieved from https://www.apa.org/topics/ stress/talking.

[315] Centers for Disease Control and Prevention. (2021 January 5). Risk and Protective Factors. Accessed on November 12, 2021. Retrieved from https://www.cdc.gov/violenceprevention/aces/riskprotectivefactors.html.

[316] Centers for Disease Control and Prevention. (2020 February 10). Teen Substance Use & Risks. Accessed on November 30, 2021. Retrieved from https://www.cdc.gov/ncbddd/fasd/features/teen-substance-use.html.

[317] Hingson, R. W., & Zha, W. (2009). Age of drinking onset, alcohol use disorders, frequent heavy drinking, and unintentionally injuring oneself and others after drinking. *Pediatrics*, 123(6), 1477–1484. https://doi.org/10.1542/peds.2008-2176.

[318] Substance Abuse and Mental Health Services Administration. (2021 November 9). Warning Signs and Risk Factors for Emotional Distress. Accessed on November 30, 2021. Retrieved from https://www.samhsa.gov/find-help/disaster-distress-helpline/warning-signs-risk-factors.

[319] Centers for Disease Control and Prevention. (2021 May 11). Alcohol Use and Your Health. Accessed on November 30, 2021. Retrieved from https://www.cdc.gov/alcohol/fact-sheets/ alcohol-use.htm.

[320] National Eating Disorders Association. (2021). Warning signs and symptoms. Accessed on November 22,2021. Retrieved from https://www.nationaleatingdisorders.org/warning-signs-and-symptoms.

they are stored safely: unloaded and locked up (e.g., in a lock box or safe). Having firearms in the home increases the likelihood of firearm-related death.[321,322] In fact, firearms are by far the most lethal means of suicide: 90% of attempted suicides with a firearm result in death, compared to less than 10% of attempted suicides overall.[323]

- *Be attentive to how children and youth spend time online.* Digital technology can help young people connect with friends and family, learn about current events, express themselves, and access telehealth and other resources.[324] At the same time, children can have negative experiences online, such as being bullied, finding harmful information, and negatively comparing themselves to others.[325] Box 3 has a list of questions you can ask yourself about your child's use of technology.
- *Be a voice for mental health in your community.* There are many ways to do this, from talking openly with friends and family about the importance of mental health, to going to school board meetings or a town hall, to volunteering with an advocacy group, to promoting greater funding and awareness of mental health programs in schools and local organizations, such as churches, libraries, parks and recreation, or sports teams.

**BOX 3.** Technology and youth mental health: Questions for families to consider

Time

- How much time is my child spending online? Is it taking away from healthy offline activities, such as exercising, seeing friends, reading, and sleeping?
- Are there healthy limits I can set on my child's use of technology, such as limiting screen time to specific times of the day or week, or limiting certain kinds of uses?

Content

- Am I aware of what devices and content my child has access to?
- Is my child getting something meaningful and constructive out of content they are looking at, creating, or sharing? How do I know?

---

321 Korioth, T. (2018). Guns in child's home raise risk of suicide, unintentional death. Accessed on November 29, 2021. Retrieved from https://publications.aap.org/aapnews/news/10383.

322 Swanson, S. A., Eyllon, M., Sheu, Y. H., & Miller, M. (2020). Firearm access and adolescent suicide risk: toward a clearer understanding of effect size. Injury prevention: *Journal of the International Society for Child and Adolescent Injury Prevention*, 27(3), 264–270. Advance online publication. https://doi. org/10.1136/injuryprev-2019-043605.

323 Conner, A., Azrael, D., & Miller, M. (2019). Suicide Case-Fatality Rates in the United States, 2007 to 2014: A Nationwide Population-Based Study. *Annals of internal medicine*, 171(12), 885–895. https://doi.org/10.7326/M19-1324.

324 Rideout, V., Fox, S., Peebles, A., & Robb, M. B. (2021). Coping with COVID-19: How young people use digital media to manage their mental health. San Francisco, CA: Common Sense and Hopelab. Retrieved from: https://www.commonsensemedia.org/sites/default/files/uploads/research/2021-coping-with-covid19-full-report.pdf.

325 Coyne, S. M., Radesky, J., Collier, K. M., Gentile, D. A., Linder, J. R., Nathanson, A. I., Rasmussen, E. E., Reich, S. M., & Rogers, J. (2017). Parenting and Digital Media. *Pediatrics*, 140(Suppl 2), S112–S116. https://doi.org/10.1542/peds.2016-1758N.

- Are there healthier ways my child could engage online? (Examples: Finding meal recipes, researching options for a family outing, video chatting with a relative, etc.)
- Is being online riskier for my child than for some other children? For example, does my child have a mental health condition that might make them react more strongly to certain kinds of stressful or emotional content?

Impact

- How does my child feel about the time they spend online?
- Is my child engaging because they want to, or because they feel like they have to?
- How can I create space for open conversations with my child about their experiences online?
- How do I feel about my own use of technology? Can I be a better role model for my child?

**Resources for Families**

*Children's Mental Health and COVID-19 Parental Resources Kit (CDC):* Resources for supporting children's social, emotional, and mental health

*HealthyChildren.org (American Academy of Pediatrics):* Parenting tips and other resources

*What's On Your Mind? (UNICEF):* Guide for talking to children about mental health

*Family Resource Center (Child Mind Institute):* Family resources on child mental health, including Media Guidelines for Kids of All Ages

*(Common Sense Media):* Information about the safety of current media and technology trends and apps for your children

*HealthCare.gov or InsureKidsNow.gov:* Infor-mation on enrolling in health insurance coverage

*MentalHealth.gov:* What to look for, how to talk about mental health, and how to get help

*Aging and Disability Networks (ACL):* Connect with advocacy and caregiver resources

## What Educators, School Staff, and School Districts Can Do

The experiences children and young people have at school have a major impact on their mental health. At school, children can learn new knowledge and skills, develop close relationships with peers and supportive adults, and find a sense of purpose, fulfillment, and belonging. They can also find help to manage mental health challenges. On the other hand, children can also have highly negative experiences at school, such as being bullied, facing academic stress, or missing out on educational opportunities (for example, due to under-resourced schools). Mental health challenges can reveal themselves in a variety of ways at school, such as in a student having trouble concentrating in class, being withdrawn, acting out, or struggling to make friends. In light of these factors, below are recommendations for how schools, educators, and staff can support the mental health of all students:

- *Create positive, safe, and affirming school environments.* This could include developing and enforcing anti-bullying policies, training students and staff on how to prevent harm (e.g., implementing bystander interventions for staff and students), being proactive about talking to students and families about mental health, and using inclusive language and behaviors.[326],[327] Where feasible, school districts should also consider structural changes, such as a later start to the school day, that support students' wellbeing.[328,329]
- *Expand social and emotional learning programs and other evidence-based approaches that promote healthy development.* Examples of social, emotional, and behavioral learning programs include Sources of Strength, The Good Behavior Game, Life Skills Training, Check-In/Check-Out, and PATHS.[330],[331],[332],[333] Examples of other approaches include positive behavioral interventions and supports and digital media literacy education.
- *Learn how to recognize signs of changes in mental and physical health among students, including trauma and behavior changes. Take appropriate action when needed.*[334] Educators are often the first to notice if a student is struggling or behaving differently than usual (for example, withdrawing from normal activities or acting out). And educators are well-positioned to connect students to school counselors, nurses, or administrators who can further support students, including by providing or connecting students with services.[335]
- *Provide a continuum of supports to meet student mental health needs, including evidence-based prevention practices and trauma-informed mental health care.* Tiered

---

[326] Morgan Stanley Alliance for Children's Mental Health. (2021 August). Tips for Supporting Students' Mental Health This Fall. Accessed on November 12, 2021. Retrieved from: https://www.morganstanley.com/assets/pdfs/reemergence-program-educator-tips-english.pdf.

[327] Centers for Disease Control and Prevention. (2018 August 7). School Connectedness. Accessed on November 12, 2021. Retrieved from https://www.cdc.gov/healthyyouth/protective/school_connectedness.htm.

[328] Adolescent Sleep Working Group, Committee on Adolescence, & Council on School Health (2014). School start times for adolescents. *Pediatrics*, 134(3), 642–649. https://doi. org/10.1542/peds.2014-1697.

[329] Centers for Disease Control and Prevention. (2020 May 29). Sleep and Sleep Disorders. Accessed on November 22, 2021. Retrieved from https://www.cdc.gov/sleep/features/schools-start-too-early.html.

[330] Stone, D.M., Holland, K.M., Bartholow, B., Crosby, A.E., Davis, S., and Wilkins, N. (2017). Preventing Suicide: A Technical Package of Policies, Programs, and Practices. Atlanta, GA: National Center for Injury Prevention and Control, Centers for Disease Control and Prevention. Retrieved from: https://www. cdc.gov/violenceprevention/pdf/suicideTechnicalPackage.pdf.

[331] National Health Promotion Associates. Botvin Life Skills Training. Accessed on November 12, 2021. Retrieved from https://www.lifeskillstraining.com/.

[332] PATHS Program Holding, LLC. PATHS Program. Accessed on November 12, 2021. Retrieved from https://pathsprogram.com/.

[333] PBIS Rewards. (nd). Check-In/Check-Out Behavior Intervention & PBIS. Accessed on November 18, 2021. Retrieved from https://www.pbisrewards.com/blog/check-in-check-out-behavior-intervention/.

[334] Substance Abuse and Mental Health Services Administration. (2021 November 5). Recognizing and Treating Child Traumatic Stress. Accessed on November 12, 2021. Retrieved from https://www.samhsa.gov/child-trauma/recognizing-and-treating-child-traumatic-stress.

[335] U.S. Department of Health & Human Services (MentalHealth.gov). (2019 March 22). For Educators. Accessed on November 12, 2021. Retrieved from https://www. mentalhealth.gov/talk/educators.

supports should include coordination mechanisms to get students the right care at the right time.[336] For example, the Project AWARE (Advancing Wellness and Resilience in Education) program provides funds for state, local, and tribal governments to build school-provider partnerships and coordinate resources to support prevention, screening, early intervention, and mental health treatment for youth in school-based settings.[337] School districts could also improve the sharing of knowledge and best practices. For example, districts could dedicate staff at the district level to implementing evidence-based programs across multiple schools). Districts could also implement mental health literacy training for school personnel (e.g., Mental Health Awareness Training, QPR training).

- *Expand the school-based mental health workforce.*[338] This includes using federal, state, and local resources to hire and train additional staff, such as school counselors, nurses, social workers, and school psychologists, including dedicated staff to support students with disabilities. For example, a lack of school counselors makes it harder to support children experiencing mental health challenges. The American School Counselor Association (ASCA) recommends 1 counselor for every 250 students, compared to a national average of 1 counselor for every 424 students (with significant variation by state).[339] The American Rescue Plan's Elementary and Secondary School Emergency Relief funds can be used for this purpose and for other strategies outlined in this document.[340]
- *Support the mental health of all school personnel.* Opportunities include establishing realistic workloads and student-to-staff ratios, providing competitive wages and benefits (including health insurance with affordable mental health coverage), regularly assessing staff wellbeing, and integrating wellness into professional development.[341] In addition to directly benefitting school staff, these measures will also help school

---

336 National Association of School Psychologists. (2020). Providing effective social–emotional and behavioral supports after COVID-19 closures: Universal screening and Tier 1 interventions. Retrieved from https://www.nasponline.org/resources-and-publications/resources-and-podcasts/covid-19-resource-center/crisis-and-mental-health-resources/providing-effective-social%E2%80%93emotional-and-behavioral-supports-after-covid-19-closures-universal-screening-and-tier-1-interventions.

337 U.S. Department of Health and Human Services. (2021 August 27). SAMHSA Awards $74.2M in Grants to Strengthen Youth Mental Health. Press Release. Retrieved from https://www.hhs.gov/about/news/2021/08/27/samhsa-awards-74-2m-in-grants-to-strengthen-youth-mental-health.html.

338 National Academies of Sciences, Engineering, and Medicine. (2021). School-Based Strategies for Addressing the Mental Health and Well-Being of Youth in the Wake of COVID-19. Washington, DC: The National Academies Press. https://doi.org/10.17226/26262.

339 American School Counselor Association. (2021). School Counselor Roles & Ratios. Accessed on November 23, 2021. Retrieved from https://www.schoolcounselor.org/About-School-Counseling/School-Counselor-Roles-Ratios.

340 Department of Education, Office of Elementary & Secondary Education. (2021 March 17). American Rescue Plan Elementary and Secondary School Emergency Relief. Retrieved from https://oese.ed.gov/offices/american-rescue-plan/american-rescue-plan-elementary-and-secondary-school-emergency-relief/.

341 U.S. Department of Education, Office of Special Education and Rehabilitative Services. (2021). Supporting Child and Student Social, Emotional, Behavioral, and Mental Health Needs. Washington, DC. Retrieved from https://www2.ed.gov/documents/students/supporting-child-student-social-emotional-behavioral-mental-health.pdf.

personnel maintain their own empathy, compassion, and ability to create positive environments for students.[342]

- *Promote enrolling and retaining eligible children in Medicaid, CHIP, or a Marketplace plan, so that children have health coverage that includes behavioral health services.* The Connecting Kids to Coverage National Campaign also has outreach resources for schools, providers, and community-based organizations to use to encourage parents and caregivers to enroll in Medicaid and CHIP to access important mental health benefits. Families can be directed to HealthCare.gov or InsureKidsNow.gov. Schools can use Medicaid funds to support enrollment activities and mental health services.[343]
- *Protect and prioritize students with higher needs and those at higher risk of mental health challenges,* such as students with disabilities, personal or family mental health challenges, or other risk factors (e.g., adverse childhood experiences, trauma, poverty).[344]

**Resources for Educators, School Staff, and School Districts**

*Supporting Child and Student Social, Emotional, Behavioral, and Mental Health Needs* (Dept. of Education): Guidance for schools, school districts, and education departments

*National Center for School Mental Health:* Resources to promote a positive school climate

*StopBullying.gov:* Learn about what bullying is, who is at risk, and how you can help

*Turnaround for Children Toolbox:* Tools to drive change towards a more equitable, whole-child approach to school

*Design Principles for Schools:* Framework for redesigning schools with a focus on supporting students' learning and social and emotional development

*Safe Schools Fit Toolkit (National Center for Healthy Safe Children):* Resources and guides to build safe and healthy schools

*Mental Health Technology Transfer Center Network*: School mental health resources

## What Health Care Organizations and Health Professionals Can Do

Our health care system today is not set up to optimally support the mental health and wellbeing of children and youth. In addition to changing government policy (see recommendations for Governments on page 33), we must reimagine how health care organizations and health

342 Lever, N., Mathis, E., & Mayworm, A. (2017). School Mental Health Is Not Just for Students: Why Teacher and School Staff Wellness Matters. *Report on emotional & behavioral disorders in youth*, 17(1), 6–12.

343 Schubel, J. (2017 April 18). Medicaid Helps Schools Help Children. Center on Budget and Policy Priorities. Accessed on November 12, 2021. Retrieved from https://www.cbpp.org/research/health/medicaid-helps-schools-help-children.

344 U.S. Department of Education. (2020 June 25). Disability Discrimination. Accessed on November 12, 2021. Retrieved from https://www2.ed.gov/policy/rights/guid/ocr/disability.html.

professionals prevent, identify, and address mental health challenges. Below are some steps health care organizations and health professionals can take:

- *Recognize that the best treatment is prevention of mental health challenges. Implement trauma-informed care (TIC) principles and other prevention strategies to improve care for all youth, especially those with a history of adversity.* In addition to working in the clinic, for example to educate families on their role in healthy child development, health care professionals should work with other sectors (e.g., schools, child care, justice, social services, public health) on prevention strategies. For instance, health care professionals can refer patients to resources such as economic supports, school enrichment programs, and legal supports.[12]
- *Routinely screen children for mental health challenges and risk factors, including adverse childhood experiences (ACEs).[345] Screenings can be done in primary care, schools, emergency departments, and other settings.* For example, primary care providers can conduct screenings during well-visit appointments, annual physicals, or routine vaccinations using principles of trauma-informed care. Screenings should account for the diverse ways in which mental health challenges can manifest, such as changes in physical health, sleep patterns, and behaviors. It's critical that screening services link to appropriate follow-up care. The American Academy of Pediatrics offers tools and resources for screening processes. California's ACEs Aware initiative offers ACEs screening tools for children, adolescents, and young adults.
- *Identify and address the mental health needs of parents, caregivers, and other family members.* The mental health of children and youth is closely linked to the mental health and wellbeing of their families. Screening parents and caregivers for depression, intimate partner violence, substance use, and other challenges can be combined with broader assessments of food insecurity, housing instability, and other social determinants of health.[346]
- *Combine the efforts of clinical staff with those of trusted community partners and child-serving systems (e.g., child welfare, juvenile justice).* For example, hospital-based violence intervention programs (HVIPs) identify patients at risk of repeat violent injury and link them to hospital- and community-based resources to address risk

---

345 Watson P. (2019). How to screen for ACEs in an efficient, sensitive, and effective manner. *Paediatrics & Child Health*, 24(1), 37–38. https://doi.org/10.1093/pch/pxy146.

346 American Academy of Pediatrics. (2021 July 28). Interim Guidance on Supporting the Emotional and Behavioral Health Needs of Children, Adolescents, and Families During the COVID-19 Pandemic. Retrieved from https://www.aap.org/en/pages/2019-novel-coronavirus-covid-19-infections/clinical-guidance/interim-guidance-on-supporting-the-emotional-and-behavioral-health-needs-of-children-adolescents-and-families-during-the-covid-19-pandemic/.

factors for violence.[347,348,349,350] Another example initiative is school-hospital partnerships, such as behavioral health urgent care clinics supported by schools.[351] New payment and delivery models, such as the Centers for Medicare & Medicaid Services Innovation Center's Integrated Care for Kids (InCK) Model, can be used to support the mental health-related needs of children across settings.[352]

- *Build multidisciplinary teams to implement services that are tailored to the needs of children and their families.* Enlist children and families as partners and engage them in all stages of decision-making, from screening to treatment.[353] Recognize that a variety of cultural and other factors shape whether children and families are able or willing to seek mental health services. Accordingly, services should be culturally appropriate, offered in multiple languages (including ASL), and delivered by a diverse mental health workforce. Additionally, support the wellbeing of mental health workers and community leaders, building their capacity to support youth and their families.

**Resources for Health Care Organizations and Health Professionals**

*Mental Health Initiatives* (American Academy of Pediatrics): Information and guidance on supporting the healthy mental development of children, adolescents, and families. For example, see here for information on developing age-appropriate screening processes.

*HealthySteps Model* (Zero to Three): A primary care model that brings together child development experts, specialists, and pediatric primary care providers to promote healthy child development

*Evidence-Based Practices Resource Center* (Substance Abuse and Mental Health Services Administration): Information to incorporate evidence-based practices into communities and clinical settings

---

347 Juillard, C., Cooperman, L., Allen, I., Pirracchio, R., Henderson, T., Marquez, R., Orellana, J., Texada, M., & Dicker, R. A. (2016). A decade of hospital-based violence intervention: Benefits and shortcomings. The journal of trauma and acute care surgery, 81(6), 1156–1161. https://doi.org/10.1097/ TA.0000000000001261.

348 Bell, T. M., Gilyan, D., Moore, B. A., Martin, J., Ogbemudia, B., McLaughlin, B. E., Moore, R., Simons, C. J., & Zarzaur, B. L. (2018). Long-term evaluation of a hospital-based violence intervention program using a regional health information exchange. *The journal of trauma and acute care surgery*, 84(1), 175–182. https://doi.org/10.1097/ TA.0000000000001671.

349 The White House Briefing Room. (2021 April 7). FACT SHEET: More Details on the Biden-Harris Administration's Investments in Community Violence Interventions. Accessed on November 12, 2021. Retrieved from https://www.whitehouse.gov/briefing-room/statements-releases/2021/04/07/fact-sheet-more-details-on-the-biden-harris-administrations-investments-in-community-violence-interventions/.

350 U.S. Department of Justice, Office for Victims of Crime. (2021 May 19). OVC FY 2021 VOCA Victim Assistance Formula Grant. Accessed on November 12, 2021. Retrieved from https://ovc.ojp.gov/funding/opportunities/o-ovc-2021-19002.

351 NPR. (2021 June 11). How A Hospital And A School District Teamed Up To Help Kids In Emotional Crisis. Accessed on November 12, 2021. Retrieved from https://www.npr.org/sections/health-shots/2021/05/26/1000400903/n-y-hospital-schools-aim-to-improve-kids-access-to-mental-health-provider.

352 Centers for Medicare & Medicaid Services. (2021 May 04). Integrated Care for Kids (InCK) Model. Accessed on November 12, 2021. Retrieved from https://innovation.cms.gov/innovation-models/integrated-care-for-kids-model.

353 Walking The Talk. (nd). A toolkit for engaging youth in mental health: Create Youth-friendly spaces. Accessed on November 12, 2021. Retrieved from: http://www.yetoolkit.ca/ content/create-youth-friendly-spaces.

| |
|---|
| *Behavioral Health Integration Compendium* (American Medical Association): Steps for integrating behavioral health care into a clinical practice<br>*Telemental Health Resource Center* (Western Regional Children's Advocacy Center): Information and tools to set up telehealth programs for mental health<br>*ACEs Screening Tools* (California's ACEs Aware Initiative): Offers tools to screen children, adolescents, and adults for ACEs<br>*Trauma Screening Tools* (Childhood Trauma Toolkit, Centre for Addiction and Mental Health): ACEs questionnaire and developmental trauma symptom screening checklist |

## What Media Organizations, Entertainment Companies, and Journalists Can Do

*Note: See next section for recommendations specific to technology platforms such as social media companies.*

Media organizations, entertainment companies, and journalists can have a powerful impact on young people. In some cases, this impact can be positive. For example, television programs can keep children and adolescents informed about current events and teach them valuable lessons.[354] On the other hand, false, misleading, or exaggerated media narratives can perpetuate misconceptions and stigma against people with mental health or substance use problems.[355,356] In addition, media coverage of traumatic events, such as bombings and natural disasters, can contribute to psychological distress among consumers.[357,358,359,360,361] Particularly in times of global crisis, such as the COVID-19 pandemic, people can come away from news stories

[354] Impact of media use on children and youth. (2003). *Paediatrics & child health*, 8(5), 301–317. https://doi. org/10.1093/pch/8.5.301.

[355] McGinty, E. E., Webster, D. W., & Barry, C. L. (2013). Effects of news media messages about mass shootings on attitudes toward persons with serious mental illness and public support for gun control policies. *The American journal of psychiatry*, 170(5), 494–501. https://doi.org/10.1176/appi.ajp.2013.13010014.

[356] Klin, A., & Lemish, D. (2008). Mental disorders stigma in the media: review of studies on production, content, and influences. *Journal of health communication*, 13(5), 434–449. https://doi.org/10.1080/10810730802198813.

[357] Pfefferbaum, B., Nixon, S. J., Tucker, P. M., Tivis, R. D., Moore, V. L., Gurwitch, R. H., Pynoos, R. S., & Geis, H. K. (1999). Posttraumatic stress responses in bereaved children after the Oklahoma City bombing. *Journal of the American Academy of Child and Adolescent Psychiatry*, 38(11), 1372–1379. https://doi. org/10.1097/00004583-199911000-00011.

[358] Holman, E. A., Garfin, D. R., & Silver, R. C. (2014). Media's role in broadcasting acute stress following the Boston Marathon bombings. *Proceedings of the National Academy of Sciences of the United States of America*, 111(1), 93–98. https:// doi.org/10.1073/pnas.1316265110.

[359] Johnston, W. M., & Davey, G. C. (1997). The psychological impact of negative TV news bulletins: the catastrophizing of personal worries. *British journal of psychology* (London, England: 1953), 88 (Pt 1), 85–91. https://doi. org/10.1111/j.2044-8295.1997.tb02622.x.

[360] Thompson, R. R., Jones, N. M., Holman, E. A., & Silver, R. C. (2019). Media exposure to mass violence events can fuel a cycle of distress. *Science advances*, 5(4), eaav3502. https://doi. org/10.1126/sciadv.aav3502.

[361] Stainback, K., Hearne, B. N., & Trieu, M. M. (2020). COVID-19 and the 24/7 News Cycle: Does COVID-19 News Exposure Affect Mental Health? *Socius: Sociological Research for a Dynamic World;* (6). https://doi. org/10.1177/2378023120969339.

feeling anxious and powerless.[362] Below are steps media organizations can take to protect the mental health of viewers while staying true to their role in informing the public:

- *Recognize the impact media coverage of negative events can have on the public's mental health.* The solution isn't to hide or downplay negative news, but rather to avoid misleading consumers, and to be more attentive to how stories are framed. Example best practices include:
  - Being fact-based in reporting and avoiding language that shocks, provokes, or creates a sense of panic.
  - Being more cautious about showing distressing content, particularly graphic images or video, without context or warnings for viewers. Help viewers decide whether they want to engage with the content.[363]
  - Giving audiences context, including highlighting uncertainties and conflicting reports. When discussing preliminary research—such as papers that have not yet been peer-reviewed—outlets should be forthright about the preliminary nature of the findings, get independent experts to weigh in, and identify areas of uncertainty.
  - Offering the public ways to make a positive difference (for example, ways to donate funds or supplies to victims of a natural disaster).
  - Including positive messages and stories of hope and healing (particularly when covering pandemics, natural disasters, and incidents of mass violence).
- Normalize stories about mental health and mental illness across all forms of media, taking care to avoid harmful stereotypes, promote scientifically accurate information, and include stories of help, hope, and healing. Example best practices[364] include:
- Avoiding harmful stereotypes about mental illness, such as the idea that people who have a mental illness are prone to violence or that mental illness causes violence. Research shows this is not the case.[365]
  - Avoiding demeaning language (e.g., "crazy," "psycho," "looney," "wacko," "nut," "junkie"). This includes using person-centered language, or language that focuses on the person rather than a disease label.[366] For example, instead of referring to someone as a "schizophrenic," refer to them as a "person living with schizophrenia."

---

[362] Su, Z., McDonnell, D., Wen, J., Kozak, M., Abbas, J., Šegalo, S., Li, X., Ahmad, J., Cheshmehzangi, A., Cai, Y., Yang, L., & Xiang, Y. T. (2021). Mental health consequences of COVID-19 media coverage: the need for effective crisis communication practices. *Globalization and health*, 17(1), 4. https://doi.org/10.1186/s12992-020-00654-4.

[363] Mental Health Media Guide. (nd). Step 5: Support Your Audience Before, During, and After Viewing. Accessed on November 12, 2021. Retrieved from https://mentalhealthmediaguide.com/guide-front-page/tips-by-step/support-your-audience-before-during-after-viewing/.

[364] Stanford University, Department of Psychiatry and Behavioral Sciences. (nd). Media & Mental Health Initiative (MMHI). Accessed on November 12, 2021. Retrieved from https://med. stanford.edu/psychiatry/special-initiatives/mediamh.html.

[365] Choe, J. Y., Teplin, L. A., & Abram, K. M. (2008). Perpetration of violence, violent victimization, and severe mental illness: balancing public health concerns. *Psychiatric services* (Washington, D.C.), 59(2), 153–164. https://doi.org/10.1176/ ps.2008.59.2.153.

[366] Crocker, A. F., & Smith, S. N. (2019). Person-first language: are we practicing what we preach?. *Journal of multidisciplinary healthcare*, 12, 125–129. https://doi. org/10.2147/JMDH.S140067.

  - Include stories of people seeking help, getting treatment, and successfully recovering. These can also include examples of people getting help from friends, family neighbors, or even strangers (not just mental health professionals).[367]
  - Direct consumers to mental health resources (as part of any mental health-related TV episode, movie, news story, podcast, or other media).
  - Craft more authentic stories by consulting with subject matter experts and people with personal experience of mental illness or mental health challenges.
- Whenever depicting suicide or suicidal ideation, adhere to best practices such as the National Recommendations for Depicting Suicide.[368] For example:
  - Convey that suicide is complex and often caused by multiple factors, not a single event.
  - Show that help is available. For example, in TV shows or movies, show characters reaching out to health professionals, talking to supportive peers, friends, or family, or calling or texting a crisis hotline.

**Resources for Media Organizations, Entertainment Companies, and Journalists**

*Mental Health Media Guide:* A guide to mental health storytelling developed by a coalition of mental health experts and entertainment industry leaders

*National Center on Disability and Journalism Resources:* Effective, sensitive ways to talk about disability in the media

*National Recommendations for Depicting Suicide (National Action Alliance):* Guidance for content creators to tell more balanced and authentic stories involving suicide

## What Social Media, Video Gaming, and Other Technology Companies Can Do

Over the past two decades, more and more of our lives have moved onto social media platforms and other digital public spaces. The COVID-19 pandemic has rapidly accelerated this trend. During the pandemic, the time teenagers spent in front of screens for activities not related to school more than doubled, from 3.8 to 7.7 hours per day.[369] In 2020, 81% of 14- to 22-year-olds said they used social media either "daily" or "almost constantly."[138]

---

[367] Metzl, J. M., & MacLeish, K. T. (2015). Mental illness, mass shootings, and the politics of American firearms. *American journal of public health*, 105(2), 240–249. https://doi. org/10.2105/AJPH.2014.302242.

[368] National Action Alliance for Suicide Prevention. (2019). National Recommendations for Depicting Suicide. Accessed on November 12, 2021. Retrieved from https://theactionalliance. org/resource/national-recommendations-depicting-suicide.

[369] Nagata, J. M., Cortez, C. A., Cattle, C. J., Ganson, K. T., Iyer, P., Bibbins-Domingo, K., & Baker, F. C. (2021). Screen Time Use Among US Adolescents During the COVID-19 Pandemic: Findings From the Adolescent Brain Cognitive Development (ABCD) Study. *JAMA pediatrics*, 10.1001/jamapediatrics.2021.4334. Advance online publication. https://doi.org/10.1001/jamapediatrics.2021.4334.

In these digital public spaces, which privately owned and tend to be run for profit, there can be tension between what's best for the technology company and what's best for the individual user or for society. Business models are often built around maximizing user engagement as opposed to safeguarding users' health and ensuring that users engage with one another in safe and healthy ways.[370,371] This translates to technology companies focusing on maximizing time spent, not time well spent.

In recent years, there has been growing concern about the impact of digital technologies, particularly social media, on the mental health and wellbeing of children and young people.[372,373,374] Part of the challenge with research on this topic is that digital technology involves a vast range of devices, platforms, products, and activities, so it's hard to generalize. Researchers also have limited access to data to inform potential research.

Many researchers argue that digital technologies can expose children to bullying, contribute to obesity and eating disorders, trade off with sleep, encourage children to negatively compare themselves to others, and lead to depression, anxiety, and self-harm.[139,187,375,376,377,378] Several studies have linked time spent on social media to mental health challenges such as

---

370 New Public. (2021 January 11). Building better digital public spaces, "Civic Signals: The qualities of flourishing digital spaces," Research Overview. Accessed on November 12, 2021. Retrieved from https://newpublic.org/signals and https://docs. google.com/presentation/d/1lO4skPVekwciJGFYxxJBIBitFzzDSC0zL1-AvhgfeNs/.

371 5Rights Foundation. (2021). Pathways: How digital design puts children at risk. Accessed on November 12, 2021. Retrieved from https://5rightsfoundation.com/uploads/Pathways-how-digital-design-puts-children-at-risk.pdf.

372 Council on Communications and Media. (2016). Media and Young Minds. *Pediatrics*, 138(5), e20162591. https://doi. org/10.1542/peds.2016-2591.

373 Hill D. L. (2020). Social Media: Anticipatory Guidance. *Pediatrics in review*, 41(3), 112–119. https://doi.org/10.1542/ pir.2018-0236.

374 Haidt, J., & Twenge, J. (2021). Social media use and mental health: A review. Unpublished manuscript, New York University. https://docs.google.com/document/d/1w-HOfseF2wF9YIpXwUUtP65-olnkPyWcgF5BiAtBEy0/edit.

375 Hagan, J. F., Shaw, J. S., & Duncan, M. P. (2017). *Bright Futures: Guidelines for Health Supervision of Infants, Children, and Adolescents.* 4th ed. Elk Grove Village, IL: American Academy of Pediatrics. https://brightfutures.aap.org/Bright%20Futures%20 Documents/BF4_HealthySocialMedia.pdf.

376 Chang, A. M , Aeschbach, D., Duffy, J. F., & Czeisler, C. A. (2015). Evening use of light-emitting eReaders negatively affects sleep, circadian timing, and next-morning alertness. *Proceedings of the National Academy of Sciences of the United States of America*, 112(4), 1232–1237. https://doi.org/10.1073/pnas.1418490112.

377 Sumner, S. A., Ferguson, B., Bason, B., Dink, J., Yard, E., Hertz, M., Hilkert, B., Holland, K., Mercado-Crespo, M., Tang, S., & Jones, C. M. (2021). Association of Online Risk Factors With Subsequent Youth Suicide-Related Behaviors in the US. *JAMA network open*, 4(9), e2125860. https://doi.org/10.1001/ jamanetworkopen.2021.25860.

378 Swedo, E. A., Beauregard, J. L., de Fijter, S., Werhan, L., Norris, K., Montgomery, M. P., Rose, E. B., David-Ferdon, C., Massetti, G. M., Hillis, S. D., & Sumner, S. A. (2021). Associations Between Social Media and Suicidal Behaviors During a Youth Suicide Cluster in Ohio. *The Journal of adolescent health*, 68(2), 308–316. https://doi.org/10.1016/j. jadohealth.2020.05.049.

anxiety and depression.[26,379,380,381,382,383] Meanwhile, others have cast doubt on the idea that technology or social media use is a major factor in youth wellbeing.[384,385, 386,387,388,389]

Importantly, the impact of technology almost certainly varies from person to person, and it also matters what technology is being used and how.[390] So, even if technology doesn't harm young people on average, certain kinds of online activities likely do harm some young people. For example, some research has linked "passive" social media use (such as scrolling through posts and auto-play video) to declines in wellbeing (versus more "active" use such as commenting on posts or recording videos).[391]

There can also be benefits to certain online activities, such as connecting meaningfully with friends and family, learning a new skill, or accessing health care, and these also vary from person to person.[392] For example, LGBTQ+ young people may be more vulnerable than other

---

379 McCrae, N., Gettings, S. & Purssell, E. (2017). Social Media and Depressive Symptoms in Childhood and Adolescence: A Systematic Review. *Adolescent Res Rev*, 2: 315–330. https://doi. org/10.1007/s40894-017-0053-4.

380 Allcott, H., Braghieri, L., Eichmeyer, S., & Gentzkow, M. (2020). "The Welfare Effects of Social Media." *American Economic Review*, 110 (3): 629-76. https://www.aeaweb.org/ articles?id=10.1257/aer.20190658.

381 Ra, C. K., Cho, J., Stone, M. D., De La Cerda, J., Goldenson, N. I., Moroney, E., Tung, I., Lee, S. S., & Leventhal, M. (2018). Association of Digital Media Use With Subsequent Symptoms of Attention-Deficit/Hyperactivity Disorder Among Adolescents. *JAMA*, 320(3), 255–263. https://doi.org/10.1001/ jama.2018.8931.

382 American Psychiatric Association. (2018 June). Internet Gaming. Accessed on November 12, 2021. Retrieved from https://www.psychiatry.org/patients-families/internet-gaming.

383 Przybylski, A. K., Weinstein, N., & Murayama, K. (2017). Internet Gaming Disorder: Investigating the Clinical Relevance of a New Phenomenon. *The American journal of psychiatry*, 174(3), 230–236. https://doi.org/10.1176/appi. ajp.2016.16020224.

384 Orben, A., & Przybylski, A. K. (2019). The association between adolescent well-being and digital technology use. *Nature human behaviour*, 3(2), 173–182. https://doi.org/10.1038/ s41562-018-0506-1.

385 Coyne, S. M., Rogers, A. A., Zurcher, J. D., Stockdale, L., & Booth M. (2020). Does time spent using social media impact mental health?: An eight year longitudinal study. *Computers in Human Behavior*, 104. https://doi.org/10.1016/j. chb.2019.106160.

386 Orben, A., Dienlin, T., & Przybylski, A. K. (2019). Social media's enduring effect on adolescent life satisfaction. *Proceedings of the National Academy of Sciences of the United States of America*, 116(21), 10226–10228. https://doi.org/10.1073/ pnas.1902058116.

387 George, M. J., Jensen, M. R., Russell, M. A., Gassman-Pines, A., Copeland, W. E., Hoyle, R. H., & Odgers, C. L. (2020). Young Adolescents' Digital Technology Use, Perceived Impairments, and Well-Being in a Representative Sample. *The Journal of pediatrics*, 219, 180–187. https://doi.org/10.1016/j. jpeds.2019.12.002.

388 Odgers, C. L., & Jensen, M. R. (2020). Annual Research Review: Adolescent mental health in the digital age: facts, fears, and future directions. *Journal of child psychology and psychiatry, and allied disciplines*, 61(3), 336–348. https://doi.org/10.1111/ jcpp.13190.

389 Valkenburg, P. M., Meier, A., & Beyens, I. (2021). Social media use and its impact on adolescent mental health: An umbrella review of the evidence. *Current opinion in psychology*, 44, 58–68. Advance online publication. https://doi. org/10.1016/j.copsyc.2021.08.017.

390 Beyens, I., Pouwels, J. L., van Driel, I. I., Keijsers, L., & Valkenburg, P. M. (2020). The effect of social media on well-being differs from adolescent to adolescent. *Scientific reports*, 10(1), 10763. https://doi.org/10.1038/s41598-020-67727-7.

391 Verduyn, P., Lee, D. S., Park, J., Shablack, H., Orvell, Bayer, J., . . . Kross, E. (2015). Passive Facebook usage undermines affective well-being: Experimental and longitudinal evidence. *Journal of Experimental Psychology:* General, 144(2), 480-488. http://dx.doi.org/10.1037/xge0000057.

392 Przybylski, A. K., & Weinstein, N. (2017). A large-scale test of the Goldilocks hypothesis: Quantifying the relations between digital-screen use and the mental well-being of adolescents. *Psychological Science*, 28(2), 204–215. https://doi. org/10.1177/0956797616678438.

young people to cyberbullying but also more likely to consider social media important for feeling less alone, expressing themselves, finding inspiration, and getting support.[138,393]

There is a clear need to better understand the impact of technologies such as social media on different kinds of users, and to address the harms to users most at risk. We need more research using strong data and research methods, such as longitudinal and experimental designs, behavioral (as opposed to self-reported) measures of time spent online and types of content engaged with, as well as data on subgroups of users (e.g., boys vs. girls).[394,395]

Most importantly, technology companies must step up and take responsibility for creating a safe digital environment for children and youth. Today, most companies are not transparent about the impact of their products, which prevents parents and young people from making informed decisions and researchers from identifying problems and solutions. At a minimum, the public and researchers deserve much more transparency. More broadly, below are specific recommendations for how these companies can prioritize the wellbeing of users above monetizing those users for profit:

- Prioritize user health and wellbeing at all stages of product development.[396]
    - *Elevate user safety, health, and wellbeing in the culture and leadership of technology companies.* Senior technology executives should acknowledge that their products can harm some young people and take material and measurable steps to prevent and mitigate these harms, even at the expense of engagement, scale, and profit. Leaders should be accountable for creating a safe, accessible, and inclusive digital environment for their users and designing safe products.
    - *Assess and address risks to users at the front end of product development.* Build products and services using a precautionary approach that focuses on making them safe for youth before they are deployed. Company employees at all levels, especially those involved in product development, should be expected to prioritize user health and wellbeing in their day-to-day work. For example, consider how to align performance incentives for product developers to measures of user wellbeing. Develop consistent procedures for receiving input on proposed products from youth, parents, health and youth development professionals, and civil society, for example through advisory groups. Create ways for employees to voice concerns about products without fear of retaliation.
    - *Continually measure the impact of products on user health and wellbeing and share data with the public.* Supplement traditional product success metrics, such as monthly active users, with dedicated metrics for user health and wellbeing. In addition to relying on user-reported data (e.g., surveys), consider using behavioral

---

393 Hinduja, S. & Patchin, J. W. (2020). Bullying, Cyberbullying, and LGBTQ Students. *Cyberbullying Research Center.* Retrieved from https://cyberbullying.org/bullying-cyberbullying-sexual-orientation-lgbtq.pdf.

394 Dickson, K., Richardson, M., Kwan, I., MacDowall, W., Burchett, H., Stansfield, C., Brunton, G., Sutcliffe, K., & Thomas, J. (2018). Screen-based activities and children and young people's mental health: A Systematic Map of Reviews, London: EPPI-Centre, Social Science Research Unit, UCL Institute of Education, University College London.

395 Parry, D. A., Fisher, J. T., Mieczkowski, H., Sewall, C. J. R., & Davidson, B. I. (2021). Social Media and Well-being: A Methodological Perspective. PsyArXiv Preprints. https://doi. org/10.31234/osf.io/exhru.

396 Lenhart, A., & Owens, K. (2021). The Unseen Teen: The Challenges of Building Healthy Tech for Young People. Data & Society. Retrieved from: https://datasociety.net/wp-content/ uploads/2021/05/The-Unseen-Teen-.pdf.

data (e.g., analysis of user inputs such as typed keywords). Make results publicly available. Take corrective action to address harms.
    - *Recognize that the impact of platforms and products can vary from user to user, and proactively ensure that products designed for adults are also safe for children and adolescents.* Consider many kinds of users, including users of different ages and developmental stages, when developing new products and features. Talk to those users and collect data to identify subgroups who may be harmed by certain products or ways of engaging. Use this data to inform product design and research.
- Be transparent and allow for independent researchers and the public to study the impact of company products on user health and wellbeing.
    - *Allow users to provide informative data about their online experience to independent researchers.* This should be a fully consented process that allows users to individually request personal data about their use to transfer to researchers (e.g., timestamps of when and how long use takes place; type of content seen and engaged with; whether, when, and how interactions with others took place). Companies should also allow third-party researchers to request data on behalf of users if evidence of full user consent is provided and facilitate the automated transfer of data to third-party researchers (e.g., through application programming interfaces or APIs).
    - *Directly provide researchers with data to enable understanding of (a) subgroups of users most at risk of harm and (b) algorithmic design and operation.* Data on algorithmic design and operation should be of sufficient granularity to allow researchers to understand when, why, and how users are shown different types of content.
    - *Partner with researchers and experts to analyze the mental health impacts of new products and features in advance of rollout. Regularly publish findings.* Where possible, design evaluations in ways that enable causal inference (for example, using randomized interventions).
    - *Allow a broad range of researchers to access data and previous research instead of providing access to a privileged few.* Make research results publicly available and do not bind researchers to non-disclosure agreements. Avoid conflicts of interest that cast doubt on researchers' independence.
- Build user-friendly tools that help children and adolescents engage online in healthy ways.
    - *Take a holistic approach to designing online spaces hospitable to young people.* For example, support the creation of industry-wide safety standards for online health and wellbeing, in partnership with civil society groups. Just as we have safety standards for offline activities, such as driving, we should also consider standards for online activities.[397,398] Private organizations, such as video game

---

[397] Austrialian Government, eSafety Commissioner. (nd). Safety by Design. Accessed on November 12, 2021. Retrieved from https://www.esafety.gov.au/about-us/safety-by-design/principles-and-background.

[398] Meyer, M., Adkins, V., Yuan, N., Weeks, H. M., Chang, Y. J., & Radesky, J. (2019). Advertising in Young Children's Apps: A Content Analysis. *Journal of developmental and behavioral pediatrics: JDBP*, 40(1), 32–39. https://doi.org/10.1097/ DBP.0000000000000622.

companies, have already begun sharing best practices and developing a common framework for protecting users.[399]

- *Limit children's exposure to harmful online content.* This can involve a mix of limiting access for younger users, reducing content amplification, prohibiting data collection of and targeted advertising to children, ensuring privacy settings are maximized by default, removing content quickly if it violates company policies, tightening age verification requirements and audits, enabling independent algorithm audits, and imposing consequences for users found to be circumventing age restrictions or other policies.[227] Companies should conduct research to evaluate whether these measures work. For example, children today can easily get around age limits by claiming to be older than they really are. To address this, some companies have required users to upload an ID and a selfie to verify identity and age (without storing the underlying ID or selfie data).[400]
- *Give users opportunities to control their online activity, including by opting out of content they may find harmful.* For example, some companies have built in "frictions," such as notifications that remind people to take breaks and limit screen time.[401] Other examples of frictions could include banning "auto-play" functions on videos or limiting scrolling capabilities for youth users. Also consider allowing users to opt out of content they believe may harm their mental health, such as ads involving violence, alcohol, or gambling, or content related to eating disorders.[402]
- *Develop products that actively safeguard and promote mental health and wellbeing.* New technologies create opportunities to reach large numbers of youth with educational interventions, such as directing youth to mental health tips and resources.[403] There are also emerging digital technologies—often referred to as "digital therapeutics"—that prevent, manage, and treat health conditions. More and more of these technologies are gaining clinical validation and regulatory approval.[404,405]

- *Promote equitable access to technology that supports the wellbeing of children and youth.* For example, donate digital technology and remote services (e.g., internet access) to under-resourced populations.

---

399 Fair Play Alliance. (nd). Fair Play Alliance. Accessed on November 12, 2021. Retrieved from https://fairplayalliance.org/.

400 Chen, C. A. (2021 September 21). Introducing Age Verification. Roblox. Accessed on November 12, 2021. Retrieved from https://blog.roblox.com/2021/09/introducing-age-verification/.

401 Elgersma, C. (2019 September 23). How to Use Apple's Screen Time Feature. Common Sense Media. Accessed on November 12, 2021. Retrieved from https://www.commonsensemedia.org/blog/ how-to-use-apples-screen-time-feature.

402 Davies, R. (2020 December 10). Google to let YouTube users opt out of gambling and alcohol ads. The Guardian. Accessed on November 12, 2021. Retrieved from https://www. theguardian.com/technology/2020/dec/10/google-to-allow-youtube-users-in-uk-to-opt-out-of-gambling-and-alcohol-ads.

403 World Health Organization. (2021 October 4). WHO brings vital mental health messages to gamers via digital channels. Accessed on November 12, 2021. Retrieved from https://www. who.int/news/item/04-10-2021-the-who-and-angry-birds-friends-team-up-for-world-mental-health-day.

404 Makin S. (2019). The emerging world of digital therapeutics. *Nature*, 573(7775), S106–S109. https://doi. org/10.1038/d41586-019-02873-1.

405 Hackett, A., Hung, A., Leclerc, O., & Velamoor, S. (2020 March 31). The promise of digital therapeutics. *McKinsey & Company*. Accessed on November 23, 2021. Retrieved from https://www.mckinsey.com/industries/ life-sciences/our-insights/ the-promise-of-digital-therapeutics.

| Resources for Social Media, Video Gaming, and Other Technology Companies |
|---|
| *Safety by Design* (Australia's eSafety Commissioner): Ways technology companies can minimize online threats and harms before they occur |
| *Toolkit for Technologists* (Center for Humane Technology): Principles to help create value-driven and humane technology environments |
| *The Children's Code* (UK's Information Commissioner): Standards for online services to protect children's safety, rights, and privacy online |
| *The Unseen Teen (Data & Society):* A report with challenges and recommendations on improving digital wellbeing for adolescent users |
| *The U.S. Access Board:* U.S. federal agency providing technical assistance for content creators and developers |

## What Community Organizations Can Do

Thousands of community organizations are doing heroic work every day to support the mental health of children and young people. While different groups address different parts of the problem, serve different youth populations, and implement different solutions, all community organizations can keep the following recommendations in mind as they continue their work:

- *Educate the public about the importance of mental health, and reduce negative stereotypes, bias, and stigma around mental illness.* Community groups can play a key role in fostering open dialogue about mental health at the local level and correcting misconceptions and biases. For example, community groups can partner with trusted messengers such as faith leaders and health care professionals to speak to community members about youth mental health needs. It's particularly important to address misconceptions in populations that have an outsized influence over young people, such as families, educators, health care professionals, juvenile justice officials, online influencers, and the media.
- *Implement evidence-based programs that promote healthy development, support children, youth, and their families, and increase their resilience.* Examples include youth enrichment programs (e.g., mentoring, after-school programs), skill-based parenting and family relationship approaches, and other efforts that address social determinants of youth health such as poverty, exposure to trauma, and lack of access to education and health care. A few respected programs include The Incredible Years,[406] Strengthening Families,[220] The Martinsburg Initiative,[407] and the Drug-Free Communities (DFC) Support Program.[408]

---

[406] Centers for Disease Control and Prevention. (2019). Preventing Adverse Childhood Experiences: Leveraging the Best Available Evidence. Atlanta, GA: National Center for Injury Prevention and Control, Centers for Disease Control and Prevention. Retrieved from: https://www.cdc.gov/ violenceprevention/pdf/preventingACES.pdf.

[407] The Martinsburg Initiative. (2020). The Martinsburg Initiative: A Model Solution To A National Problem. Retrieved from: https://themartinsburginitiative.com/.

[408] Centers for Disease Control and Prevention (2021). Drug-Free Communities Support Program. Accessed on October 7, 2021. Retrieved from: https://www.cdc.gov/drugoverdose/drug-free-communities/about.html.

- *Ensure that programs rigorously evaluate mental health-related outcomes.* For example, track outcomes around anxiety, depression, and suicide (including ideation, plans, and attempts), as well as around upstream risk and protective factors (e.g., social connectedness, coping skills, economic supports).[409]
- *Address the unique mental health needs of at-risk youth, such as racial and ethnic minorities, LGBTQ+ youth, and youth with disabilities.* Youth-serving organizations should think intentionally about how and to whom program services are offered. For example, actively recruit and engage populations who have historically been prevented from equal access to opportunities and may benefit the most from services. Engage with youth to understand what unique barriers prevent them from accessing mental health services. Recruit program staff directly from communities being served. Build program staff capacity to recognize personal biases, as well as structural challenges in these communities. For example, provide training on cultural and linguistic competence and related topics.
- *Elevate the voices of children, young people, and their families.* Youth are experts on their own lives, so it is important to engage youth in community-based mental health efforts. Explore youth advisory councils and other ways to involve young people in all phases of programming, from ideation to implementation. Gather feedback to understand what is and isn't working. Include youth and families directly in delivering services, for example by creating peer support programs.

**Resources for Community Organizations**

*Having conversations in your community* (MentalHealth.gov): Provides a toolkit to help communities and groups plan and facilitate dialogues about mental health.

*Preventing Adverse Childhood Experiences (ACEs)* (CDC): Guidance to equip communities with the best available evidence for the prevention of ACEs

*A Comprehensive Technical Package for the Prevention of Youth Violence and Associated Risk Behaviors* (CDC): Strategies to help communities sharpen their focus on prevention activities to stop youth violence and its consequences

*Preventing Suicide: A Technical Package of Policy, Programs, and Practices* (CDC): Strategies to help communities sharpen their focus on activities to prevent suicide

*The Community Guide on Mental Health* (Community Preventive Services Task Force, or CPSTF): Evidence-based findings to select community interventions to improve mental health

*Mentoring for Youth with Mental Health Challenges* (National Mentoring Resource Center): Research on mentoring for youth (ages 18 and younger) experiencing mental health challenges

---

[409] U.S. Department of Health and Human Services (HHS) Office of the Surgeon General, & National Action Alliance for Suicide Prevention. (2021). The Surgeon General's Call to Action to Implement The National Strategy for Suicide Prevention. HHS. https://www.hhs.gov/sites/default/files/sprc-call-to-action.pdf.

## What Funders and Foundations Can Do

Philanthropic and other funding organizations play a critical role in supporting the mental health of children and young people across the full continuum of need. For example, they can make bets on promising but untested technologies or programs for which government funding may not be available. They can also serve as reliable partners to community-based organizations across the country, and promote and build cross-sector partnerships. Below are some recommendations for how funding organizations can support youth mental health:

- *Create sustained investments in equitable prevention, promotion, and early intervention.* Prioritize interventions that address social and economic factors known to affect children's healthy development and mental health, such as poverty, discrimination, and inequality, among others.[410]
- *Incentivize coordination across grantees and foster cross-sector partnerships to maximize reach and bring together a diversity of expertise.* The scale and complexity of mental health issues among young people require collaborative approaches. Consider leveraging resources across sectors to advance practices, policies, and research that support the mental health of children, youth, and families. And support grantees in developing and sharing meaningful mental health outcome measures.
- *Scale up evidence-based interventions, technologies, and services.* Use a structured process to assess an intervention's readiness to scale and support high-quality implementation at a community level.[411] Share information and convene stakeholders to provide education and consultation to spread innovation.
- *Invest in innovative approaches and research on mental health.* For example, fund participatory research that involves young people in understanding their online experiences. Develop and test new solutions, including digitally enabled solutions that can reach young people at scale and in underserved communities. Consider different kinds of funding models, such as incubators and accelerators, that can drive funding toward promising projects at very early stages.[412,413]
- *Elevate and amplify the voices of youth and families in all stages of funding and evaluation.* Listening to young people is critical to understanding what kinds of solutions will work and what communities need to scale successful interventions. Bring young people, parents, and caregivers to the table to identify their needs and create ongoing meaningful opportunities to inform grantmaking strategies and decision-making. Engage youth from different identities and backgrounds—particularly those that come from vulnerable communities.

---

410 Dopp, A. R., & Lantz, P. M. (2020). Moving Upstream to Improve Children's Mental Health Through Community and Policy Change. *Administration and policy in mental health*, 47(5), 779–787. https://doi.org/10.1007/s10488-019-01001-5.

411 Needels, K., Richman, S., Maxwell, N., & Anderson M.A. (2020). Scaling an Intervention: Recommendations and Resources, A Guide for Funders and Grantmakers. AmeriCorps and Mathematica. Retrieved from: https://americorps.gov/sites/default/files/document/AmeriCorps_ScalingRecsAndResources_ORE_9Apr2021.pdf.

412 Headstream. (nd). Building wellness through inclusive digital experiences. Accessed on November 12, 2021. Retrieved from https://www.headstreaminnovation.com/.

413 University of California Berkeley. (nd). The Fung Fellowship. Accessed on November 12, 2021. Retrieved from https://fungfellows.berkeley.edu/about/our-story/.

**Resources for Funders and Foundations**

*Grantmakers in Health:* Resources for health funders to learn, connect, and grow

*Incorporating Youth Voice and the Lived Experience in Research (NAM):* Seminar examining the importance of including youth voices in research

*Health in Mind:* A Philanthropic Guide for Mental Health and Addiction (UPenn Center for High Impact Philanthropy): Guidance for funders on mental health and addiction

*COVID-19 Pandemic:* Supporting Mental Health (UPenn Center for High Impact Philanthropy): Guidance for funders on how to help individuals and communities struggling with the stress of COVID-19

*The Promise of Adolescence (NAM):* Report supported by the Funders for Adolescent Science Translation (FAST) Collaborative with recommendations for funders and other adolescent-serving systems on supporting young people's development

*Disability & Philanthropy Forum:* Resources to advance disability inclusion in philanthropy

## What Employers Can Do

Employers can play an outsized role in supporting the mental health of children and young people. They can directly help younger employees, such as high school students working part-time jobs or young adults starting out in the labor force after high school or college. For example, employers can provide affordable health insurance that covers mental health needs.

Employers can also support children and youth indirectly. For example, they can offer insurance coverage for employees' dependent children, offer parent-friendly benefits such as family leave and childcare, and promote work-life balance and a positive culture at work to reduce family stress.

Below are some recommendations for how employers can support the mental health of young people:

- *Provide access to comprehensive, affordable, and age-appropriate mental health care for all employees and their families, including dependent children.* Research shows that parental mental health challenges not only impact their productivity in the workplace, but can also affect the mental health of their children.[414,415] Employers should offer health insurance plans that include no or low out-of-pocket costs for

---

414 Goetzel, R. Z., Roemer, E. C., Holingue, C., Fallin, M. D., McCleary, K., Eaton, W., Agnew, J., Azocar, F., Ballard, D., Bartlett, J., Braga, M., Conway, H., Crighton, K. A., Frank, R., Jinnett, K., Keller-Greene, D., Rauch, S. M., Safeer, R., Saporito, D., Schill, A., … Mattingly, C. R. (2018). Mental Health in the Workplace: A Call to Action Proceedings From the Mental Health in the Workplace-Public Health Summit. *Journal of occupational and environmental medicine*, 60(4), 322–330. https://doi.org/10.1097/JOM.0000000000001271.

415 Weissman, M. M., Wickramaratne, P., Nomura, Y., Warner, V., Pilowsky, D., & Verdeli, H. (2006). Offspring of depressed parents: 20 years later. *The American journal of psychiatry*, 163(6), 1001–1008. https://doi.org/10.1176/ajp.2006.163.6.1001.

mental health services, and a robust network of high-quality mental health care providers.

- *Implement policies that address underlying drivers of employee mental health challenges, including both home and workplace stressors.* Employers should:
  - Offer paid family leave and sick leave where feasible. Consider additional employee benefits such as respite care for caregivers and mental health and wellness tools.
  - Help caregivers secure affordable childcare, or offer more flexible work arrangements. This can reduce stress and improve productivity.[416,417]
  - Ensure employees are aware of and can easily make use of these benefits. For example, include information on mental health benefits in emails, webinars, and during onboarding and training for all new hires.
- Create a workplace culture that affirms the importance of the mental health and wellbeing of all employees and their families.
  - Create space for employees to speak up about how they are feeling and encourage company leaders to serve as role models for discussing mental health and modeling healthy behaviors. For example, ensure that senior leaders take advantage of benefits such as paid leave and vacation days.
  - Solicit ideas from employees about how to support their mental health and wellbeing as well as that of their children and families.
  - Adopt clear messaging that promotes mental health awareness and addresses common misconceptions about mental health (for example, that mental health issues are not a sign of weakness).
  - Provide managers and supervisors with training to help recognize negative mental health symptoms in themselves and colleagues and encourage employees to seek help.[418] Mental health employee resource groups, for example, can help increase mental health awareness, build community, and offer peer support.
- *Regularly assess employees' sense of wellbeing within the workplace.* Tools such as employee surveys can help employers understand the wellbeing of employees across demographic groups (e.g., gender, race, sexual orientation), levels of seniority, business units, and geographies, and to identify opportunities for improvement. Employers should make sure to assess the wellbeing of young adults just starting out in the workforce, as well as of parents with young children.

---

[416] Forry, N. D., & Hofferth, S. L. (2011). Maintaining Work: The Influence of Child Care Subsidies on Child Care-Related Work Disruptions. *Journal of family issues*, 32(3), 346–368. https://doi.org/10.1177/0192513X10384467.

[417] Ray, T. K., & Pana-Cryan, R. (2021). Work Flexibility and Work-Related Well-Being. *International journal of environmental research and public health*, 18(6), 3254. https://doi.org/10.3390/ ijerph18063254.

[418] Centers for Disease Control and Prevention. (2021). Mental Health in the Workplace. Accessed on November 12, 2021. Retrieved from: https://www.cdc.gov/workplacehealthpromotion/tools-resources/workplace-health/mental-health/index.html.

**Resources for Employers**

*Center for Workplace Mental Health* (American Psychiatric Association Foundation): Resources to help employers create a more supportive workplace environment

*Work and Wellbeing Initiative* (Harvard-MIT Collaboration): Employer toolkit to help improve workplace conditions and list of employee assessment tools

*What Works Wellbeing* (UK): UK's independent body for wellbeing evidence, policy, and practice. For example, see example employee wellbeing snapshot survey.

*Employer's Guide to Digital Tools and Solutions for Mental Health* (One Mind PsyberGuide): Information for employers on digital mental health solutions for employees

*Generation Work* (Annie E. Casey Foundation): Research briefs, blogs, and tools to help employers of youth better understand and integrate positive youth development approaches

*Mental Health Toolkit* (Employer Assistance and Resource Network on Disability Inclusion): Background, tools and resources to help employers learn more about mental health and cultivate a welcoming and supportive work environment

*Office of Disability Employment Policy* (Department of Labor): Resources for disability-related workplace policies and practices

## What Federal, State, Local, and Tribal Governments Can Do

*Note: For actions taken by the Biden Administration from January to October 2021 to support youth mental health, see Fact Sheet: Improving Access and Care for Youth Mental Health and Substance Use conditions.*

Ultimately, youth mental health challenges cannot be addressed solely by the efforts of youth, their families, local communities, and private organizations. Federal, state, local, and tribal governments all have a role to play. While the below recommendations are not comprehensive, their implementation would mark an enormous step forward in supporting youth and their families:

- *Address the economic and social barriers that contribute to poor mental health for young people, families, and caregivers.* Priorities should include reducing child poverty and ensuring access to quality childcare, early childhood services, and education; healthy food; affordable health care; stable housing; and safe neighborhoods with amenities such as parks and playgrounds. Recent federal investments in child poverty reduction, safe school reopening, and other pandemic-related measures represent historic progress on this front, but additional investments are needed at all levels of government.[419] Emphasis should be placed on preventing adverse childhood experiences (ACEs), which are strong risk factors for mental health challenges.[12]

- *Take action to ensure safe experiences online for children and young people.* Example opportunities include but are not limited to increasing investment in research on the role of social media and technology in youth mental health; educating consumers about potential mental health risks online; requiring companies to be more transparent with researchers and the public (e.g., disclosing meaningful data for research purposes, enabling systemic auditing of social media algorithms), and developing safety standards for online services (e.g., standards for data collection, age verification, user engagement techniques such as 'nudges', and advertising aimed at kids and teens). For instance, the United Kingdom's Age appropriate design code has led companies including Instagram, TikTok, and YouTube to announce product changes to protect their users' safety, rights, and privacy.[420,421] In addition, the Australian government's Safety by Design initiatives have resulted in a set of principles for user safety, tools for companies to assess their safety practices, resources for investors and financial entities to manage online safety risks, and a pilot program with universities to embed Safety by Design materials into curricula.[422]
- *Ensure all children and youth have comprehensive and affordable coverage for mental health care.* Example opportunities include strengthening public and private insurance coverage for children and young adults (e.g., by promoting enrollment), ensuring adequate payment for pediatric mental health services, investing in innovative payment models for integrated and team-based care, increasing the participation of mental health professionals in insurance networks, and ensuring compliance with mental health parity laws.[423] Local, state, and tribal governments can access outreach and enrollment resources to help enroll and retain eligible children in Medicaid and CHIP at InsureKidsNow.gov.
- *Support integration of screening and treatment into primary care. For example, continue expanding Pediatric Mental Health Care Access programs,* which give primary care providers teleconsultations, training, technical assistance, and care

---

[419] The White House. (2021 June 11). FACT SHEET. Biden-Harris Administration Announces Child Tax Credit Awareness Day and Releases Guidance for Unprecedented American Resue Plan Investments to Support Parents and Healthy Child Development. Accessed on November 12, 2021. Retrieved from https://www.whitehouse.gov/briefing-room/statements-releases/2021/06/11/fact-sheet-biden-harris-administration-announces-child-tax-credit-awareness-day-and-releases-guidance-for-unprecedented-american-rescue-plan-inve-stments-to-support-parents-and-healthy-child-dev/.

[420] Information Commissioner's Office. (nd). Introduction to the Age appropriate design code. Accessed on November 12, 2021. Retrieved from https://ico.org.uk/for-organisations/guide-to-data-protection/ico-codes-of-practice/age-appropriate-design-code/.

[421] Lomas, N. (2021 September 1). UK now expects compliance with children's privacy design code. Tech Crunch. Accessed on November 12, 2021. Retrieved from https://techcrunch.com/2021/09/01/uk-now-expects-compliance-with-its-child-privacy-design-code/.

[422] Australian Government, eSafety Commissioner. (nd). Safety by Design. Accessed on November 29, 2021. Retrieved from https://www.esafety.gov.au/industry/safety-by-design.

[423] The White House. (2021 October 19). FACT SHEET: Improving Access and Care for Youth Mental Health and Substance Use Conditions. Retrieved from https://www. whitehouse.gov/briefing-room/statements-releases/2021/10/19/fact-sheet-improving-access-and-care-for-youth-mental-health-and-substance-use-conditions/.

coordination to support diagnosis, treatment, and referral for children with mental health and substance use needs.[424,425,426] Expanding screening for ACEs is also critical. For instance, California recently enacted a law that will significantly expand coverage for ACEs screening.[427]

- *Provide resources and technical assistance to strengthen school-based mental health programs.* Example opportunities include improving education about mental health, increasing screening of students for mental health concerns, investing in additional staff (e.g., school counselors) to support student mental health needs, improving care coordination, and financing school-based mental health services. As mentioned in the earlier section with recommendations for educators, the American Rescue Plan's Elementary and Secondary School Emergency Relief funds can be used for these purposes, along with Project AWARE (Advancing Wellness and Resilience in Education) program funds, which provide support for state, local, and tribal governments in building school-provider partnerships and coordinating resources to support prevention, screening, early intervention, and mental health treatment for youth in school-based settings.[428] In California, a recent law will ensure that all middle and high school students learn about mental health in health education classes.[429] And, in New Jersey, a recent program will provide funding for school districts to screen students for depression.[430]
- *Invest in prevention programs, such as evidence-based social and emotional learning.* Example opportunities include implementing developmentally appropriate social and emotional learning standards and programs, supporting professional development for educators, and providing funding for teachers and school leaders to work with families to support student health needs. For example, the CDC's Legacy for Children program, which promotes positive parenting among low-income mothers, has been found to improve children's behavioral, social, and emotional health.[431]

---

424 U.S. Department of Health & Human Services. (2021 August 27). Biden-Harris Administration Invests $10.7 Million in American Rescue Plan Funds to Expand Pediatric Mental Health Care Access. Press Release. Retrieved from https://www. hhs.gov/about/news/2021/08/27/biden-harris-admin-invests-nearly-11-million-for-pediatric-mental-health-access.html.

425 Massachusetts Child Psychiatry Access Program. Connecting Primary Care with Child Psychiatry. Accessed on November 12, 2021. Retrieved from https://www.mcpap.com/.

426 The White House. (2021 May 20). PRESS RELEASE. HHS Announces $14.2 Million from American Rescue Plan to Expand Pediatric Mental Health Care Access. Accessed on November 29, 2021. Retrieved from https://www.hhs.gov/about/ news/2021/05/20/hhs-announces-142-million-american-rescue-plan-expand-pediatric-mental-health-care-access.html.

427 Office of the California Surgeon General. (2021 October 8). PRESS RELEASE. New ACEs Equity Act Significantly Expands ACE Screening in California. Retrieved from https://osg.ca.gov/wp-content/uploads/sites/266/2021/10/CA-OSG-News-Release-ACEs-Equity-Act.pdf.

428 U.S. Department of Health and Human Services. (2021 August 27). SAMHSA Awards $74.2M in Grants to Strengthen Youth Mental Health. Press Release. Retrieved from https://www.hhs.gov/about/news/2021/08/27/samhsa-awards-74-2m-in-grants-to-strengthen-youth-mental-health.html.

429 California Legislation Information. (2021). SB-224 Pupil instruction: mental health education (2021-2022). Retrieved from https://leginfo.legislature.ca.gov/faces/billNavClient.xhtml?bill_id=202120220SB224.

430 Tap Into Bordentown. (2021 October 2). New Law Creates Grant Program for Depression Screening in Schools. Accessed on November 23, 2021. Retrieved from https://www.tapinto.net/towns/bordentown/sections/education/articles/new-law-creates-grant-program-for-depression-screening-in-schools.

431 Centers for Disease Control and Prevention. (2021 February 22). Behavioral and Socioemotional Outcomes Through Age 5 of the Legacy for Children™ Public Health Approach to Improving Developmental Outcomes

- *Expand the use of telehealth for mental health challenges.* Example opportunities include addressing regulatory barriers (such as limits on provision of telehealth across state lines), ensuring appropriate payment, and expanding broadband access. For instance, Colorado recently established the "I Matter" program, offering young people three free behavioral health sessions, primarily via telehealth.[432]
- *Expand and support the mental health workforce.* Example opportunities include investing in training and hiring individuals from a broader set of disciplines (e.g., peer supports, community health workers, family counselors, care coordinators), accelerating training and loan repayment initiatives, supporting the mental health and wellbeing of health workers, and recruiting a diverse workforce that reflects local communities. In the school setting, governments should invest in building a pipeline of school counselors, nurses, social workers, and school psychologists.[253]
- *Expand and strengthen suicide prevention and mental health crisis services.* Example opportunities include providing flexible funding to fund crisis care needs, increasing access to intensive outpatient and other "step-down" programs, supporting access to trauma-informed services for traumatized children, implementing the 988 mental health crisis and suicide prevention hotline, and promoting public awareness of crisis hotlines and other resources. Governments should also collaborate with the private sector and local communities to reduce access to firearms and other lethal means of suicide and promote best practices such as safe storage.
- *Improve coordination across all levels of government to address youth mental health needs.* One example is to ensure households eligible for social services and supports are receiving them. For instance, states can align renewal processes across Medicaid and the Supplemental Nutrition Assistance Program (SNAP), use data from SNAP files to complete Medicaid renewal, and allow qualified entities like schools to make presumptive eligibility determinations.[433]
- *Support continued reduction in biases, discrimination, and stigma related to mental health.* Example opportunities include enforcing laws that support the needs of at-risk youth (e.g., students with disabilities), identifying and improving policies and programs that inappropriately target or harm youth with mental health needs, and conducting targeted education campaigns to address stigma, promote new cultural norms, and increase safety and trust in local communities.
- *Support the mental health needs of youth involved in the juvenile justice system.* Example opportunities include investing in alternatives to incarceration (e.g., school, probation, and police-based diversion models for youth with mental health needs[434]),

---

among Children Born into Poverty. Accessed on November 22, 2021. Retrieved from https://www.cdc.gov/ncbddd/childdevelopment/features/legacy-for-children-keyfindings.html.

[432] Colorado Department of Human Services. (2021). I Matter Providing Free Mental Health Support for Colorado Youth. Accessed on November 23, 2021. Retrieved from https://cdhs. colorado.gov/i-matter-program.

[433] Brooks, T., Roygardner, L., Artiga, S., Pham, O, & Dolan, R. (2020 March 26). Medicaid and CHIP Eligibility, Enrollment, and Cost Sharing Policies as of January 2020: Findings from a 50-State Survey. *Kaiser Family Foundation.* Retrieved from https://www.kff.org/report-section/medicaid-and-chip-eligibility-enrollment-and-cost-sharing-policies-as-of-january-2020-findings-from-a-50-state-survey-enrollment-and-renewal-processes/.

[434] Mental Health and Juvenile Justice Collaborative for Change: A Training, Technical Assistance and Education Center and a member of the Models for Change Resource Center Partnership. (nd). Better Solutions for Youth with Mental Health Needs in the Juvenile Justice System. Retrieved from https://ncyoj.policyresearchinc.org/

expanding mental health training for staff, supporting high-quality and trauma-informed mental health care inside these systems, and improving coordination across different youth-serving agencies.[435]

- *Support the mental health needs of youth involved in the child welfare system.* Example opportunities include expanding family-centered mental health services to prevent unnecessary entry and increase reunification;[436] ensuring youth and caregivers are informed about medications; investing in peer support services; providing mental health services before, during, and after new placements and when emancipating from foster care;[437] ensuring youth have access to mental health services in community settings whenever possible; and avoiding unnecessary placements in non-family settings. Coordination should be improved across different youth-serving agencies.
- *See "Where Additional Research is Needed" section for recommendations specific to research and data on youth mental health*

## Where Additional Research Is Needed

Despite the evidence that millions of young people are suffering and in crisis, there is still a lot we don't know. Below are recommendations for the kinds of research questions and studies that should be prioritized to better understand and address youth mental health needs:

- *Improve mental health data collection and integration to understand youth mental health needs, trends, services, and evidence-based interventions.*
    - Today, data on youth mental health are collected and analyzed by multiple agencies and often take months or years to be released. The federal government should strengthen research and data integration across governments, health systems, and community organizations to ensure regular, longitudinal surveillance of national mental health trends across the age continuum. Data collection and data linkages should be improved to enable real-time surveillance (e.g., at the census tract level).
    - Data should be able to be disaggregated to enable analysis of trends (by age, gender, race, ethnicity, disability status and type, sexual orientation, socioeconomic background, family characteristics, insurance status, etc.)[438]

---

img/resources/Better_Solutions_for_Youth_with_Mental_Health_Needs_in_the_Juvenile_Justice_System-501172.pdf.

[435] Shufelt, J. L., Cocozza, J. J., & Skowyra, K. R. (2010). Successfully Collaborating With the Juvenile Justice System: Benefits, Challenges, and Key Strategies. Washington, DC: Technical Assistance Partnership for Child and Family Mental Health. https://www.air.org/sites/default/files/downloads/report/ jjresource_collaboration.pdf.

[436] Berger, L. M., & Font, S. A. (2015). The Role of the Family and Family-Centered Programs and Policies. *The Future of children*, 25(1), 155–176.

[437] Villagrana, M. (2021). Foster Care Alumni's Perceptions of Mental Health Services Received While in Foster Care. *Child Adolesc Soc Work J*. https://doi.org/10.1007/s10560-021-00803-7.

[438] The White House. (2021 January 20). Executive Order On Advancing Racial Equity and Support for Underserved Communities Through the Federal Government. Retrieved from https://www.whitehouse.gov/briefing-room/presidential-actions/2021/01/20/executive-order-advancing-racial-equity-and-support-for-underserved-communities-through-the-federal-government/.

- *Foster public-private research partnerships.* For example, academic partners, community-based organizations, technology companies, health care companies, and others can partner to conduct novel studies using nontraditional data sources (e.g., data from wearables and online platforms) to better understand needs, track outcomes, and evaluate risk and protective factors for youth mental health.
- *Increase investments in basic, clinical, and health services research to identify treatment targets for mental health conditions and develop innovative, scalable therapies.* For example, conduct research to optimize stepped-care approaches to treatment for youth populations (e.g., different kinds of cognitive-behavioral therapy such as self-guided, computerized, and group-based vs. solely individual therapy).[439]
- *Prioritize data and research with at-risk youth populations, such as racial, ethnic, and sexual and gender minority youth, individuals from lower socioeconomic backgrounds, youth with disabilities, youth involved in the juvenile justice system, and other groups.*[440] Researchers and research sponsors should ensure that these populations are represented in basic, translational, effectiveness, and services research studies. This will help improve understanding of disparities in risk and trajectories for mental illnesses, responsiveness to interventions, and access to, and engagement with, quality mental health services.
- *Advance dissemination and implementation science to scale up and improve compliance with evidence-based mental health practices in systems that serve children, youth, and their families.* For example, appropriate funding agencies can prioritize demonstration projects of effective evidence-based interventions in and across schools or other systems (e.g., primary care offices, clinics, treatment facilities, family services, child welfare settings, juvenile justice settings). Translate findings into actionable policy proposals and disseminate them effectively to improve adoption of best practices.
- *Conduct research to expand understanding of social media and digital technology's impact on youth mental health and identify opportunities for intervention.* For example, explore the impact of frequent exposure to social comparisons, hateful speech, and graphic content on children and youth, and which groups are most- and least-affected. Also, identify opportunities for families to engage with youth around social media as a means of connection, and offer guidance in handling difficult interactions and content. Explore how pre-existing mental health status and environmental conditions in young people's lives inform how they engage with and experience content online, and empower young people with effective strategies (e.g., mood management) to actively manage their online experiences.

---

[439] Williams, C., & Martinez, R. (2008). Increasing Access to CBT: Stepped Care and CBT Self-Help Models in Practice. *Behavioural and Cognitive Psychotherapy*, 36(6), 675-683. doi:10.1017/S1352465808004864.

[440] Teplin, L. A., Abram, K. M., Washburn, J. J., Welty, L. J., Hershfield, J. A., & Dulcan, M. K. (2013 February). The Northwestern Juvenile Project: Overview. U.S. Department of Justice, Office of Justice Programs, Office of Juvenile Justice and Delinquency Prevention. Retrieved from https://ojjdp.ojp.gov/ sites/g/files/xyckuh176/ files/pubs/234522.pdf.

## Conclusion

As we learn the lessons of the COVID-19 pandemic, and start recovering and rebuilding, we have an opportunity to offer a more comprehensive, more fulfilling, and more inclusive vision of what constitutes public health. And for a generation of children facing unprecedented pressures and stresses, day in and day out, change can't come soon enough.

It won't come overnight. Many of the recommendations offered in this Advisory require structural buy-in and change.

But everyone has a role to play in combating this mental health pandemic. Without individual engagement, no amount of energy or resources can overcome the biggest barrier to mental health care: the stigma associated with seeking help. For too long, mental and emotional health has been considered, at best, the absence of disease, and at worst, a shame to be hidden and ignored.

If we each start reorienting our priorities to create accessible space in our homes, schools, workplaces, and communities for seeking and giving assistance, we can all start building a culture that normalizes and promotes mental health care.

This is the moment to demand change—with our voices and with our actions.

Only when we do will we be able to protect, strengthen, and support the health and safety of all children, adolescents, and young adults—and ensure everyone has a platform to thrive.

## Acknowledgments

This Advisory was prepared by the Office of the Surgeon General (OSG) with contributions from the following interagency partners:

**Department of Health and Human Services**
Administration for Children and Families (ACF)
Administration for Community Living (ACL)
Behavioral Health Coordinating Council Subcommittee on Children and Youth
Centers for Disease Control and Prevention (CDC)
National Center for Injury Prevention and Control (NCIPC)
National Center for HIV, Viral Hepatitis, STD, and TB Prevention (NCHHSTP)
Division of Adolescent and School Health (DASH)
Centers for Medicare and Medicaid Services
Center for Medicaid and CHIP Services
Food and Drug Administration (FDA)
Office of Pediatric Therapeutics
Health Resources and Services Administration (HRSA)
Maternal and Child Health Bureau (MCHB)
Indian Health Service (IHS)
National Institutes of Health (NIH)
National Institute of Mental Health (NIMH)
National Institute on Drug Abuse (NIDA)

*Eunice Kennedy Shriver* National Institute of Child Health and Human Development (NICHD)

Office of the Assistant Secretary for Health (OASH)

Office of Minority Health (OMH)

Office of the Assistant Secretary for Planning and Evaluation (ASPE)

Office of Human Services Policy (HSP)

Office of Behavioral Health, Disability, and Aging Policy (BHDAP)

Substance Abuse and Mental Health Services Administration (SAMHSA)

Additional Partners

Department of Education

Office of Special Education and Rehabilitative Services (OSERS)

Department of Justice (DOJ)

Office of Justice Programs (OJP)

White House Domestic Policy Council (DPC)

White House Office of Science and Technology Policy (OSTP)

*Note: Examples and external resources in this advisory are provided for informational purposes only, and their inclusion does not constitute an endorsement by any government office or agency.*

## Chapter 8

# Supporting Your Teen's Mental Health: Tips for Parents*


## Family and Youth Services Bureau


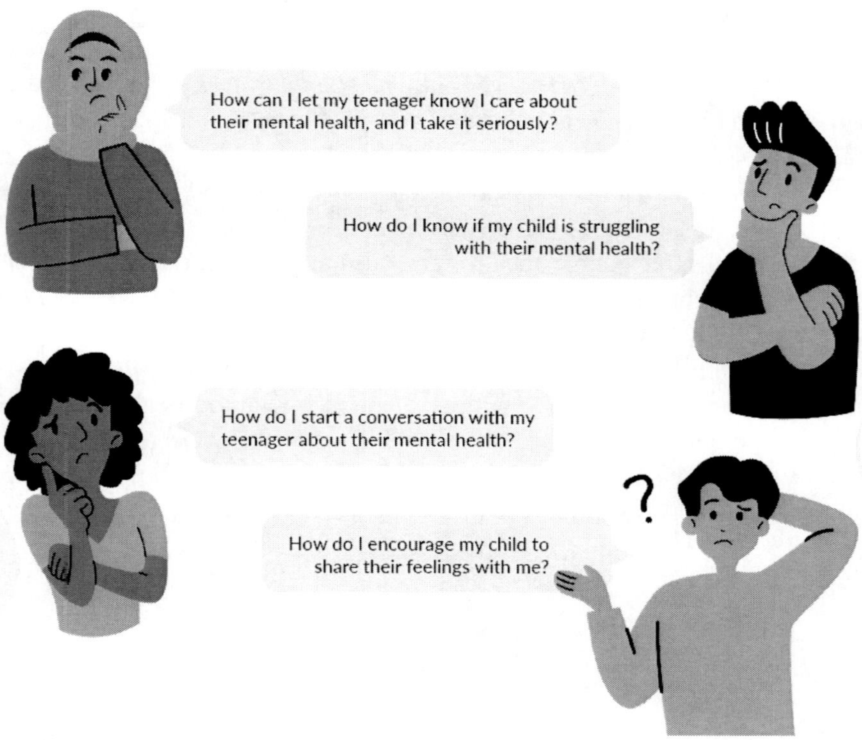

How can I let my teenager know I care about their mental health, and I take it seriously?
How do I know if my child is struggling with their mental health?
How do I start a conversation with my teenager about their mental health?
?
How do I encourage my child to share their feelings with me?


As a parent or caregiver, you play a critical role in supporting your teen's mental health. According to recent data from the Centers for Disease Control and Prevention (CDC):

- 37% of high school students reported they experienced poor mental health during the COVID-19 pandemic, and 44% reported feeling persistently sad or hopeless over the past year.

---

* This is an edited, reformatted and augmented version of This is an edited, reformatted and augmented version a Family and Youth Services Bureau Publication, dated February 2021.


In: Understanding Youth Mental Health
Editor: Michael A. Post
ISBN: 979-8-89530-700-7

- Over the past decade, rates of suicide among young people have increased. According to Youth Risk Behavior Surveillance data, almost one in five high school students reported having seriously considered suicide in the past year.
- Lesbian, gay, and bisexual youth and female youth reported greater levels of poor mental health.

The good news is that there are many ways parents and caregivers can help!

The U.S. Surgeon General's Advisory on Protecting Youth Mental Health has many recommendations for parents on how to address mental health challenges and help youth become resilient and thrive:

- *Be a role model by taking care of your own mental and physical health.* You can show your child/youth you look for help when you need it and demonstrate positive ways of dealing with stress.
- *Help children and youth develop strong, safe, and stable relationships with you and other supportive adults.* Children build resilience through stable relationships with supportive adults. Encourage open communication, show interest in the activities they enjoy, accept them for who they are, praise them for things they do well, and encourage them to ask for help when they need it.
- *Encourage children and youth to build healthy social relationships with peers.* You can give them healthy opportunities to interact with peers (sports, after-school programs, volunteering) and help them learn how to manage peer pressure. Have clear conversations with your teen about their values and teach them how to be comfortable and confident expressing their needs and boundaries.

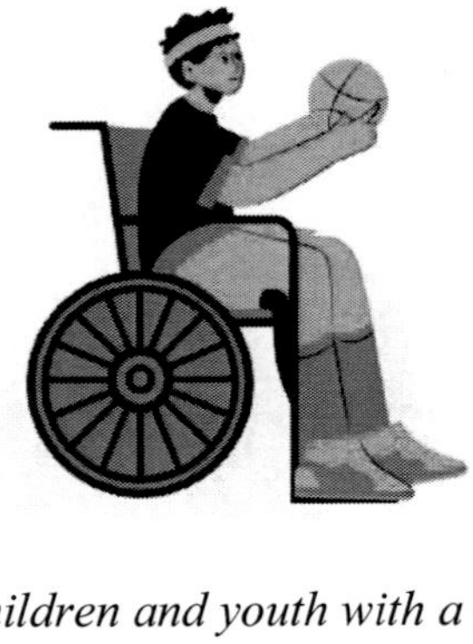

- *Do your best to provide children and youth with a supportive, stable, and predictable home and neighborhood environment.* You can try to help children stick to a regular and predictable daily schedule, such as regular dinnertime and bedtime, be thoughtful about whether and how to discuss stressful topics with them and minimize their exposure to violence.
- *Try to minimize negative influences and behaviors in young people's lives.* Talk with them about the risks of alcohol, tobacco, and drug use.
- *Ensure children and youth have regular check-ups with a pediatrician, family doctor, or other health care professional.* Health care professionals can help you monitor your child's health, give you advice on how to prevent problems, and diagnose and treat physical and mental illnesses.

- *Look out for warning signs of distress and seek help when needed.* Talk with your child's doctor, a nurse, a school counselor, or other professional.

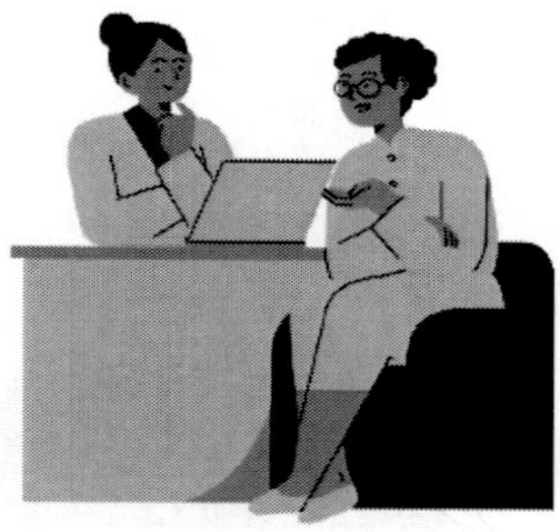

## Warning Signs

- Irritability
- Anger
- Withdrawal or loss of interest in favorite activities
- Difficulty sleeping
- Mood swings
- Difficulty concentrating
- Excessive worry
- Changes in appetite
- Changes in their appearance, performance at school, or other behaviors
- *Minimize your child's access to means of self-harm, including firearms and prescription medications.* Keep medications out of reach for youth. If you choose to keep firearms in the home, ensure they are stored safely: unloaded and locked up in a lock box or safe.
- *Pay attention to how youth spend time online.* Digital technology has many positive applications for youth, but it can also contribute to harmful experiences like bullying or negatively comparing themselves to others.
- *Be a voice for mental health in your community.* You can promote awareness of mental health among your friends and family and within the organizations you are a part of such as schools, community organizations, and churches.

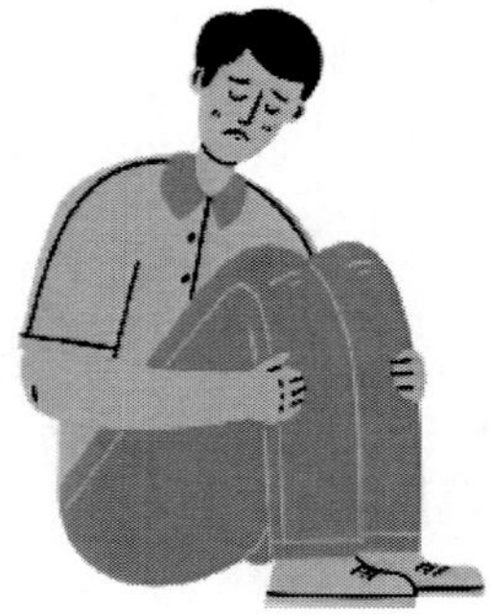

*Most importantly, talk with your teen about mental health and how important it is to get help when they need it.* Tell them that mental health is just as important as physical health, everyone struggles with difficult emotions at some point in their lives, and it's important not to be alone with their feelings. Here are some tips on having those conversations.

Starting the conversation:

- Plan what you want to say.
    - Make note of any symptoms or behaviors that worry you.
    - Find information online from a trusted source or consult with your teen's doctor or a mental health professional if you need information for your conversation.
    - Practice your conversation.
- Choose a comfortable time and place to talk.
    - Make sure you're not rushed or distracted by other things.
    - Pick a time when you feel calm.
    - Talk with your teen while you're doing something together, like going for a walk or having a meal.

During your talk:

- Expect that your teen might be hesitant to talk with you. Reassure your teen
- that it's safe for them to be open with you.
- Speak at a developmentally appropriate level in a clear,
- straightforward manner.
- Listen attentively! Let them speak and give them your full attention.
- Take them seriously. Don't overreact or dismiss what they're saying. It's important to validate your teen's emotions.
- Let them know that mental health is something many people struggle with.
- If you don't know the answer to something, tell them you'll help them find out.
- Some ideas for what to say:
    - *"I've noticed you don't seem like your usual self. Would you like to talk about it?"*
    - *"Can you tell me more about what is going on?"*
    - *"I'm here to listen. How can I help?"*

- *"If you would feel more comfortable speaking with a mental health professional, I'd love to help you find someone."*
- *"I'm concerned about your safety. Can you tell me if you have thoughts about harming yourself or others?"*

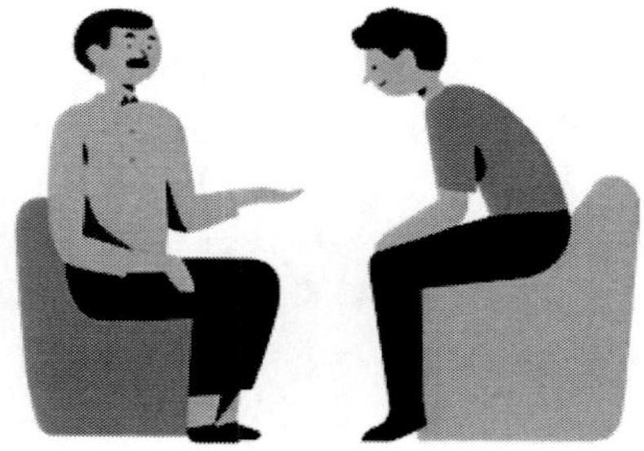

After your talk:

- Check in regularly with your teen.
- Talk to your teen's doctor, school nurse, or other health care provider about any challenge your teen is experiencing and ask for advice.
- If your teen needs additional help, consider seeking a mental health specialist.
- Talk to your teen's provider about medication and treatment plans.
- Learn more! Below are some resources you may find helpful.

## Mental Health Resources and Hotlines

Information for you:

- What Is Children's Mental Health (CDC)
- Emotional Wellness (healthychildren.org)
- Mental health and well-being (UNICEF)
- Family Resource Center (Child Mind Institute)
- Resources for Parents, Educators &
- Communities (Netsmartz)
- Parents' Ultimate Guides (Common Sense Media)
- Resources (mentalhealth.gov)

Information for your teen:

- *We Think Twice Mental Health page*
  We Think Twice has quizzes, articles, and infographics geared especially for teens.
- YouthEngaged4Change
  This site offers articles, inspiring stories, videos, and blogs about adolescent mental health and well-being.

- NIH: Meditation and Mindfulness: What You Need To Know
  This article is about meditation and mindfulness (how it works and why it's good for you).
- NIH: Your Healthiest Self: Wellness Toolkits This site provides strategies and checklists with steps you can take to improve emotional health and well-being.
- GirlsHealth.Gov: Your Feelings
  The "Your Feelings" section of this website offers guidance for teenage girls on recognizing a mental health problem, getting help, and talking to parents.

Finding a mental health specialist:

- If you have health insurance, see their list of providers.
- Ask for a recommendation or referral from your teen's primary care provider.
- Talk with other family members or friends about
- professionals they like.
- Ask your teen's school counselor for a recommendation.
- Search the internet for nonprofit, government, or mental health organizations in your area. Use search terms like "counselors," "psychologists," "psychiatrists," or "social service organizations."
- Use an online directory to find a mental health provider near you who has skills in the issues your teen is facing. You can also use filters to help you narrow your search. For example, you can find a provider of a particular gender, age, ethnicity, or religion. You can also search for one who speaks a particular language.
- Learn about the different types of mental health providers and what each one does. Some are able to prescribe medication, and some are not.
  - Doctors (with Doctor of Medicine (MD) or Doctor of Osteopathic Medicine (DO) degrees), physician assistants, and some psychiatric-mental health nurses can prescribe medication.
  - Most psychologists, licensed clinical social workers (LCSWs), licensed professional counselors (LPCs), or licensed clinical professional counselors (LCPCs) cannot prescribe medication.

Keep in mind:

- *Specialty:* Look for a provider who specializes in your teen's main area of need. If your teen is struggling with anxiety, try to find a mental health professional who specializes in anxiety disorders.
- *Severity:* Your teen's primary care provider will be able to tell you more about any symptoms your child is experiencing. They may recommend that your teen see a psychiatrist, psychologist, or both.
- *Health insurance coverage:* Your insurance provider or Medicaid may have a list of mental health providers they cover. They may only cover certain types of mental health providers and may have limits on the number of visits.
- MentalHealth.gov: For Young People Looking for Help
  Information about signs of mental health issues and how to get help.

- CDC: How Right Now: Finding What Helps This CDC page covers lots of emotions like stress, grief, and loss, and discusses ways to cope and ways to get support.
- National Academies of Medicine: Tools for Youth and Teens National Academies of Medicine has stories showing how teens use different coping techniques to feel better.

Hotlines:

- General Emergency Services
  Call or text 911.
- 988 Suicide and Crisis Lifeline
  Call or text 988 or chat 988lifeline.org for free and confidential support for people in distress. For TTY Users: Use your preferred relay service or dial 711 then 988.
- **LOVEIS:** National Dating Abuse Helpline
  Call 866-331-9474, text "LOVEIS" to 22522, or use TTY: 800-787-3224 to access 24/7 support if you or someone you know may be experiencing or is at risk of experiencing dating abuse. Remember that dating abuse is a pattern of behaviors used to gain or maintain power and control over a partner—physical violence is just one example of dating abuse.
- **LOVEIS:** National Dating Abuse Helpline – Deaf Services
  Deaf advocates are available to answer your call about dating abuse 24/7. Call 855-812-1001 by video phone.
- National Human Trafficking Hotline
  Call 888-373-7888 or text "HELP" to 233733 for 24/7, confidential support if you or someone you know may be a victim of human trafficking. TTY: 711.
- National Runaway Safeline
  Call 800-786-2929 (800-RUNAWAY) or text 66008 for 24/7 confidential and non-judgmental support for youth considering running away from their living situation.
- SAMHSA's National Treatment Referral Routing Service
  Call 800-662-4357 (800-662-HELP) or text your zip code to 435748 (HELP4U) or use TTY: 800-487-4889 for free, confidential, 24/7 treatment referrals and information services (in English and Spanish) for individuals and families facing mental or substance use disorders.
- StrongHearts Native Helpline
  Call 844-762-8483 (844-7NATIVE) to access a free, confidential and anonymous, culturally appropriate 24/7 domestic, dating and sexual violence helpline for Native Americans.
- The Trevor Project
  Call 866-488-7386 or text 678678 for 24/7 free and confidential support for LGBTQ youth. The Trevor Project provides trained counselors for young people in crisis, feeling suicidal, or in need of a safe and judgment-free place to talk.

## Chapter 9

# Advancing Mental Health Supports for Youth of Color Experiencing Homelessness and Other Youth Populations Critically in Need of Services and Supports*


## U.S. Department of Health and Human Services


To: Runaway and Homeless Youth Program Grantees Adolescent Pregnancy Prevention Program Grantees

Re: National Minority Mental Health Awareness Month

July is National Minority Mental Health Awareness Month, which is a good time to highlight the importance of mental health and how essential it is to overall well-being. As part of our efforts to raise awareness, the U.S. Department of Health and Human Services' (HHS), Administration for Children and Families (ACF), Administration for Children, Youth and Families, Family and Youth Services Bureau (FYSB); the Office of Minority Health (OMH); and the Substance Abuse and Mental Health Services Administration (SAMHSA) are pleased to release this joint letter, which shares our commitment to highlighting critical resources to support the mental health of youth of color experiencing homelessness and other youth populations critically in need of services and supports.

We know from the National Institute of Mental Health (NIMH) that in the United States, there can be notable differences in the experience of mental illness, access to quality health care, and health outcomes based on gender and gender identity, sexual orientation, age, race, ethnicity, and geography. In addition, recent data and information provide evidence that many of our nation's youth, including those from underserved and marginalized communities, are experiencing significant mental health challenges.

Other reports have shared additional concerning data. For example, the:

- *White House Fact Sheet released on May 23, 2023, Actions to Protect Youth Mental Health, Safety & Privacy Online,* noted that the United States is experiencing an unprecedented youth mental health crisis. The document shared that "the number of children and adolescents with anxiety and depression has risen nearly 30% in recent

* This is an edited, reformatted and augmented version a Family and Youth Services Bureau Publication.


In: Understanding Youth Mental Health
Editor: Michael A. Post
ISBN: 979-8-89530-700-7

years; between 2011 and 2021, the number of teens and young adults with depression more than doubled; and nearly 1 in 3 high school girls reported having seriously considered suicide."

- *Centers for Disease Control and Prevention, Youth Risk Behavior Survey Data Summary & Trends Report (2011-2021),* which provides 2021 surveillance data and 2011-2021 trend data on health behaviors and experiences among high school students in the United States, noted that the percentage of Black students who were injured in a suicide attempt increased from 2011 to 2021.
- *Surgeon General's Advisory on Protecting Youth Mental Health* reported in 2021 that the COVID-19 pandemic most heavily affected those who were already vulnerable, including youth with disabilities; racial and ethnic minority youth; youth who identify as lesbian, gay, bisexual, transgender, queer, or questioning (LGBTQ+); and other marginalized communities.
- *NIMH Director's Message* conveyed that as of 2018, suicide became the second leading cause of death in Black children aged 10-14, and the third leading cause of death in Black adolescents aged 15-19. The address also reflected that "one factor that may be contributing to increases in the risk of suicide in Black youth may be disparities in access to mental health services." Similarly, it conveyed that "Black youth continue to be less likely to receive mental health treatment for depression when needed, compared to White youth."

Moreover, youth of color face unique challenges due to compounding issues deeply rooted in systemic and historical inequities and marginalization. Through data, research, and important conversations with youth with lived experiences, including pregnant and parenting youth and those that identify as LGBTQI+, we recognize that these youth are particularly at risk for experiencing homelessness, and have a significant need for high-quality, compassionate responses and culturally and linguistically appropriate solutions.

Given the tremendous need to prevent and support youth experiencing mental health challenges, we are writing to underscore the importance of several critical resources, including hotlines, we believe should be at the forefront of your program's strategies when developing and expanding mental health supports for youth of color experiencing homelessness and other youth populations critically in need of services and supports.

As a leader in your community, we ask that you use and disseminate the resources we are sharing and take steps to collaborate with your state, territory, tribal, faith-based, and community organizations as well as local businesses and other youth-serving and health care entities (e.g., primary care providers, schools) related to this issue. Creating a community response plan, or strengthening existing community response plans, establishes a coordinated strategy for communities to ensure youth experiencing mental health challenges have access to the vital supports needed. As these plans are developed, and as existing plans are strengthened, they can support meaningful engagement with culturally and linguistically relevant community-based organizations to address the systematic barriers to health care access and other critical supports.

When developing collaborations and strategies, we invite you to use tools such as the Behavioral Health Implementation Guide for the National Standards for Culturally and

Linguistically Appropriate Services (CLAS) in Health and Health Care and research that promotes the use of an equity lens.

It is our desire to help Runaway and Homeless Youth (RHY) and Adolescent Pregnancy Prevention (APP) programs and other partners across the human services spectrum increase access to mental health services for youth. This is one of many actions we are taking to underscore how having mental health resources can be the key to achieving long-term success for youth of color experiencing homelessness and other youth populations critically in need of services and supports. We are pleased to join many organizations and communities nationwide in acting from every angle to offer help.

We thank you for the work you are doing and your willingness to share tools, including hotlines that are free, confidential, and available to all in multiple languages 24/7, 365 days a year. We look forward to communicating again in the future as we expand ways to help youth experiencing homelessness and mental health challenges, find the care they need.

Should you have questions or would be willing to share how your program has implemented actions to advance mental health supports for youth of color experiencing homelessness and other youth populations critically in need of services and supports in your programs, please contact: Linda Reese-Smith at linda.reesesmith@acf.hhs.gov and Curtis Porter at curtis.porter@acf.hhs.gov.

Rebecca Jones Gaston, MSW
Commissioner
Administration on Children, Youth and Families
Administration for Children and Families
U.S. Department of Health and Human Services

RDML Felicia Collins, MD, MPH, FAAP
Deputy Assistant Secretary for Minority Health
Director, Office of Minority Health
U.S. Department of Health and Human Services

Kimberly A. Waller
Associate Commissioner
Family and Youth Services Bureau
on Children, Youth and Families Administration
Administration for Children and Families
U.S. Department of Health and Human Services

Anita Everett, MD, DFAPA
Director, Center for Mental Health Services
Substance Abuse and Mental Health Services Administration
U.S. Department of Health and Human Services

## Free and Confidential Critical Mental Health Hotlines and Additional Resources

- The Substance Abuse and Mental Health Services Administration's (SAMHSA) FindSupport.gov offers support for issues with mental health, drugs, or alcohol.
- *The SAMHSA National Helpline, 1-800-662-HELP (4357)* (also known as the Treatment Referral Routing Service) or TTY: 1-800-487-4889, is a confidential, free, 24-hour-a-day, 365-day-a-year information service, in English and Spanish, for individuals and family members facing mental and/or substance use disorders. This service provides referrals to local treatment facilities, support groups, and community-based organizations. Also visit the online treatment locator, or send your zip code via text message to: 435748 (HELP4U) to find help near you. Read more about the HELP4U text messaging service.
- *The 988 Suicide & Crisis Lifeline* (formerly known as the National Suicide Prevention Lifeline) offers 24/7 call, text and chat access to trained crisis counselors who can help people experiencing a suicidal, substance use, and/or mental health crisis, or any other kind of emotional distress. People can also dial 988 if they are worried about a loved one who may need crisis support. 988 serves as a universal entry point so that no matter where you live in the United States, you can reach a trained crisis counselor who can help. If you or someone you know is struggling or in crisis, help is available. Call or text 988 or chat 988lifeline.org. Visitors can press "2" for Spanish or "3" to receive specialized LGBTQI+ youth counseling. To access more information, please visit: behavioral health and homelessness resources.
- *The National Runaway Safeline (NRS)* crisis hotline offers online services 24 hours a day, 365 days a year to youth at risk of running away, those who have run away or are homeless, and their families. NRS helps in the following ways:
  - *Crisis Intervention:* Front line staff and volunteers are trained to use a solution-based crisis intervention model.
  - *Information and Referrals:* NRS locates local resources and makes appropriate referrals to meet each caller's needs.
  - *Three-Way Conference Calls:* NRS initiates calls between youth and their parents or guardians, staying on the line to mediate the discussion. NRS also initiates calls between youth and social service protection agencies, and between adults and organizations that can help resolve their problems.
  - *Message Relay:* When youth and their parents or guardians are not yet ready for one-on-one interactions, they may take the first step toward reconnecting with each other by leaving messages with NRS.
  - *Free Trip Home:* NRS has a partnership with Greyhound Bus Lines to offer runaway and homeless youth a free bus ticket home.
  - *Advocacy:* The NRS front line team advocates for youth and ensures they get support and guidance from authorities, school administrators, social service agencies, and medical and legal professionals.

    CALL: 1-800-RUNAWAY<br>
    CLICK: 1800RUNAWAY.org<br>
    TEXT: 66008

- The Health Resources and Services Administration (HRSA) has a maternal mental health hotline that pregnant and parenting youth can use. To reach the National Maternal Mental Health Hotline, call or text 1-833-943-5746 (1-833-9-HELP4MOMS). TTY users can use a preferred relay service or dial 711 and then 1-833-943-5746. This hotline service is offered 24/7 and provides free, confidential support before, during, and after pregnancy. Parents and their loved ones who contact the Hotline will speak to professional counselors who speak English and Spanish. Interpreter services are also available in 60 languages. Counselors will immediately provide real-time support, information, and resources. Counselors will also provide referrals to local or telehealth providers if you need longer-term care and support. Counselors are licensed or certified and have training in how to provide culturally appropriate and trauma-informed support.
- *The National Human Trafficking Hotline* provides assistance to individuals in crisis through safety planning, emotional support, and/or immediate connections to emergency services through our network of trained service provider and law enforcement partners.

## Mental Health Resources

- Issue Brief: Runaway and Homeless Youth, Mental Health, and Trauma-Informed Care
- Issue Brief: Understanding and Addressing Mental Health Issues of African American Youth Experiencing Homelessness
- Issue Brief: Trauma-Informed Care for the Full Range of RHY Services
- Youth.gov—RHY and Behavioral Health Resources
- Administration for Children and Families, Behavioral Health webpage includes a range of federal resources, including resources specifically for teens and young adults, parents and caregivers, tribes, and providers.
- NIMH Get Involved webpage includes resources on Child and Adolescent Mental Health for raising awareness on several mental health topics such as anxiety, teen depression, signs of bipolar disorder in teens and young adults.
- Indian Health Service Mental Health—Behavioral Health Resources
- HHS Center for Faith-based and Neighborhood Partnerships Mental Health: Youth Mental Health and Well-being in Faith and Community Settings: Practicing Connectedness

## Resources for Providers

- National Clearinghouse on Homeless Youth and Families, Runaway and Homeless Youth Screening and Assessment Toolkit Resource Page
- SAMHSA's Mental Health and Substance Use in Young Adults Resource
- SAMHSA's Parent and Caregiver Resources
- SAMHSA's National Child Traumatic Stress Network

- National Clearinghouse on Homeless Youth and Families (NCHYF) Mental Health Partners Resource
- Office of Minority Health – Improving Cultural Competency for Behavioral Health Professionals E-Learning Program
- Office of Minority Health/SAMHSA – Behavioral Health Implementation Guide for the National Standards for Culturally and Linguistically Appropriate Services in Health and Health Care
- Expanding Access to and Use of Behavioral Health Services for People At Risk for or Experiencing Homelessness

## Adolescent Pregnancy Prevention Mental Health Resources

- Family and Youth Services Bureau, Adolescent Pregnancy Prevention, Youth Mental Health Resources
- Family and Youth Services Bureau, Dealing with Grief Resources
- Family and Youth Services Bureau, We Think Twice Resources: We Think Twice is a movement designed with teens, for teens, with tools and resources to help you make healthy decisions, set goals, manage money, improve leadership skills, look out for your mental health, and resist peer pressure.

## Related Special Reports

- Protecting Youth Mental Health: The U.S. Surgeon General's Advisory
- Ring the Alarm: The Crisis of Black Youth Suicide in America. A Report to Congress from the Congressional Black Caucus Emergency Taskforce on Black Youth Suicide and Mental Health.

## Related Resources

- *After an Attempt: A Guide for Taking Care of Your Family Member After Treatment in the Emergency Department*
  Aids family members in coping with the aftermath of a relative's suicide attempt. Describes the emergency department treatment process, lists questions to ask about follow-up treatment, and describes how to reduce risk and ensure safety at home.
- *Family Therapy Can Help: For People in Recovery from Mental Illness or Addiction*
  Explores the role of family therapy in recovery from mental illness or substance abuse.
- Explains how family therapy sessions are run and who conducts them, describes a typical session, and provides information on its effectiveness in recovery.

## Relevant Fact Sheets, Roadmaps, and Information Memorandum

- *Fact Sheet: President Biden to Announce Strategy to Address Our National Mental Health Crisis, As Part of Unity Agenda in his First State of the Union*
- *The HHS Roadmap for Behavioral Health Integration*
- *The White House Executive Order on Further Advancing Racial Equity and Support for Underserved Communities Through the Federal Government*
- *SAMHSA and Administration for Children and Families (ACF) issued a joint Information Memorandum (IM)* in 2019 calling for increased collaboration between domestic violence, mental health, and substance use disorder treatment service providers and systems. Working at the intersections of domestic violence, substance use, and mental health, this IM highlights the prevalence of domestic violence among individuals receiving services in mental health and substance use disorder treatment settings and offers information about training, resources, and strategies for improved collaboration between systems to effectively respond to survivors, youth and children experiencing the traumatic effects of domestic violence.

# Index

## L



## M



## N



## O



## P

## T

## U



## V



## W



## Y